Psychosocial Interventions for Social Issues in Contemporary India

U. Vindhya
Editor

Psychosocial Interventions for Social Issues in Contemporary India

Springer

Editor
U. Vindhya
Hyderabad, Telangana, India

ISBN 978-981-96-6552-5 ISBN 978-981-96-6553-2 (eBook)
https://doi.org/10.1007/978-981-96-6553-2

This Springer imprint is published by the registered company Springer Nature Singapore Pte Ltd.
The registered company address is: 152 Beach Road, #21-01/04 Gateway East, Singapore 189721, Singapore

Dedicated to the memory of Bhargavi V. Davar
For whom mental well-being was a social justice issue, and striving for which she was such an inspiring crusader

Contents

List of Contributors

Somya Agarwal Centre for Mental Health Law and Policy, Indian Law Society, Pune, India

Nimisha Ajaikumar Centre for Mental Health Law and Policy, Indian Law Society, Pune, India

Padma Bhate-Deosthali ICRW, New Delhi, India

Nalini Bikkina School of Humanities and Social Sciences, GITAM, Visakhapatnam, India

Nayreen Daruwalla Society for Nutrition, Education and Health Action, Mumbai, India

Vanessa D'Souza Society for Nutrition, Education and Health Action, Mumbai, India

Sharanya Gautam Society for Nutrition, Education and Health Action, Mumbai, India

Sangeeta Goswami Institute of Positive Mental Health & Research, MIND India, Guwahati, Assam, India

Sumati Guntaka KL University, Guntur, India

Nikhil Jain Centre for Mental Health Law and Policy, Indian Law Society, Pune, India

Kaustubh Joag Centre for Mental Health Law and Policy, Indian Law Society, Pune, India

Jacquleen Joseph The Jamsetji Tata School of Disaster Studies, Tata Institute of Social Sciences, Mumbai, India

Aparna Joshi Tata Institute of Social Sciences (TISS), Mumbai, India

Jasmine Kalha Centre for Mental Health Law and Policy, Indian Law Society, Pune, India

Gargi Khandekar Society for Nutrition, Education and Health Action, Mumbai, India

Palak Korde Centre for Mental Health Law and Policy, Indian Law Society, Pune, India

Isha Lohumi Centre for Mental Health Law and Policy, Indian Law Society, Pune, India

Anna Madill University of Leeds, Leeds, UK

David Osrin Wellcome Trust Fellow at University College London, London, England

Shanti Pantvaidya Society for Nutrition, Education and Health Action, Mumbai, India

Soumitra Pathare Centre for Mental Health Law and Policy, Indian Law Society, Pune, India

Sangeeta Rege CEHAT, Mumbai, Maharashtra, India

Roomana N. Siddiqui Department of Psychology, Aligarh Muslim University, Aligarh, India

Shobna Sonpar Kullu, India

Sunayana Swain School of Public Policy and Governance, Tata Institute of Social Sciences, Hyderabad, India

U. Vindhya Independent Researcher, and Former Professor, Tata Institute of Social Sciences, Hyderabad, Telangana, India

Chapter 1
What Is This Book About? Principles and Practice of Psychosocial Interventions

U. Vindhya

Abstract This chapter provides an overview of what the book is about: the varied kinds of psychosocial interventions carried out for some of the most pressing issues of contemporary social concern in India—agrarian distress, disasters, violence against women, suicide, social conflict, and socio-economic inequalities and disparities. As the term 'psychosocial' implies, the interventions weave together the psychological and the social. The interventions are aimed at mitigation of distress at the level of the individual. But they are informed by an understanding of the broader social structural forces and the contexts of inequalities and power imbalances that contribute to the distress, and are laced with the overarching perspectives of social justice, human rights, and inclusion. Located broadly at the tri-junction of psychology, social work, and social sciences in general, the interventions in this volume demonstrate the processes and outcomes of what has been/can be done in order to alleviate distress and enhance the psychological and social functioning and well-being of individuals.

Keywords Psychosocial · Psychological distress · Social justice · Social issues in India

In the past three decades or so, there has been heightened awareness about psychosocial interventions in the context of what are known as 'humanitarian settings', that is, people and places affected by disasters and armed conflicts (International Federation of Red Cross & Red Crescent Societies, 2009; Tol et al., 2015). Whether the settings are political and ethnic conflicts or large-scale natural disasters such as earthquakes, floods and cyclones, these situations challenge and disrupt human capacity for coping with crises. Psychosocial interventions for exposure to conflict, war, and disasters that cause immense damage, destruction and human suffering involve therefore, responding to their negative consequences for restoration of psychosocial well-being. A significant turning point in psychosocial programming and practice was

U. Vindhya (✉)
Independent Researcher, and Former Professor, Tata Institute of Social Sciences, Hyderabad, Telangana, India
e-mail: u.vindhya@gmail.com

U. Vindhya (ed.), *Psychosocial Interventions for Social Issues in Contemporary India*,
https://doi.org/10.1007/978-981-96-6553-2_1

the tsunami in 2004 in the case of natural disasters (e.g., Bhugra & Ommeren, 2009), and the Bhopal gas disaster in 1984 that was a major milestone in law, policy, and psychosocial relief services for industrial and transport accidents in India (e.g., Murthy, 2014). Similarly, since 2020, it was the enormous public health crisis wrought by the Covid-19 pandemic with its burden of physical health concerns as well as its psychosocial impact that posed an unprecedented challenge to planning and delivery of psychosocial interventions worldwide (Saladino et al., 2020).

This book however, is not directly about either armed conflicts or industrial, or natural disasters. The issues covered in this volume, for which interventions have been carried out, are what can broadly be termed as social issues in contemporary India. The only exception is that of Covid-19, that, as mentioned earlier, can perhaps be described as an extraordinary crisis with public health, social and psychological ramifications. As a veritable field of long-standing and complex social issues, India has had a long history of grappling with a magnitude of these social challenges, ranging from poverty and associated socio-economic disparities and inequities, to caste and gender inequalities, and to communal and ethnic conflagrations, amongst many others. These have been examined primarily through the prisms of sociological, political, and economic levels of analyses. The psychological distress associated with social and economic inequalities and inequities, and caused by the loss of life, uprooting and displacement due to violent conflicts as in caste and communal riots, has not been so much the object of scrutiny. Therefore, on the one hand, the role of the psychological—emotion, cognition, behaviour, well-being—in social issues is not explicitly examined. On the other hand, the usage of psychosocial interventions in the discipline of psychology and related fields has been for the most part confined to mental disorders and substance abuse.

Hence, a central motivation for putting together this volume, is to bring to the (psychology) table, interventions for social issues ranging from violence against women, agrarian distress, to socio-economic inequalities and disparities, that are not generally addressed frontally in psychology curriculum and research in our country. By exploring and examining how the psychological and the understanding of the social are combined in the conceptualization, design and implementation of interventions for a variety of social issues, the chapters in this volume demonstrate the necessity and efficacy of such interventions that alleviate or attempt to alleviate individual suffering, pain and distress determined and impacted by social structural forces. It is hoped that students, researchers, practitioners of psychology, social work and allied disciplines, as well as those in the development sector, will be enabled to draw fresh insights from this explicating of the processes and outcomes of the interventions covered in this volume, and thereby expand and enrich the field of designing and implementing psychosocial interventions for social issues in India.

This volume does not make any claim however, to cover all social issues in contemporary India, nor is it a comprehensive review or assessment of psychosocial interventions that engage with such issues. It aims to provide only a small sampling of the range of social issues and the kind of interventions, designed and implemented to address them from a psychosocial lens. More importantly, the chapters in this volume underline the necessity of taking into consideration the *social origins* of psychological distress, and for planning interventions that address directly or indirectly, the broader social and cultural determinants of distress, and that are embedded in the specific social context in which people live. In short therefore, the primary impetus for this book is to bring together varied interventions for wide-ranging social issues, and unravel the rationale as well as the process, and in some cases, the outcomes too of these interventions.

The Psychological and the Social: Towards Defining Psychosocial Interventions

The term 'psychosocial intervention' (PSI) has been in fairly wide circulation in the humanitarian and development sectors. However, there has been disagreement and debate about a precise definition of psychosocial intervention (van Ommeren et al., 2006). It was in 2007 that a taskforce of international humanitarian agencies called the Interagency Standing Committee (IASC) of the United Nations Office of Humanitarian Coordination Assistance (UNOCHA) was formed in order to address the lack of consensus among humanitarian agencies on what constitutes such interventions and to come up with a set of guidelines for implementing psychosocial support in humanitarian settings (van Ommeren & Wessells, 2007). The guidelines used the umbrella term 'mental health and psychosocial support' (MHPSS) to refer to support that "aims to protect or promote psychosocial wellbeing and/or prevent or treat mental disorder" (IASC, 2007). Although mental health and psychosocial support are fused in this definition, practitioners in humanitarian settings have noted that there is often a divide between those who use 'mental health' interventions on the one hand and those who tend towards 'psychosocial support' on the other. The former, it is noted, is used to describe clinical interventions delivered by health staff in order to reduce psychiatric symptoms, while the term psychosocial support is used to indicate community-based interventions, aimed at enhancing and strengthening safety and social support systems, and livelihoods, all of which are, in turn, expected to foster positive mental health, reduce risk for mental disorders, and support recovery (Tol et al., 2015). However, as these scholars point out, despite this implicit distinction being made, there is often overlap in the specific actions undertaken, such as for example, counselling and ensuring social support and connectedness, which are commonly seen across different psychosocial interventions.

Despite the perception that there is lack of a commonly agreed definition of psychosocial interventions (Hodges et al., 2011), a broad consensus currently is the understanding that psychosocial intervention refers to any intervention that focuses on psychological or social factors and actions rather than on pharmacological/medical ones in order to improve psychological and social functioning, produce change, promote well-being, and prevent harm either to self and/or to others (England et al., 2015; WHO, 2024). Thus, a basic definition of psychosocial interventions refers to programs that improve psychological well-being through social programs (van Ommeren & Wessells, 2007) with the key goal being to reduce psychological dysfunction and impaired everyday functioning, by employing a repertoire of techniques (Kazdin, 2018).

As the term implies, PSI involve the *psychological*—the typical mental health interventions that aim to reduce psychological distress, improve psychological well-being outcomes, and directed primarily at the micro-level of the individual; and the *social*—that are directed at the macro-level and could range from interventions in the societal (laws, public policy), and community (public education, coordination of services, training and capacity-building of frontline workers) domains. What distinguishes PSI from other interventions such as medical interventions (e.g., pharmacological) on the one end, and exclusively social interventions (e.g., food and relief distribution) on the other end, is, as its name implies, its ability to encompass a wide range of actions, straddling several domains from the macro to the micro, and intending to capitalize on both psychological and social actions in order to produce change in psychological, social, and even in biological outcomes (e.g., PSI for terminal and chronic illnesses such as cancer (Park et al., 2019) and dementia (McDermott et al., 2018). The effectiveness of such interventions, be it for natural disasters, or war and displacement, or problematic substance use, to name just a few of the applications, lies perhaps in the wide repertoire of services and support they offer wherever relevant. These range from active listening and emotional support—the very immediate responses needed, to providing information or psychoeducation, rendering psychological first aid or humane, supportive and practical help, to crisis intervention, advocacy and outreach, building multisectoral linkages for referral and increasing social resources, and integrating them with existing services such as health, social protection, rehabilitation or educational services. By thus employing an array of interpersonal and community-based activities, the overarching goal of these interventions is to improve functioning and well-being (Goldstein, 2009). A review of interventions in humanitarian settings found that the most frequently used and effective interventions were doing basic counselling for individuals and families, strengthening community resources and support, creating child-friendly spaces and structured recreational and creative activities, and psychoeducation and raising awareness about mental health (Tol et al., 2011).

The specific emphasis on which element—psychological or social—is to be focused upon, might have to do with the disciplinary mandate and theoretical inclination. The psychosocial framework, that originated in social work practice and programme, laid emphasis on the goals of PSI to restore, maintain and enhance the personal and social functioning of individuals through "mobilizing strengths, supporting coping capacities, building self-esteem, modifying dysfunctional patterns of thinking, feeling and relating to others; linking people to necessary resources, and alleviating environmental stressors" (Goldstein, 2009, p. 14). The inclination in psychology and the mental health disciplines, on the other hand, and in line with their disciplinary orientation has been on various types of mental and physical health issues, or even in the case of humanitarian settings, on the psychiatric consequences of exposure to trauma caused by disasters and armed conflicts, such as symptoms related to post-traumatic stress and depression and on interventions including cognitive and behavioural therapeutic approaches, psychoeducation, family therapy, social skills training, to name a few, in order to alleviate the psychological distress of the individual. A key focus of interventions in disasters for psychologists and professionals from related fields has been obviously on mental health needs with the coinage of terms such as 'disaster mental health' and 'psychological first aid' gaining widespread global currency (e.g., Shultz & Forbes, 2014).

The sheer diversity of these interventions in terms of techniques/activities as well as in settings and contexts where they are delivered also makes it rather difficult to pinpoint precisely the nature of psychosocial interventions. As mentioned earlier, the techniques range from "*the explicitly psychological*" (Galappatti, 2003) services such as psychological counselling, to the more *social* such as improving linkages and networking with state and community resources through providing of information, facilitating socio-economic support and inclusion such as supported employment and the like. Diversity exists for the kind and nature of problems too for which psychosocial interventions are applied. For instance, the psychosocial strategies and actions adopted in the wake of the civil war (1983–2009) and in the post-tsunami recovery efforts in Sri Lanka ranged from the overtly psychological or medically therapeutic services such as counselling and assessment for PTSD, to skills training for improving material security (Galappatti, 2003). Similarly, the settings in which these interventions are delivered also vary from the individual as a focus of intervention as in the case of mental health and substance use disorders to the larger population as in the case of a disaster such as an earthquake and so on.

Regardless of the nature of the problem and the setting in which the intervention is delivered, a fundamental aim of these interventions may be described as improving well-being and building resilience. However, a common understanding of what constitutes *psychosocial well-being* itself may be difficult to arrive at, given that individual experience may be subjective, and that it is also largely determined by the social context in which individuals are embedded. Nevertheless, three core domains have been identified as the essence of psychosocial well-being: (a) human *capacity* (knowledge, capability, and skills; (b) social *ecology* (social support systems and connections that ensure and enhance cohesive social bonds and connectedness); and *culture* and *values* (norms and behaviours that are linked to value systems) (International Federation of Red Cross & Red Crescent Societies, 2009). Given that any kind of crisis and adverse circumstances not only disrupt people's lives, but also drain individual resources from these core domains, psychosocial well-being, according to this framework, is contingent upon external interventions and support in order to shore up and rebuild both individual and communal psychosocial well-being.

In addition, psychosocial well-being is recognized as a cross-cutting issue, with linkages to, in case of environmental disasters for instance, to shelter, relocation, distribution of food and other relief materials, health care, as well as to providing of psychological first aid and emotional support to deal with loss of loved ones and property, and displacement. Practitioners and researchers in the humanitarian sector therefore have called for an integrated cross-sector response to material, mental, biological, social and cultural well-being in humanitarian settings and to include psychosocial support in overall relief and rehabilitation activities (Padmavati et al., 2020; Williamson & Robinson, 2006; World Health Organization (WHO), 2006).

Regardless however, of the type of outcome of the intervention one chooses, be it protected/enhanced well-being or prevented/reduced psychopathological symptoms, the nature or process of the intervention is equally important (van Ommeren et al., 2006). It is this nature and process of intervention that is the primary focus of the set of chapters in this book, and although some do refer to the outcomes achieved, a major emphasis has been on unravelling and understanding of how the intervention was done and in the process, gain insights into the nature and complexity of the social issue itself.

Conceptual Framework and Principles in Practice

This volume has a set of two papers in each thematic category illumining different dimensions and facets of the intervention. Except for the Covid-19 and the public health crisis it brought in its wake, that is of recent times, the other issues taken up in the volume are of long-standing nature and persistence. Agrarian distress/farmers' suicides, violence against women, intergroup conflict, socio-economic disparities and inequities are some examples of contemporary social issues in India that are not only of enduring nature, but also call for multifactorial interventions.

Practitioners in humanitarian settings have noted that despite some consensus and coordination between various agencies in arriving at a definition and understanding of psychosocial interventions, the focus has always been on concrete actions, and less on building a theoretical perspective. Hence the literature does not touch upon explicitly on 'principles and theory' (Wessels & van Ommeren, 2008).

In this volume too, although the theoretical framework is not made explicit in all the chapters, if there is one common conceptual scaffolding that ties all the chapters together, it is that they are broadly informed by social justice, public health and human rights perspectives. That is, the understanding and recognition that privileges, resources and advantages are not equally and equitably distributed, that some sections of the population are disproportionately affected by social and economic disadvantage; but that all have equal rights to fair allocation of resources, care and justice (Bhugra, 2016)—is an overarching perspective that runs through all the chapters. Social justice, as an ideological standpoint informing research and practice, is currently perhaps a buzz word both in popular discourse and in academic rhetoric. While not explicitly using the term, as mentioned above, the practice of the interventions included in this volume are nevertheless imbued by the philosophy and vision of social justice. The philosophy includes the recognition of inequities and injustice within social structures, the resulting impact on people's well-being, and undertaking of action in order to ensure rights to care and well-being of those sections which are particularly vulnerable to these injustices. For instance, the chapters of Sangeeta Rege and Padma Deosthali, and of Nayreen Daruwalla et al. on interventions for violence against women; Swain and Vindhya on farmers in agrarian distress; Jasmine Kalha et al. on common mental health conditions; Nikhil Jain et al. on suicide prevention in youth and promotion of their psychological well-being; of Shobna Sonpar on human rights accountability in conflict situations such as in Kashmir and imparting knowledge and training on rights and entitlements, have at their centre the rights of the victims/survivors to care and justice. In addition to the centrality of rights, many of the chapters focus on interventions that are community-driven and locally relevant, thereby reinforcing the importance of community participation, another key pillar of social justice.

Again, although none of the chapters in this book explicitly use the term 'critical psychology' while giving an indication of their theoretical orientation, the volume as a whole, takes a critical psychological lens. As the editor, whose primary disciplinary background is in psychology, I have been influenced by the framework of critical psychology that challenges mainstream psychology in several fundamental ways. While mainstream psychology is that which is taught in most universities and which is practised by most clinicians and researchers (Fox et al., 2009), critical psychology "alerts us to (its) limitations … and promises to put social issues on the agenda…" (Parker, 2007). As stated by Fox et al. (2009) in their introduction to the approaches in critical psychology, its key themes centre around "pursuing social justice, promoting the welfare of communities in general and of oppressed groups in particular, and transforming the status quo of both society and psychology" (p. 5).

The chapters in this volume, turn our attention to the social structural context in India: the context of inegalitarianism in particular—of the perpetuation and reinforcing of inequalities and disparities of varied kinds—that generates psychological distress. The social issues covered in this volume may be characterized as manifestations of inequalities, conflicts and imbalances within societal systems and structures. One might argue that such issues require structural solutions that address root causes of the problem and make systemic changes to the underlying structures through measures such as social and economic policies and programs, legal frameworks and governance, and not through individual-level interventions. Furthermore, it can also be argued that interventions with individuals to alleviate the consequences of social adversities might be a "reductionist diversion of attention from the need for wider societal change" (Johnson, 2017, p. 245).

While it is certainly essential to ground social problems in structural solutions, what is equally important perhaps is also not to lose sight of the necessity of individual-level interventions that can be complementary to the structural approaches. To put it simply, as the chapters in this volume demonstrate, they target social structural issues, but the point of intervention is the individual. More specifically, a common thread binding the interventions elaborated in these chapters is the shared recognition that while pervasive systemic inequalities and inequities might be the underlying cause of individual distress, a diversity of interventions are necessary to alleviate psychosocial distress and enhance well-being. As the range of interventions elaborated in the chapters shows, they are framed against the backdrop of an understanding of structural inequalities and power imbalances, thereby bridging in a sense, the structural and the individual.

The focus, therefore, of the chapters in this volume, is not so much on the determinants of distress but on intervention strategies and actions, and also on prevention (as in the case of suicide risk), that can ameliorate the psychological distress associated and determined by the social structural context. The underlying emphasis in the chapters in this volume, in line with the central premise of critical psychology, is thus on the understanding of psychosocial well-being as an issue of social justice, that is, the risks of well-being are seen to be intrinsically linked to social inequalities and power imbalances in society.

Although the relationship between social and structural factors and mental health and well-being is fairly well-established (e.g., Lund, 2020; Lund et al., 2018; Oswald et al., 2024), as the social determinants of health model attests, the social remains 'the poor relative in the biopsychosocial triad' when it comes to evidence-based interventions (Johnson, 2017). It is further made complex as the range of potential targets for social interventions is 'dauntingly wide' (Johnson, 2017), going beyond mental health services at the individual and family levels, and extending to the broader domains of social policy, law, and restructuring of the social order. To reiterate, the chapters in this volume, taken together, indicate the importance of recognizing the impact of the political and socio-economic context, and of cultural norms and values—on psychosocial well-being.

Another motivation for this book arises from the dearth of research in community psychology in India, a sub-field that comes closest to the focal theme of this book. While mainstream psychology in India has for the most part focused on the individual-level microsystem, sub-fields such as community psychology are a recent entrant (Bhatia & Sethi, 2007). However, as the architects and advocates of the critical psychology approach emphasise, community psychology offers concepts and methods in order to understand the linkages between social injustice and psychological experience (Evans et al., 2014; Prilleltensky & Nelson, 2008).

So, how do the perspective and principles of social justice work on the ground? In terms of putting the social justice perspective into concrete practice, the chapters reflect, simply stated, "one's responsibility to care for others [for] the common good of society" (Robinson, 2010, p. 134). This responsibility is seen both in micro-actions such as empathetic listening to supporting and implementing on the ground social policies and other rights-based initiatives that protect the vulnerable and disadvantaged, whether it is women affected by violence, or farmers in agrarian distress, or those caught in ethnic/political conflict, or vulnerable youth at risk of suicide or substance addiction. Furthermore, some of the ethical guidelines proposed for social justice work in psychology (Hailes et al., 2020) are reflected in this volume, as for instance, in critical reflection and mitigation of relational power dynamics (in the chapters of Rege & Bhate Deosthali, and Daruwalla et al. on violence against women); prioritization of concerns of socially and economically disadvantaged communities and awareness about the impacts of the system on individual and community well-being (Daruwalla et al. on urban, low-income settlements; Kalha et al. on community outreach with rural populations; Jain et al. on promotion of well-being and suicide prevention in vulnerable youth; Swain & Vindhya on farmers in agrarian distress; Siddique on conflict between a majoritarian religious group and one that occupies the minority position); and engaging with socio-political systems (Sonpar on peace-building in the context of protracted political conflict and violence) and cultural norms (Daruwalla et al. on prevention strategies for violence against women). And finally, the implicit recognition underlying the initiation and implementation of the interventions are informed by the fundamental conviction that the situations that lead to distress also ought to be *prevented*.

A Quick Tour of the Book

The contributors to this volume are from several disciplines ranging from psychology, social work, psychiatry, public health, as well as from the social sciences, and include both academics/researchers and practitioners with rich and extensive experience on the field. The chapters report on interventions carried out in different regions across India from Gujarat and Maharashtra in the west to Kashmir in the north and Assam in the north-east, and to Andhra Pradesh in the south. Furthermore, a repertoire of methods is seen across the chapters in order to engage with the target population that go beyond the conventional one-on-one format of psychological counselling.

The volume begins with two review chapters of the psychosocial initiatives in the context of the most recent issue—the unprecedented public health crisis of the Covid-19. The pandemic with its profound impact on a range of dimensions had not only exacerbated existing health inequalities, but had sharply brought into focus the inadequacies of the existing mental health care system in India (Yadavendu, 2023). In this volume, the chapter of Jacquleen Joseph focuses on a review of the initiatives undertaken in the first few months of 2020, immediately following the nation-wide lockdown in March 2020, while Aparna Joshi's chapter traces the longer term. As both the chapters show, the number of initiatives taken by the government as well as NGOs have been several and extensive—from the guidelines and advisories issued by the Ministry of Health and Family Welfare, to the online capacity building of health workers in providing psychosocial support, creation of toll-free helpline, and digital well-being platform such as MANAS, and to the free online counselling provided by several NGOs across the country. While such digital interventions, following the pandemic, have now "come to stay" as Joseph argues in her chapter, she cautions about challenges such as following an individualistic approach, implementing them as a stand-alone service, contrary to the multidisciplinary approach of the MHPSS, and not taking into consideration issues of digital divide in countries such as ours, that may very well dent their efficacy. In order to address such challenges, Joseph underscores the integration of standalone MHPPS interventions with humanitarian interventions, and for strengthening the social intervention component in these programs. Joshi too, in her chapter argues that the pandemic experience has served as a wakeup call to the necessity of prioritizing mental health and well-being in our intervention programs, and that that it is an opportune moment to reconceptualize the notion of mental well-being away from its rigid biomedical framework and integrate it instead in a broader, inclusive and rights-based public health and development model. Thus, both these chapters are in line with similar calls given by public health researchers (e.g., Rangaswamy et al., 2022) for action to integrate mental health in universal health coverage plans, for enhancing access to psychosocial interventions and addressing the needs of neglected populations.

Violence against women (VAW) remains one of the most directly visible indicators of gendered inequalities in India. Despite the proliferation of interventions in the last three to four decades, by the activism of women's groups for macro-level initiatives such as changes in law and policy, provision of services, and counselling and psychosocial support at the individual level, the prevalence figures are persistently and distressingly high. A major gap in the literature in India on psychosocial interventions for VAW, is paucity of assessment of their effectiveness. Research and documentation on their processes and outcomes remain both fragmented and sparse, with much of the information remaining as 'oral histories' of organizations, as Rege and Deosthali, have argued, in this volume. Their chapter traces the evolution of interventions for VAW from the 1970s—the socio-political context of emergence and upsurge of several social movements in post-independence India, including that of autonomous women's groups, and unravels in the process, the manner in which 'feminist counselling', a mode of intervention that bridges the structural and the personal, came to be crystallized for addressing VAW. The chapter also presents an evaluation of the impact of the 'Dilaasa' model, located in the public health care context, and initiated by CEHAT, a Mumbai-based NGO. The Dilaasa intervention can be characterized as the original prototype of One Stop Centres, that were later introduced as a state-sponsored scheme in 2013 in the country for providing integrated services to women and girls affected by violence.

The other chapter in the volume dealing with VAW, of Daruwalla et al., emphasises different levels of prevention of violence including deep involvement with the community for addressing risk factors such as socio-cultural norms—the toughest of them all—that condone violence and gender inequality. Using a socio-ecological framework and a theory of change, and set in the sprawling and teeming low-income settlements of Mumbai, the authors emphasize a multidisciplinary, locally relevant and community-led psychosocial approach involving primary, secondary, and tertiary strategies for violence prevention.

Both the chapters speak about efforts made by their organizations to conduct evaluations of the impact of their interventions to equip themselves with insights about what works as well as provide them with a roadmap for the future. Both the chapters underscore the necessity of providing of an extensive range of support services for survivors of violence including engaging with multiple stakeholders such as the police and courts as a key plank for securing redress and justice for the survivors. Rege and Deosthali emphasize in their assessment of the interventions that effectiveness of the intervention has been most pronounced at the individual level with reduction of personal distress of the survivor, but rather bumpy when it comes to liaison and coordination with state agencies for redressal and justice. Daruwalla et al. point to challenges in acceptance by the community, threats of reprisal from the survivor's family following disclosure of violence, and the need to take utmost care while asking sensitive questions about intimate details of their marital lives.

Psychosocial interventions for mental disorders and problematic substance use have been the staple interventions emanating from the mental health disciplines and the chapters in this category (of Jasmine Kalha et al., Nalini Bikkina et al., and of Sangeeta Goswami and Ann Madill) demonstrate the widespread prevalence of common mental health conditions, and of substance addiction, and importantly, the effectiveness of simple techniques of intervention. Common mental health conditions such as depression and anxiety are currently regarded as a major public health problem, contributing the most to the burden of mental health on Disability Adjusted Life Years (DALY) in terms of 91 million people out of around 197.3 million affected by mental disorders of varying severity (India State-Level Disease Burden Initiative Mental Disorders Collaborators, 2020). The studies of Kalha et al. and Bikkina et al., based in the states of Gujarat and Andhra Pradesh, confirm the extant research on the high prevalence of common mental disorders—the range of anxiety and depressive disorders—and how these mental health concerns are often disguised and an undetected form of psychological distress. However, the care gap remains alarmingly huge, with an overwhelming majority unable to access mental health care. Aligned to a rights and recovery-based framework, and in line with the increasing evidence of recruiting lay health workers to reduce this gap, the study of Kalha et al. report on the implementation of a community-led intervention. Designed as a five-tiered community volunteer model to address the mental health and social care needs of the population, the intervention has been effectively upscaled to cover a larger population across districts in Gujarat and five other states. Apart from delineating the process and outcomes of the intervention, the chapter also captures the voices of the community workers, designated as *Champions*, and *Community Facilitators*, to reflect about the impact of the intervention on their own lives as well as on the lives of the community.

The study of Bikkina et al. set in a primary health care centre in Visakhapatnam city in northern Andhra Pradesh, shows the significantly high prevalence of common health conditions. But perhaps more importantly, the fairly equal distribution of categories of concerns expressed by those consulting the health facility—of physical health, psychological problems, and interpersonal/social issues such as domestic violence—underscores the fact that it is not physical health alone, but rather a range of underlying issues of distress that manifest as physical health complaints, driving people to consult the health centre. The study also demonstrates how a simple psychosocial intervention such as Brief Counselling can be effective in a setting such as a primary healthcare facility. The most frequently used counselling interventions, reflecting the needs of the sample, were *ventilation*, followed by *problem-solving* indicating the need for a non-threatening, non-judgmental space for people to ventilate their concerns, and *psychoeducation* for problem-resolution. The significance of this study is also essentially the setting in which it was conducted—primary care, that is the first point of contact with the health care system (World Health Organization, 2008). While the WHO vision of "comprehensive primary health care which links health to issues of social justice, equity, participation and broader social development" (Rifkin & Walt, 1986) may seem idealistic in the current scenario in India, the chapter shows up the interconnected links of psychological distress with social and economic inequalities, in line with the social determinants of health model.

The chapter by Sangeeta Goswami and Ann Madill highlights the gravity of substance abuse among the youth population in particular in the north-eastern state of Assam, as a serious public health concern. The risk factors for the issue are located both in the geo-political context of the state (easy availability of substances due to its proximity to the international border), as well as in socio-economic factors common to several regions such as rapid urbanization, changing lifestyles, peer pressure and so on. Based on the lived experiences of users, the intervention used creative methods such as making posters and films to capture their experiences, and traced their journey from recreational use, to addiction, and eventually to supported recovery, in order to develop what the authors term as a multi-route, multidirectional pathways to recovery model. The outcomes of the intervention, according to the authors, have been useful in providing evidence-based information to the government and coming up with a set of policy recommendations on substance abuse in the region. These recommendations include increased family and community education and peer-to-peer support in educational institutions.

Another public health crisis in recent decades has been that of suicide, with India currently having the dubious distinction of reporting the highest number of suicide deaths in the world (Armstrong & Vijayakumar, 2018; Vijayakumar et al., 2022). A rather striking feature of the occurrence of suicide in India as well as in other 'developing' countries is that the relationship between mental illness and suicide is not as pronounced as it is in the economically developed countries in the west (Vijayakumar, 2016). Rather, the phenomenon of suicide in India is seen to be impacted by broader social, economic, and cultural factors ranging from agricultural crisis, indebtedness, economic upheavals, the gradual dissolution of cohesive social bonds, and changing social relations in the context of globalization and the technological changes that have come in its wake in recent decades (Dandona, 2023; Rajguru & Balhara, 2023). In addition, psychosocial stressors such as high pressure of competition, interpersonal relationship conflicts, caste discrimination, examination pressure/failure, alcoholism, and chronic physical illness are identified as some of the predominant factors pushing individuals to end their lives (Amudhan et al., 2020; Mathew et al., 2021; Vijayakumar, 2010). The increasing suicide rate thus points to the urgent and compelling need to address its prevention, and the framing of the first-ever prevention policy in India, the National Suicide Prevention Strategy in 2022 is a step in the direction of addressing this significant burden of suicide (Dandona & Kumar, 2023).

The two chapters of Nikhil Jain et al. and of Sunayana Swain and Vindhya in this volume focus on two vulnerable groups—youth and farmers respectively. It has been noted that despite the high incidence rate of suicide in India, the number of intervention studies remains low and hence, intervention research needs to be accorded top priority (Rappai et al., 2020; Vijayakumar et al., 2022). Although the target groups in the two chapters in this volume are different, the authors demonstrate the effectiveness of the intervention and build a strong case for an integrated community-based model of intervention that is locally relevant, socially and culturally appropriate, and cost effective.

The reported high incidence of suicide in the 15–29 years age group makes suicide prevention initiatives among youth an even more pressing need. The chapter by Jain and colleagues elaborates on the process and outcomes of a universal mental health promotion programme with adolescent students in public schools in Gujarat. Employing a range of creative and expressive activities such as small group work, role plays, a variety of IEC materials, and situating them in a supportive and culturally-attuned environment, the intervention was able to effectively realize the goals of reduction in suicidal ideation and depression.

Similarly, Swain and Vindhya in their chapter show that users of the intervention in the suicide-affected region of Vidarbha in Maharashtra, reported high levels of satisfaction with the services and in particular with the home-based psychosocial support provided by community health workers that enabled prompt identification of people with symptoms of mental illness, and creating better awareness about mental health and help-seeking behaviour. Given thus the complex multi-faceted dimensions of this problem, both the chapters show that focusing on multi-component interventions and targeted approaches is more effective than taking the mental health intervention approach alone.

While intergroup conflicts and peace-building efforts are located in specific historical, social, political and economic contexts, the role of social psychological processes in their eruption, and escalation, as well as in negotiation and mediation of peaceful resolution of conflict is no less significant (Bar-Tal, 2022; Somasundaram, 2007). The final set of chapters of Roomana Siddiqui and Shobna Sonpar focus on the extremely challenging issue of intergroup conflicts and advocacy initiatives for peace-building. Exposure to situations such as war and ethnic conflict, as well as to sudden, large-scale natural disasters have both individual effects and searing impacts on the community and society as a whole. Traditionally, psychology has focused on the individual-level microsystem of interventions that focus on individual-level emotion, behavior, and well-being (Rosado-Solomon et al., 2023) but the nature of long-simmering socio-political conflicts in broadly collectivistic societies like ours is such that the problems at the community level too have to be understood and addressed if the interventions are to be meaningful and relevant. Sonpar's chapter in this volume addresses the long-lasting negative impact at the collective level on social processes, relationships, institutions, dynamics, and practices that has been variously referred to in the literature as 'tearing of the social fabric', collective trauma', 'cultural bereavement', and 'loss of communality'.

Roomana Siddique's chapter provides a brief overview of the social psychological concepts such as prejudice, threat perception, relative deprivation, collective memory, that explain the emergence and maintenance of intergroup conflicts, and communal conflicts, in particular in India. Pointing to the near absence of attention to psychosocial interventions in this regard in mainstream psychology in India, she emphasises the necessity of understanding of the origins and dynamics of intergroup conflicts, in order to plan for interventions.

Taking a larger canvas, Sonpar in her chapter on peace-building initiatives elaborates on the historical evolution and trajectories of the development of psychosocial interventions for sustainable peace in the context of intractable political conflict. She provides a useful account of the *components* of these interventions with relevant examples from settings of long-lasting conflicts such as in Sri Lanka, Northern Ireland, and Kashmir in India. These illustrative examples show the diversity and overlapping levels of the interventions, that do not rely only on professional mental health experts such as clinical psychologists and psychiatrists but are anchored in multidisciplinary approaches. Importantly, Sonpar also draws attention to the challenge of practitioners and researchers in taking a 'neutral' or 'apolitical' stand in these conflicts, given the stance of value-neutrality, that is so prized in mainstream psychology.

A recent scoping review of MHPSS interventions in humanitarian settings found six broad themes related to goals and outcomes of these programs that is, those seeking to (1) promote individual resilience and psychosocial well-being and prevent mental health and psychosocial problems; (2) reduce particular mental health symptoms; (3) build capacity of personnel in order to identify, intervene and monitor mental health and psychosocial problems; (4) enhance the environment for development and flourishing of children and adolescents; (5) macro-level outcomes such as peace-building between groups in post-conflict settings and support of peaceful co-existence between and within communities; and (6) protect specific vulnerable groups such as women, people with disabilities, children and the elderly, and work on issues such as reduction of risk of gender-based violence (Augustinavicius et al., 2018, p. 6). As these researchers note, such a review is necessary and useful for facilitating conceptualization and designing of interventions as well as to reflect on accountability to key stakeholders. It may be pertinent to note here that each of the chapters in the present volume demonstrate commitment and accountability to at least one or more of the above-mentioned goals.

Finally, a chapter that unfortunately, could not be completed is that of the late Bhargavi Davar on a community-based program, driven by the understanding of mental well-being as an issue of social justice. Foregrounding the right to mental health care and inclusion, the chapter was to present the process and outcomes of the implementation of a psychosocial intervention for mental health in an urban low-income setting by the Bapu Trust Seher programme. We reproduce below a few lines from the abstract that Bhargavi had sent but could not complete the chapter intended for this volume, due to illness that tragically cut short her life mid-way.

> Realizing social justice as a mental health strategy: Experiences from the Bapu Trust Seher program
>
> Bhargavi Davar, Founder-Director, Bapu Trust, Pune

….The Bapu Trust for Research on Mind & Discourse developed the 'Seher' program using iterative research learning and developing a design for deep community engagement. Situated in the low-income communities (bastis) of Pune city, and at scale, providing services to approximately 800,000 population through 5 wellness centres, the Seher program used an intervention design called the 'Eight Point Recovery Framework'. It is this framework that proved to have scalable features across different bastis, as well as allowing for knowledge to be captured through trainings. The EPRF (as it is called) is the scalable part of the program, now packaged into trainings for partners to implement. The paper will describe the elements of this framework, using data from the program and case studies, which establish our claim that 'realizing social justice is in itself a mental health strategy'.

Prilleltentsky and Nelson (2008), the pioneering figures in critical psychology, distinguish between *ameliorative* practices, that is, those that "tend to the wounded, care for the disabled, and treat the infirm" and *transformative* practices that are aimed instead to "change systems that wound and marginalize so many in the first place" (p. 16). Critical psychologists fault those in mainstream psychology for being confined to ameliorative practices, by focusing on the individual and individual-centred techniques such as therapy for psychological distress, without being mindful of the structural and systemic factors that cause the distress. However, what emerges from these chapters is that interventions need to engage with both the levels—of ameliorative practices, bringing succour and relief to the individual, while focusing at the same time on the need for transformation at the broader level.

To conclude this opening chapter, the triad of social justice, human rights, and public health perspectives, as mentioned earlier, underpin the psychosocial interventions elaborated in the following chapters and are at the heart of this volume. These perspectives are also tied essentially to the core values and philosophy of the Sustainable Development Goals (SDGs) launched by the United Nations in 2015. While 'sustainable development' may have become a commonly heard buzzword in recent times, the chapters do point, as the SDGs do, to the need for prioritization of access to justice; inclusiveness; and accountability of governance systems for sustainable development to be real and not merely empty rhetoric. By doing so, the chapters taken together, also emphasise the two-way conversation necessary between psychology and the social sciences for understanding of and intervention in what are termed as social and structural issues.

And finally, the issues taken up for intervention in this volume vary, the disciplinary emphasis and inclination may be different, but what remains a common thread, to reiterate once again, is the *principle of social responsibility and care* for those in distress, and acknowledgement of their *rights to care and justice.*

References

Amudhan, S., Gururaj,G., & Varghese, M. (2020). A population-based analysis of suicidality and its correlates: Findings from the National Mental Health Survey of India, 2015–16. *The Lancet Psychiatry, 7*, 41–51.

Armstrong, G., & Vijayakumar, L. (2018). Suicide in India: A complex public health tragedy in need of a plan. *The Lancet Public Health, 3*(10), e459–460. https://doi.org/10.1016/S2468-2667(18)30142-7

Augustinavicius, J. L., Greene, M. S., Lakin, D. P., & Tol, W. A. (2018). Monitoring and evaluation of mental health and psychosocial support programs in humanitarian settings: A scoping review of terminology and focus. *Conflict and Health, 12*(9), 1–10.

Bar-Tal, D. (2022). Introduction: Conflicts and social psychology. In D. Bar-Tal (Ed.), *Intergroup conflicts and their resolution: A social psychological perspective.* Psychology Press.

Bhatia, S., & Sethi, N. (2007). History and theory of community psychology in India: An international perspective. In S. M. Reich, M .Reimer, I. Prilleltensky, & M. Montero (Eds.), *International community psychology*. Springer.

Bhugra, D. (2016). Social discrimination and social justice. *International Review of Psychiatry, 28*(4), 336–341. https://doi.org/10.1080/09540261.2016.1210359

Bhugra, D., & Ommeren, M. (2009). Mental health, psychosocial support and the tsunami. *International Review of Psychiatry, 18*(3), 213–216.

Dandona, R., & Kumar, G. A. (2023). India's National Suicide Prevention Strategy: Considerations to enhance desired outcomes. *The Lancet Psychiatry, 10*(3), 162–163. https://doi.org/10.1016/S2215-0366(22)00434-5

England, M. J., Butler, A. S., & Gonzalez, M. (Eds.). (2015). *Psychosocial interventions for mental and substance use disorders: A framework for establishing evidence-based standards.* The National Academies Press.

Evans, S. D., Rosen, A. D., & Nelson, G. (2014). Community psychology and social justice. In C. V. Johnson, H. L. Friedman, J. Diaz, Z. Franco, & B. K. Nastasi (Eds.), *The Praeger handbook of social justice and psychology: Fundamental issues and special populations* (pp. 143–163). Praeger/ABC-CLIO.

Fox, D., Prilleltensky, I., & Austin, S. (2009). Critical psychology for social justice: Concerns and dilemmas. In D. Fox, I. Prilleltensky & S. Austin (Eds.), *Critical psychology: An introduction* (2nd ed., pp. 3–19). Sage.

Galappatti, A. (2003). What is a psychosocial intervention? Mapping the field in Sri Lanka. *Intervention, 1*(2), 3–17.

Goldstein, E. (2009). *Psychosocial framework.* Oxford Bibliographies.

Hailes, H., Ceccholini, C. J., Gutowski, E., & Liang, B. (2020). *Ethical guidelines for social justice in psychology.* Research and Practice. Advance online publication. https://doi.org/10.1037/pro0000291

Hodges, L. J., Walker, J., Kleiboer, A. M., Ramirez, A. J., Richardson, A., Velikova, G., & Sharpe, M. (2011). What is a psychological intervention? A metareview and practical proposal. *Psychooncology, 20*(5), 470–478.

Inter-Agency Standing Committee. (2007). *IASC guidelines on mental health and psychosocial support in emergency settings.* http://www.who.int/mental_health/emergencies/guidelines_iasc_mental_health_psychosocial_june_2007.pdf

International Federation of Red Cross and Red Crescent Societies. (2009). *Psychosocial interventions: A handbook.* International Federation Reference Centre for Psychosocial Support.

India State-Level Disease Burden Initiative Mental Disorders Collaborators. (2020). The burden of mental disorders across the states in India: The Global Burden of Disease Study 1990–2017. *The Lancet Psychiatry, 7,* 148–161.

Johnson, S. (2017). Social interventions in mental health: A call to action. *Social Psychiatry and Psychiatric Epidemiology, 52*, 245–247. https://doi.org/10.1007/s00127-017-1360-6

Kazdin, A. (2018). *Innovations in psychosocial interventions and their delivery: Leveraging cutting-edge science to improve the world's mental health.* Oxford University Press.

Lund, C. (2020). Reflections on the next ten years of research, policy and implementation in global mental health. *Epidemiology and Psychiatric Sciences*, 29, e77. https://doi.org/10.1017%2FS204579601900074X

Lund, C., Brooke-Sumner, C., Baingana, F., Baron, E. C., Breuer, C., Chandra, P., Haushofer, J., Herrman, H., Jordans, M., Kieling, C., Medina-Mora, M. E., Morgan, E., Omigbodun, O., Tol, W., Patel, V., & Saxena, S. (2018). Social determinants of mental disorders and the Sustainable Development Goals: A systematic review of reviews. *Lancet Psychiatry, 5*(4), 357–369.

Mathew, A., Saradamma, R., Krishnapillai, V., & Muthubeevi, S. B. (2021). Exploring the family factors associated with suicide attempts among adolescents and young adults: A qualitative study. *Indian Journal of Psychological Medicine, 43*(2), 113–118.

McDermott, O., Charlesworth, G., Hogervorst, E., Stoner, C., Moniz-Cook, E., Aimee Spector , A., Csipke, E., & Orrell, M. (2018). Psychosocial interventions for people with dementia: A synthesis of systematic reviews. *Aging Ment Health, 4*, 393–403.

Murthy, R. S. (2014). Mental health of survivors of 1984 Bhopal disaster: A continuing challenge. *Industrial Psychiatry, 2*(2), 86–93. https://doi.org/10.4103%2F0972-6748.151668

Oswald, T. K., Nguyen, M. T., Mirza, L., Lund, C., Jones, H. G., Crowley, G., Aslanyan, D., Dean, K., Scchofield, P., Hotopf, M., & Das-Munshi, J. (2024). Interventions targeting social determinants of mental disorders and the Sustainable Development Goals: A systematic review of reviews. *Psychological Medicine, 54*(8), 1475–1499.

Padmavati, R., Raghavan, V., Rera, H., Kearns, M., Rao, K., John, S., & Thara, R. (2020). Learnings from conducting mental health research during 2004 tsunami in Tamil Nadu, India. *BMC Public Health, 20*(1), 1627–1631. https://doi.org/10.1186/s12889-020-09733-y

Park, C. L., Pustejovsky, J. E., Trevino, K., Sherman, A., Esposito, C., Berendsen, M., & Salsman, J. M. (2019). Effects of psychosocial interventions on meaning and purpose in adults with cancer: A systematic review and meta-analysis. *Cancer, 125*(14), 2383–2393.

Parker, I. (2007). Critical psychology: What is it and what it is not. *Social and Personality Psychology Compass.* https://doi.org/10.1111/j.1751-9004.2007.00008.x

Prilleltensky, I., & Nelson, G. (2008). Community psychology: Advancing social justice. In D. Fox, I.Prilleltensky, & S. Austin (Eds.), *Critical psychology: An introduction* (pp. 126–143). Sage.

Rajguru, A. J., & Balhara, Y. P. S. (2023). Increasing trend of deaths due to suicide attributable to mental disorders and substance use (disorders) in India. *Asian Journal of Psychiatry, 88*, 103722. https://doi.org/10.1016/j.ajp.2023.103722

Rangaswami, T., Grover, S., Tyagi, V., & Bhan, A. (2022). How did the mental health care system in India respond to Covid-19 pandemic? *Schizophrenia Bulletin Open, 3*(1), 1–6. https://doi.org/10.1093/schizbullopen/sgac043

Rappai, R., Cherian, A. V., Lukose, A., & Vijayakumar, L. (2020). Suicide research in India: An overview of four decades. *Asian Journal of Psychiatry, 53*, Article 102191. https://doi.org/10.1016/j.ajp.2020.102191

Reisch, M. (2014). Introduction. In M. Reisch (Ed.), *The Routledge international handbook of social justice.* https://doi.org/10.4324/9781315857534

Rifkin, S. B., & Walt, G. (1986). Why health improves: Defining the issues concerning 'comprehensive primary health care' and 'selective primary health care.' *Social Science and Medicine, 6*, 559–566.

Robinson, F. (2010). After liberalism in world politics? Towards an international political theory of care. *Ethics and Social Welfare, 4*(2), 130–144.

Rosado-Solomon, E. H., Koopman, J., Lee, W., & Cronin, M. A. (2023). Mental health and mental illness in organizations: A review, comparison, and extension. *The Academy of Management Annals, 17*(2), 751–797.

Substance Abuse and Mental Health Administration (SAMSHA). (2014, September 17). *Working definition of recovery.* http://store.samhsa.gov/shin/content/PEP12-RECDEF/PEP12RECDEF.pdf

Saladino, V., Algeri, D., & Auriemma, V. (2020). The psychological and social impact of Covid-19: New perspectives of well-being. *Frontiers in Psychology, 11*, A 577684, 1–6. https://doi.org/10.3389/fpsyg.2020.577684
Shultz, J.M., & Forbes, D. (2014). Psychological first aid. *Disaster Health, 2*(1), 3–12. https://doi.org/10.4161%2Fdish.26006
Somasundaram, D. (2007). Collective trauma in Northern Sri Lanka: A qualitative psychosocial-ecological study. *International Journal of Mental Health Systems, 1*(1), 5.
Taylor, J. E., & Charlton, D. (2018). *The farm labor problem: A global perspective*. Academic Press.
Tol, W. A., Barbui, C., Galappatti, A., Silove, D., Betancourt, T. S., Souza, R., Golaz, A., & van Ommeren, M. (2011). Mental health and psychosocial support in humanitarian settings: Linking practice and action. *Lancet, 378*, 1581–1591.
Tol, W. A., Purgato, M., Bass, J. K., Galappatti, A., & Eaton, W. (2015). Mental health and psychosocial support in humanitarian settings: A public mental health perspective. *Epidemiology and Psychiatric Sciences, 24*, 484–494.
van Ommeren, M., & Wessells, M. (2007). Interagency agreement on mental health and psychosocial support in emergency settings. *Bulletin of the World Health Organization, 85*(11), 822–823. https://doi.org/10.2471%2FBLT.07.047894
van Ommeren, M., Morris, J., & Saxena, S. (2006). Integrated programme planning and psychosocial concepts in humanitarian response: A response to Williamson and Robinson. *Intervention, 4*, 26–28.
Vijayakumar, L. (2010). Indian research on suicide. *Indian Journal of Psychiatry, 52*(1), S291–S296.
Vijayakumar, L. (2016). Suicide prevention: Beyond mental disorder. *Indian Journal of Psychological Medicine, 38*, 514–516.
Vijayakumar, L., Chandra, P., Kumar, M. S., Pathare, S., Banerjee, D., Goswami, T., & Dandona, R. (2022). The national suicide prevention strategy in India: Context and considerations for urgent action. *The Lancet Psychiatry, 9*(2), 160–168. https://doi.org/10.1016/S2215-0366(21)00152-8
Wessels, M., & van Ommeren, M. (2008). Developing inter-agency guidelines on mental health and psychosocial support in emergency settings. *Intervention, 6*(3–4), 199–218.
Williamson, J., & Robinson, M. (2006). Psychosocial interventions or integrated programming for well-being? *Intervention, 4*(1), 4–25.
World Health Organization (WHO). (2006). Report of the psychosocial support programme in tsunami-affected populations in India. *International Review of Psychiatry, 18*(3), 299–308.
World Health Organization (WHO). (2008). *The World Health Report 2008: Primary health care—Now more than ever*. WHO.
World Health Organization (WHO). (2024). *Psychological interventions implementation manual: Integrating evidence-based psychological interventions into existing services*. WHO.
Yadavendu, V. K. (2023). Looking beyond the lamp post: Health inequality in the times of COVID-19. *International Journal of Social Determinants of Health and Health Services, 53*(4), 478–487.

U. Vindhya was formerly with Tata Institute of Social Sciences, Hyderabad, the Centre for Economic and Social Studies, Hyderabad, and Andhra University, Visakhapatnam. Her research interests lie at the intersections of psychology, feminism, social justice and human rights, with focus on gender and mental health, violence against women, trafficking, feminist counselling, and the psychological dynamics of women's political activism. Her publications include Feminist Psychologies: Identities, Relations, and Well-being in India (2024) and the co-edited Handbook of International Feminisms: Perspectives on Psychology, Women, Culture and Rights that won the 2012 Distinguished Publication Award from the Association for Women in Psychology (USA). She has led several research projects sponsored by the World Bank, Gates Foundation, ICRW, UGC, and ICSSR amongst others. She is the recipient of several awards and fellowships including the South Asian Visiting Scholarship (Oxford University, UK); Fulbright Visiting Lecturership (USA); and Visiting Professorships in Eotvos Lorand University, Hungary and University of Gothenburg, Sweden.

Chapter 2
Rise to Stardom: Mental Health and Digital Interventions in the Context of COVID 19

Jacquleen Joseph

Abstract The phrase "No one is left untouched by a disaster" has been true at a global scale in the context of COVID 19. The recognition of the shared phenomenon of psychological suffering and the spread of technology like that of smartphones among others has brought digital mental health services to the forefront (signified in the title as *Rise to Stardom*) as an innovative approach. Since it addresses key challenges of access and scale-up of interventions during disasters, it is more likely to stay. Thus, it becomes imperative to reflect on the opportunities and challenges that each disaster and the emerging interventions, poses to the progress in multidisciplinary mental health sciences. This chapter is based on the review of secondary literature and eight digital mental health services in the Indian context, sampled from the items available in response to a google search for digital mental health services in June 2020, that is in the first phase of COVID 19. The predominance of digital mental health intervention challenges the progress in mental health sciences during disasters, as most services are stand-alone and individualistic in its approach, psychologically oriented and overshadows the emphasis on the social origin of distress. Finally, the chapter puts forth a twofold strategy of integrating standalone services and strengthening of social interventions by drawing from existing social science understanding of vulnerability to distress and illness, and its social origin, to address the pressing needs on the ground.

Keywords Digital mental health services · Disasters · COVID 19 · Mental health sciences · Social science

---

J. Joseph (✉)
The Jamsetji Tata School of Disaster Studies, Tata Institute of Social Sciences, Mumbai, India
e-mail: jacquleenjoseph@tiss.ac.in; josephjacquleen@gmail.com

U. Vindhya (ed.), *Psychosocial Interventions for Social Issues in Contemporary India*,
https://doi.org/10.1007/978-981-96-6553-2_2

Introduction

The phrase "No one is left untouched by a disaster" needs no more substantiation in the context of COVID 19 pandemic. The uncertainties attached to the virus, its treatment, the legal enforcement of lockdown, compulsory assessment, detention, quarantine, and the socio-economic consequences, has made psychological suffering an everyday shared phenomenon. The recognition of the shared psychological suffering has elicited renewed interest and commitment to Mental Health and PsychoSocial Support (MHPSS) interventions, at a global scale and the chapter signifies the same as "Rise to Stardom" in its title. It also provides hope for a better future that recognizes mental health in par with physical health and ensures better allocation of resources, reduced feelings of otherness and stigma, experienced by people living with mental ill-health (Editorial, *The Lancet Psychiatry*, 2020a; 2020b; Wind et al., 2020). However, the literature on the historical evolution of disaster mental health research and practice shows a contrary trend especially with regard to the plight of people living with mental illness (Editorial, *The Lancet Psychiatry*, 2020c; Howell, 2012; Raphael & Maguire, 2009). The politics underlying the transition of the tabooed subject, seeming to become a priority are complex and multi-layered (Foucault, 1991; Pupavac, 2002; UNHCR, 2022; Young, 1997). The political processes unleashed as part of the everyday is maximized in the context of disasters and is beyond the scope of this chapter (Abramowitz & Kleinman, 2008; Howell, 2012; Pupavac, 2002). Furthermore, this chapter deliberately disengages from the extensive theoretical debates (Agamben, 1998; Foucault, 1991; Pupavac, 2001, 2002, 2004a, 2004b, 2005, 2006a, 2006b, 2008, 2012; Rehberg, 2015) of the past and focuses on pragmatic solutions for evidence informed services during COVID 19 and future disasters. This pragmatic focus is justified by drawing from the so-called "breakthrough in professional reflexivity" (Abramowitz & Kleinman, 2008; Wind et al., 2020) to be able to overcome the disillusionment created by the counterproductive theoretical debates. However, these theoretical critiques re-iterate the need to look at MHPSS interventions in the context of COVID 19 with caution, as they are the sign of things to come, hastened by the window of opportunity opening up in the context of disasters.

Digital or virtual interventions like helplines, telephonic/online/video counselling, chat based counselling via Facebook, Instagram, Twitter and Live chat, mental health Applications and platforms, Interactive Voice Response System (IVRS) based telephonic outpatient follow-up and e-prescription services, digital programmes and Artificial Intelligence based self-help tools and voice/video therapy sessions, among others have emerged as a promising possibility and have been widely used across contexts owing to the social distancing enforced by the pandemic (Banerjee et al., 2021; Gonsalves et al., 2023; Roy et al., 2021; Wind et al., 2020). This perspective paper reflects on the implications of COVID 19 and the emerging digital mental health interventions, for the larger field of MHPSS in the context of disasters and humanitarian emergencies. The chapter first reflects on the historical evolution of the disaster MHPSS, its unique contributions to the field of mental health sciences, and the various undercurrents in the wake of different disasters that have shaped the sector the way it stands today. The paper then moves on to reflect on the evolution of the digital mental health interventions, and the nature of digital mental health interventions in the context of COVID, highlighting the challenges and opportunities it brings forth to the sector of Disaster MHPSS. The way forward section highlights the key priorities and strategies to be upheld, to ensure the progression of the field of MHPSS during disasters and humanitarian emergencies, by integrating the scholarship from multiple disciplines constituting the mental health sciences.

The Paradigm Shift from Traumatic Stress Perspective to That of Mental Health Sciences

Mental health is recognized to be a multidimensional concept or phenomenon informed by the lived experiences of people living with mental illness and scholarship in multiple disciplines, referred to as the mental health sciences. But the dominance of psychiatry and related clinical fields, in everyday practice and research, is the reality. However, early disaster research that focuses on the social consequences of disasters has been a significant contributor to the integration of alternative disciplinary perspectives in practice. Thus, the field of disaster MHPSS has been more multidisciplinary than the everyday mainstream practice of mental health (in theory if not in practice). The consensus around the Interagency Standing Committee guidelines (IASC, 2006) for MHPSS and the recognition of psychosocial consequences along with mental health consequences, has been a significant milestone in acknowledging the social context of individual experiences during disasters and emergencies. However, the much-revered consensus known as the "breakthrough in professional reflexivity" (Abramowitz & Kleinman, 2008) was not a new phenomenon of the twenty-first century. It is one among the multiple social science assertions against the politics of mental health and social control, since the second half of the twentieth century. The work of disaster researchers in the 50s and 60s (Baker, 1962; Dynes, 1969; Lifton, 2012; Quarantelli, 1954) brought about a sociological turn to the trauma and psychopathology centric research and practice of the 40s and 50s (Adler, 1943; Lindemann, 1944; Tyhurst, 1951; Wolfenstein, 2018). These social researchers acknowledged the nature of stressors (death, destruction, injury and loss) and its implications for individual and collective trauma. Thus, these researchers also brought to the forefront, the impact of disaster events on communities and societies, the mass response to it, and the interpretations and meanings, not limited to that of an individual (Raphael & Maguire, 2009).

In the 1970s and 80 s, though there was a specific focus on mental health impacts of human-induced disasters (Abrahams et al., 1976; Editorial, *The Lancet Psychiatry*, 2020c; Kinston & Rosser, 1974; Milne, 1977; Taylor & Frazer, 1982) both sociological and mental health approaches were utilized to study disasters such as the Buffalo Creek Disaster (Erikson, 1976; Gleser et al., 1978; Titchener et al., 1976), and victims of political terrorism (Ochberg & Soskis, 1982). These studies unearthed the powerful social influences in individual experience and outcomes.

With the conceptualization of the Traumatic stress syndromes (Horowitz, 1976), the establishment of the diagnosis of Post-Traumatic Stress Syndrome in Diagnostic and Statistical Manual (DSM) III in 1980, and the increasing number of research on human-induced disasters, there was a reversal of the sociological turn, bringing the traumatic stress syndrome and focus on individuals back to priority. This was also the period that saw the institutionalization of mental health within the humanitarian architecture (World Health Organization [WHO], United Nation [UN] & Non-Governmental Organizations [NGOs]), the emergence of new institutions such as the International Society for Traumatic Stress and the emphasis on developing interventions. Thus, the preliminary versions of today's evidence informed trauma interventions such as psychological first aid, psychological debriefing (Raphael, 1977), bereavement counselling (Singh & Raphael, 1981), psychotherapeutic outreach (Lindy et al., 1983), and Critical Incident Stress Debriefing (Mitchell, 1983) were also conceptualized and implemented during this period. The resurgence of the critique of traumatic stress perspective (Kleber et al., 2013; Summerfield, 1999, 2001) and specifically that of PTSD, gave way to professional reflexivity to acknowledge social context briefly in the 1990s, only to be replaced by the focus on trauma post 9/11.

The recent breakthrough in professional reflexivity and commitment to multidisciplinarity in the twenty-first century has been once again made possible by the shared psychological suffering of the so-called "normal", the convergence of informal helpers, the consolidation of the UN Cluster System and the inability of the traditional individualistic approaches to be able to reach out to the large populations needing services at the time of disasters such as the 2004 Tsunami (Joseph, 2016). The recent professional reflexivity has also led to the resurgence of the public mental health and ecological approaches in the context of disasters and humanitarian emergencies (Campion et al., 2020; Kleber, 2019; Galway et al., 2019).

Though disaster MHPSS is multidisciplinary in its conception, the field of practice is largely co-opted by mainstream mental health clinical practice that is trauma focussed and individualistic in its approach. The 20th-century social sciences research on the social contexts of trauma have not made much progress and have been narrowly conceptualized and operationalized in the field of practice, as social support programmes at the level of the individual (Rehberg, 2015). The social science perspective emphasizes the need to address the social origins of distress rather than locating distress within the individual (Silove, 2005). Thus, it prioritizes alternate ways of responding to suffering over the therapeutic processing of emotions based on the assumption of the emotional vulnerability of individuals (Bracken, 2002). For example, Barton refers to disasters and humanitarian emergencies like that of COVID 19, as collective stress situations in which "many members of a social system fail to receive expected conditions of life from a system" (Barton, 1969, p. 38). Thus, the locus of action is not the mental health clinics, professional or individual clients, but the social context of the disaster setting. It conceptualizes stakeholders beyond mental health professionals to include communities, political actor, policymakers, bureaucrats and humanitarian workers, in addressing the support and pragmatic basic needs of the so-called "normal" and that of the people living with mental illness. However concerted efforts would be required from within non-clinical mental health sciences to discover, evaluate and refine social interventions that address distress and ill-health experienced by individuals and collectives.

As every subsequent disaster has the potential to skew the balance between the traumatic stress and social science perspective, as witnessed in the past (Raphael & Maguire, 2009), it becomes imperative to analyse the factors that structure MHPSS interventions in each disaster.

In the context of COVID 19, the social factors contributing to distress are more than obvious not just in Low or Middle Income Countries (LMIC). However, there is a threat of the available solution or technology shaping the definition of the problem uniformly across contexts. This would overshadow the significant social issues of economic vulnerability, marginalization, deprivation, access and social exclusion that are specific to LMIC and specific vulnerable groups such as the people living with mental illness in most contexts. Thus, in the given context of differential vulnerability in the LMIC context, the paper explores the nature of digital mental health interventions and the extent to which they take into consideration the social context that contributes to distress and ill-health. To address this purpose the paper draws from the review of secondary literature on the evolution of digital mental health services and eight digital mental health services in the Indian context, sampled from the items available in response to a Google search for digital mental health services in June 2020. Search results for digital mental health services that had adequate information in the areas being explored and those that represented various mental health stakeholders were purposefully chosen to constitute a comprehensive picture of the opportunities and challenges posed by digital mental health services in response to COVID 19 in the Indian context.

The Evolution of the Digital Mental Health Services as the Key Mental Health Response to COVID 19: Opportunity and Challenges

The movement for Global Mental Health (Patel, 2012) emphasizes the need to address the global burden of mental illness and treatment gap, by reconsidering the traditional approaches to service delivery within institutions. This led to the development and evaluation of several psychological interventions that could be delivered by community workers and trained volunteers, especially for the treatment of common mental disorders such as depression, anxiety, self-harm and suicides. The impetus for mechanistically informed psychological interventions, innovations in traditional mental health service delivery and the emergence of new low-cost technology of smartphones, internet services and cloud-based calling, set the base for digital mental health services. The identification of an unmet need and the low-cost technology to bridge the gap, created the market opportunity for psychological interventions in the recent past, resulting in a range of products that replaces the older version of telepsychiatry (Wind et al., 2020). Table 2.1 captures some of the digital mental health services in India in the context of COVID 19.

Though digital services seem to be a perfect solution to the social distancing enforced by COVID 19, the mental health discipline has been sceptical of its efficacy, access and promise as a mode of mental health service delivery since long (Barton, 1969; Holmes et al., 2018; O'Connor & Portzky, 2018). The review of the various digital mental health interventions in LMIC too indicated its continued growth, however a closer look at their efficacy is not very conclusive and needs serious evaluation (Carter et al., 2021; Gonsalves et al., 2023).

The past trends in the field of disaster MHPSS such as the introduction of crisis counselling, Critical Incident Stress Debriefing (CISD)/Critical Incident Stress Management (CISM), psychological first aid, Mental Health Gap Action Programme (mhGAP), task shifting approach, among others has demonstrated the mainstream mental health discourse's potential to co-opt the field of practice in disasters, although the underlying principles shaping practice in the context of disasters are quite different. Thus, digital mental health services are here to stay, especially because they promise a solution to the key challenges encountered in the context of disasters: limited or non-existent mental health human resource in the remote contexts hit by disasters and the need to scale up, to address the needs of large populations requiring services. Thus, it becomes imperative to reflect on the implications of digital mental health services on the larger field of disaster MHPSS, especially the fine equilibrium between social and mental health interventions.

Based on the review of a sample of digital mental health services in the Indian context, this chapter identifies the key challenges in the field of practice to be: the individualistic approach; primarily brief and one-time stand-alone services; and the issue of access among a large majority who really need the services. Most services are universal and some target specific vulnerable groups such as children and women facing violence. The conception of vulnerable groups is very universal and static in the field of clinical practice, with almost all the world's population fitting into one or the other category. The intersectionality in vulnerability to distress and mental illness, in line with the syndemics approach[1] (Singer, 2009; Singer & Snipes, 1992; Sharma, 2017), is to be understood in identifying and delivering targeted interventions to the most vulnerable in each disaster context (Holmes et al., 2020).

In the given context of differential vulnerability to COVID 19 in the LMIC context, the predominance of universal digital mental health services (customized only using technologies such as Artificial Intelligence and Machine Learning) poses a threat of overshadowing the recognition of social origin of distress; pathologizing of normal reactions to abnormal situations; disproportionate focus on the subjective reactions such as fleeting emotions expressed over social media that is easily monitored, but

[1] "The term syndemic refers to synergistic health problems that affect the health of a population within the context of persistent social and economic inequalities" (Mendenhall et al., 2017, p. 951). "the most unique feature of the syndemic approach to understanding various disease states and the way in which they cluster is the emphasis on the situation and circumstances in which individuals live" (Sharma, 2017).

Table 2.1 The nature of digital mental health services in the Indian context during COVID 19

	Nature of digital mental health services	Organization/ category	Point of initiation of digital mental health services/other competencies
1	Online Counselling and Mental Health Facility for Mental Health Issues	Department of Applied Psychology, University of Mumbai / Academic	During COVID 19 Pandemic/ Academic Programmes in Psychology and allied activities
2	PAN INDIA FREE PSYCHOLOGICAL CRISIS INTERVENTIONS THROUGH VOLUNTEER COUNSELLORS Video Counselling Mind Care App	Master Mind Foundation/NGO	2005 Pre COVID 19 Pandemic/ Disaster Relief, Tree Plantation, Workshops, Seminars and Training
3	Mental Health Consultation and Guidance—Telephone Counselling with 60 psychologists on call	Tamil Nadu Psychology Association/ Professional Association	During COVID 19 Pandemic/ Networking and Publications
4	IVRS Based Telephone Outpatient Follow-up Services (Only for previously registered patient) along with e-prescription services Psychosocial Support and Mental Health Services during Disaster—TOLL FREE HELPLINE PSYC-CARE—A platform to support health workers involved in providing psychological help in the context of COVID-19	NIMHANS	During COVID 19 /Apex centre for mental health and neuro sciences education in the country
5	COVID 19 Counselling and Therapeutic Support—Telephonic counselling and Chat based counselling via Facebook, Instagram, Twitter, and live chat	ARPAN/NGO	Pre COVID-19/Child Sexual Abuse Related Services—Personal Safety Education, Counselling, Training and Advocacy, Online Courses
6	TOLL FREE Helpline NO	Maharashtra Government and Bhrihumumbai Municipal Corporation along with MPower/ Government	During COVID/ Mpower offers Workshops, Youth Mental Health First Aid, Support Groups, and Movement for Combating Stigma and Awareness Generation

(continued)

Table 2.1 (continued)

	Nature of digital mental health services	Organization/ category	Point of initiation of digital mental health services/other competencies
7	Paramarsh Free helpline No for telephonic/online Counselling of COVID 19 related Psychological Issues	Indian Association of Clinical Psychologists/ Professional Association	During COVID/Networking and Publication
8	COVID 19 Self Care Guide Mental Health Platform that offers digital programmes, AI based self-help tools and voice/ video therapy sessions	Inner Hour/Start Up	Pre COVID 19/Paid Counselling Services (20% discount during COVID 19), Employee Happiness Programmes, Webinars

a less precise and skewed indicator of distress of individuals and larger collectives; not reaching out to the most vulnerable and needy who are alienated and at the periphery of technology's reach, among others. However, the opportunities that the digital mental health services offer are many, if one utilizes it taking to cognizance the limitations it puts forth and attempts to bridge the same. The key window of opportunity that this disaster opens up is the integration of a whole range of private practitioners and mental health professionals who were far from the hinterlands of disasters, into the disaster mental health and psychosocial support interventions field. They could be networked and streamlined to provide specialized and non-specialized services to groups at risk of psychological distress and illness during future disasters. However, to complete this integration, more work is required regarding interdisciplinary capacity building and research to evolve, evaluate and refine current digital mental health services in the context of disasters and emergencies. This would provide more space for professional reflexivity and ensure that the distinct principles of disaster mental health and psychosocial interventions are upheld, thus contributing to the furtherance of the multidisciplinary mental health sciences in the context of disasters.

Way Forward

This section builds on the "breakthrough in professional reflexivity" (Abramowitz & Kleinman, 2008) achieved in the context of disaster MHPSS. The strategies put forth for operationalizing the concept of the multidisciplinary mental health sciences in the context of disasters are two-fold:

(1) Integration of Stand-Alone Mental Health and Psychological Interventions with Pragmatic Humanitarian Interventions: Standalone mental health and psychological services are contrary to the multidisciplinary moorings of mental health sciences. Moreover, as standalone mental health and psychological services are most

likely to ignore the situations and circumstances in which individuals live, their effectiveness especially in the context of disasters need to be revisited. The conception of the reactions to disasters as normal reactions to an abnormal context, reiterates the need for integration of standalone services with at least pragmatic services to begin with. The integration could be achieved at different levels and scale. It could range from the level of departments within an organization to between organizations in line with the multi-team systems and can be at the scale of any administrative unit. Box 1 below summarizes the changes made to the nature of psychological interventions provided to medical staff in response to the challenges faced in the acceptance of services offered, highlights the reflexivity of mental health professionals in the context of COVID 19 and the approach of integration (Bracken, 2002). Such professional reflexivity could be fostered through orientation and capacity building of mental health professionals regarding the significance of multi-disciplinarity especially in the context of disasters. The networking of standalone interventions could foster collaborations leading to integration, capacity building, evolution of guidelines to ensure quality of services and collation of data to establish the efficacy of the digital mental health and psychological interventions in LMIC context.

Box 1: Reflexivity Among Mental Health Professionals During Covid 19, in The Second Xiangya Hospital, China

In response to psychological suffering perceived among the medical staff the following set of interventions were designed: building a psychological intervention medical team to provide online courses to medical staff to deal common psychological problems; a psychological assistance hotline team, which provided guidance and supervision to solve psychological problems; and psychological interventions, which provided various group activities to release stress.

However, the team encountered the following hurdles in the implementation of the psychological intervention: refusal of help despite obvious signs of psychological distress, concerns for the families' well-being over and above one's well-being and risk of infection, attribution of distress to the constraints encountered in the work environment such as inadequate rest, lack of protective devices, challenges of handling uncooperative patients, among others. Thus instead of attributing the implementation challenges to the lack of psychological mindedness of the medical staff, the reflexivity of the mental health team re-structured the psychological interventions as follows: Enhancing the work environment by providing a place for rest, food and daily living supplies, helping staff connect to family members to alleviate family's concerns, capacity building of staff to identify and respond to psychological problems in patients, making available assistance of hospital security staff to handle uncooperative patients, developing protocols for use and management of protective equipment to address worries about shortage, making available training and leisure activities for self-care, and reaching out to staff at the rest areas to listen to their difficulties and stories and provide support accordingly.

(2) Strengthening and Establishing Efficacy of Social Interventions within Disaster Mental Health and Psychosocial Support Services: Though the so called "breakthrough in professional reflexivity" was with regard to the equal footage of social interventions, with mental health and psychological interventions, it never materialized in practice. In the context of COVID 19 too, though the social origin of distress is acknowledged, very little emphasis is placed on interventions to address the same (Gunnell et al., 2020; Holmes et al., 2020; Kawohl & Nordt, 2020; Klomek, 2020). The co-option by main-stream clinical practice resulting in the narrow definition of social interventions in terms of individual level social support programmes (James et al., 2012) is a key challenge in current practice. There has been very minimal focus on understanding and addressing social origin or determinants of distress among individuals and collectives, similar to that of the syndemic approach in health sciences. The focus should shift from the emotions experienced by individuals that dominate current day practice, to that of understanding and addressing social stressors contributing to distress among those vulnerable to distress and mental illness. To strengthen the social interventions dimension of MHPSS, one has to start with the collation of social interventions that have implications for psychological distress, collate the evidence base of social interventions, design and roll out research to establish the efficacy of macro social interventions like policy interventions, economic relief packages and recovery programmes, in addressing distress. The key challenge is with regard to the amenability of such complex interventions to the efficacy logic of RCTs and the dilution of its essence in reducing complex social interventions to mechanistically informed interventions. However, this is a challenge to be addressed by social science practitioners and researchers, as mental health professionals with their clinical training are not always best suited to design and implement social support programmes (van Ommeren et al., 2005).

Conclusion

In the context of disasters, the tabooed subject of Mental Health gains prominence and this chapter attempts to unravel the pragmatic consequences of the same for those needing services especially in the LMIC. Though disaster MHPSS interventions are much more multi-disciplinary in its conception, social interventions and the public mental health approach that address the social origin of distress among collectives in the context of disasters and emergencies are limited. Thus, the predominance of the individualistic approaches during disasters and emergencies limits the ability of the sector to reach out to large populations in distress. The paper reflects on the emerging digital mental health services in the context of disasters and emergencies in the light of the significant gaps and challenges faced by the sector. Though they seem to be a perfect innovation in the context of social distancing during the current crisis, they are not the solution to the challenges of scale and access that the sector is grappling with. However, professional reflexivity emerging from the knowledge of the challenges can make a difference to MHPSS services in the context of disaster and emergencies. The chapter identifies a twofold strategy for operationalizing the concept of the multidisciplinary mental health sciences in the context of disaster and emergencies: integration of standalone MHPSS services with pragmatic humanitarian interventions; and strengthening the social interventions component within MHPSS services, designed along with robust research to demonstrate its efficacy. Drawing in from the existing social science understanding of mental health, especially regarding the context of vulnerability and its contribution to distress and illness, in line with the syndemic approach, can help in making a difference in mental health services, especially to the most vulnerable including Persons Living with Mental Illness (PLWMI) and the larger populations in distress, in the context of disasters and emergencies.

References

Abrahams, M. J., Price, J., Whitlock, F. A., & Williams, G. (1976). The Brisbane floods, January 1974: Their impact on health. *Medical Journal of Australia, 2*(25–26), 936–939.

Abramowitz, S., & Kleinman, A. (2008). Humanitarian intervention and cultural translation: A review of the—IASC Guidelines on Mental Health and Psychosocial Support in Emergency Settings. *Intervention Journal of Mental Health and Psychosocial Support in Conflict Affected Areas, 6*(3), 219–227.

Adler, A. (1943). Neuropsychiatric complications in victims of Boston's Cocoanut Grove disaster. *Journal of the American Medical Association, 123*(17), 1098–1101.

Agamben, G. (1998). *Homo sacer: Sovereign power and bare life*. Stanford university Press. Available from https://doi.org/10.1515/9781503603158-001/html

Baker, G. W., Chapman, D. W., & Jacobsen, C. F. (1962). *Man and society in disaster* (No Title). Basic Books.

Banerjee, D., Vajawat, B., & Varshney, P. (2021). Digital gaming interventions: A novel paradigm in mental health? Perspectives from India. *International Review of Psychiatry, 33*(4), 435–441.

Barton, A. H. (1969). *Communities in disaster: A sociological analysis of collective stress situations* (No Title). Anchor.

Bracken, P. (2002). *Trauma: Culture, meaning and philosophy*. Whurr Publishers.

Carter, H., Araya, R., Anjur, K., Deng, D., & Naslund, J. A. (2021). The emergence of digital mental health in low-income and middle-income countries: A review of recent advances and implications for the treatment and prevention of mental disorders. *Journal of Psychiatric Research, 133*, 223–246.

Campion, J., Javed, A., Sartorius, N., & Marmot, M. (2020). Addressing the public mental health challenge of COVID-19. *The Lancet Psychiatry, 7*(8), 657–659.

Chen, Q., Liang, M., Li, Y., Guo, J., Fei, D., Wang, L., & Zhang, Z. (2020). Mental health care for medical staff in China during the COVID-19 outbreak. *The Lancet Psychiatry, 7*(4), e15–e16.

Dynes, R. R. (1969). *Organized behavior in disaster: Analysis and conceptualization* (No. 3). Disaster Research Center, Ohio State University.

Editorial. (2020a). Send in the therapists? *The Lancet Psychiatry, 7*(4), 291.

Editorial. (2020b). Isolation and inclusion. *The Lancet Psychiatry, 7*(5), 371.
Editorial. (2020c). Mental health and COVID-19: Change the conversation. *The Lancet Psychiatry., 7*(6), 463.
Erikson, K. T. (1976). Disaster at Buffalo Creek: Loss of communality at Buffalo Creek. *The American Journal of Psychiatry, 133*(3), 302–305.
Foucault. M. (1991). Governmentality. In G. Burchell, C. Gordon, & P. Miller (Eds.), *The Foucault effect: Studies in governmentality.* University of Chicago Press.
Galway, L. P., Beery, T., Jones-Casey, K., & Tasala, K. (2019). Mapping the solastalgia literature: A scoping review study. *International Journal of Environmental Research and Public Health, 16*(15), 2662.
Gleser, G. C., Green, B. L., & Winget, C. N. (1978). Quantifying interview data on psychic impairment of disaster survivors. *The Journal of Nervous and Mental Disease, 166*(3), 209–216.
Gonsalves, P. P., Bhat, B., Sharma, R., Jambhale, A., Chodankar, B., Verma, M., & Patel, V. (2023). Pilot randomised controlled trial of a remotely delivered online intervention for adolescent mental health problems in India: Lessons learned about low acceptability and feasibility during the COVID-19 pandemic. *Bjpsych Open, 9*(1), Article e7.
Gunnell, D., Appleby, L., Arensman, E., Hawton, K., John, A., Kapur, N., & Yip, P. S. (2020). Suicide risk and prevention during the COVID-19 pandemic. *The Lancet Psychiatry, 7*(6), 468–471.
Holmes, E. A., Ghaderi, A., Harmer, C. J., Ramchandani, P. G., Cuijpers, P., Morrison, A. P., & Craske, M. G. (2018). The Lancet Psychiatry Commission on psychological treatments research in tomorrow's science. *The Lancet Psychiatry, 5*(3), 237–286.
Holmes, E. A., O'Connor, R. C., Perry, V. H., Tracey, I., Wessely, S., Arseneault, L., & Bullmore, E. (2020). Multidisciplinary research priorities for the COVID-19 pandemic: A call for action for mental health science. *The Lancet Psychiatry, 7*(6), 547–560.
Horowitz, M. J. (1976). *Stress response syndromes* (p. 386). Aronson.
Howell, A. (2012). The demise of PTSD: From governing through trauma to governing resilience. *Alternatives, 37*(3), 214–226.
Inter-Agency Standing Committee. (2006). IASC guidelines on mental health and psychosocial support in emergency settings. *Geneva, Switzerland: IASC 2006.*Available from https://ci.nii.ac.jp/naid/10030164622/
James, L. E., Noel, J. R., Favorite, T. K., & Jean, J. S. (2012). Challenges of postdisaster intervention in cultural context: The implementation of a lay mental health worker project in postearthquake Haiti. *International Perspectives in Psychology, 1*(2), 110–126.
Joseph, J. (2016). Disaster mental health vs. psychosocial well Bebing: The need for a true paradigm change, *Austin Journal of Emergency and Critical Care Medicine, 3*(2), 1–3 [ISSN: 2380–0879].
Kawohl, W., & Nordt, C. (2020). COVID-19, unemployment, and suicide. *The Lancet Psychiatry, 7*(5), 389–390.
Kinston, W., & Rosser, R. (1974). Disaster: Effects on mental and physical state. *Journal of Psychosomatic Research, 18*(6), 437–456.
Kleber, R. J., Figley, C. R., & Gersons, B. P. (Eds.). (2013). *Beyond trauma: Cultural and societal dynamics.* Springer Science & Business Media. Available from https://doi.org/10.1007/978-1-4757-9421-2
Kleber, R. J. (2019). Trauma and public mental health: A focused review. *Frontiers in Psychiatry, 10*, Article 397907.
Klomek, A. B. (2020). Suicide prevention during the COVID-19 outbreak. *The Lancet Psychiatry, 7*(5), 390.
Lifton, R. J. (2012). *Death in life: Survivors of Hiroshima.* University of North Carolina Press.
Lindemann, E. (1944). Symptomatology and management of acute grief. *American Journal of Psychiatry, 101*(2), 141–148.
Lindy, J. D., Green, B. L., Grace, M., & Titchener, J. (1983). Psychotherapy with survivors of the Beverly Hills Supper Club fire. *American Journal of Psychotherapy, 37*(4), 593–610.

Mendenhall, E., Kohrt, B. A., Norris, S. A., Ndetei, D., & Prabhakaran, D. (2017). Non-communicable disease syndemics: Poverty, depression, and diabetes among low-income populations. *The Lancet, 389*(10072), 951–963.
Milne, G. (1977). Cyclone tracy: II the effects on darwin children. *Australian Psychologist, 12*(1), 55–62.
Mitchell, J. T. (1983). When disaster strikes: The critical incident stress debriefing process. *Journal of Emergency Medical Services,*8, 36–39.
O'Connor, R. C., & Portzky, G. (2018). Looking to the future: A synthesis of new developments and challenges in suicide research and prevention. *Frontiers in Psychology, 9*, 391532. Available from https://doi.org/10.3389/fpsyg.2018.02139/full
Ochberg, F. M., & Soskis, D. A. (1982). *Victims of terrorism* (No Title). Westview Press.
Patel, V. (2012). Global mental health: From science to action. *Harvard Review of Psychiatry, 20*(1), 6–12.
Perry, R. W., & Quarantelli, E. L. (2005). *Disaster and collective stress—In: What is a disaster?: New answers to old questions.* Xlibris Corporation.
Pupavac, V. (2001). Therapeutic governance: Psycho-social intervention and trauma risk management. *Disasters, 25*(4), 358–372.
Pupavac, V. (2002). Pathologizing populations and colonizing minds: International psychosocial programs in Kosovo. *Alternatives, 27*(4), 489–511.
Pupavac, V. (2004a). International therapeutic peace and justice in Bosnia. *Social & Legal Studies, 13*(3), 377–401.
Pupavac, V. (2004b). Psychosocial interventions and the demoralization of humanitarianism. *Journal of Biosocial Science, 36*(4), 491–504.
Pupavac, V. (2005). Human security and the rise of global therapeutic governance: Analysis. *Conflict, Security & Development, 5*(2), 161–181.
Pupavac, V. (2006). Humanitarian politics and the rise of international disaster psychology. *Handbook of International Disaster Psychology, 1*, 15–34.Available from https://doi.org/10.13140/2.1.1715.4883
Pupavac, V. (2006). *Refugees in the' 'sick role': Stereotyping refugees and eroding refugee rights.* UNHCR, Evaluation and Policy Analysis Unit. Available from https://www.unhcr.org/research/working/44e198712/refugees-sick-role-stereotyping-refugees-eroding-refugee-rights-vanessa.html
Pupavac, V. (2008). Refugee advocacy, traumatic representations and political disenchantment. *Government and Opposition, 43*(2), 270–292.
Pupavac, V. (2012). Global disaster management and therapeutic governance of communities. *Development Dialogue, 58*, 81–97.
Quarantelli, E. L. (1954). The nature and conditions of panic. *American Journal of Sociology, 60*(3), 267–275.
Raphael, B. (1977). The Granville train disaster: Psychological needs and their management. *Medical Journal of Australia, 1*(9), 303–305.
Roy, A., Singh, A. K., Mishra, S., Chinnadurai, A., Mitra, A., & Bakshi, O. (2021). Mental health implications of COVID-19 pandemic and its response in India. *International Journal of Social Psychiatry, 67*(5), 587–600.
Maguire, R. B. (2009). Disaster mental health research: Past, present, and future. In Y. Neria, S. Galea, F. H. Norris (Eds.), *Mental health and disasters* (pp. 7–28). Cambridge University Press (cited 2021 August 27).
Raphael, B., & Maguire, P. (2009). Disaster mental health research: Past, present, and future. *Mental health and disasters* (pp. 7–28). Cambridge University Press. Available from https://www.cambridge.org/core/product/identifier/9780511730030%23c88387-2-1/type/book_part
Rehberg, K. (2015). Revisiting therapeutic governance: The politics of mental health and psychosocial programs in humanitarian settings. *American Journal of Medical Research, 2*(2), 130–169.
Sharma, A. (2017). Syndemics: Health in context. *Lancet, 389*(10072), 881.

Silove, D. (2005). The best immediate therapy for acute stress is social. *Bulletin of the World Health Organization, 83*(1), 75–76.

Singer, M., & Snipes, C. (1992). Generations of suffering: Experiences of a treatment program for substance abuse during pregnancy. *Journal of Health Care for the Poor and Underserved, 3*(1), 222–234.

Singer, M. (2009). *Introduction to syndemics: A critical systems approach to public and community health.* Wiley.

Singh, B., & Raphael, B. (1981). Postdisaster morbidity of the bereaved: A possible role for preventive psychiatry? *The Journal of Nervous and Mental Disease, 169*(4), 203–212.

Summerfield, D. (1999). A critique of seven assumptions behind psychological trauma programmes in war-affected areas. *Social Science & Medicine (1982), 48*(10), 1449–1462.

Summerfield, D. (2001). The invention of post-traumatic stress disorder and the social usefulness of a psychiatric category. *BMJ, 322*(7278), 95–98.

Swinburn, B. A., Kraak, V. I., Allender, S., Atkins, V. J., Baker, P. I., Bogard, J. R., & Dietz, W. H. (2019). The global syndemic of obesity, undernutrition, and climate change: The Lancet Commission report. *The Lancet, 393*(10173), 791–846.

Taylor, A. J. W., & Frazer, A. G. (1982). The stress of post-disaster body handling and victim identification work. *Journal of Human Stress, 8*(4), 4–12.

Titchener, J. L., Kapp, F. T., & Winget, C. (1976). The Buffalo Creek syndrome: Symptoms and character change after a major disaster. In *Emergency and disaster management: A mental health sourcebook* (pp. 283–94). Bowie, MD: The Charles Press Publishers.

Tyhurst, J. S. (1951). Individual reactions to community disaster: The natural history of psychiatric phenomena. *American Journal of Psychiatry, 107*(10), 764–769.

UNHCR. (2022). Strengthening mental health and psychosocial support in UNHCR: Achievements in 2021 and priorities for 2022 and beyond. Available from https://reliefweb.int/report/world/strengthening-mental-health-and-psychosocial-support-unhcr-achievements-2021-and-priorities-2022-and-beyondf and Accessed on 30th June 2025.

Van Ommeren, M., Saxena, S., & Saraceno, B. (2005). Mental and social health during and after acute emergencies: Emerging consensus? *Bulletin of the World Health Organization, 83*(1), 71–75.

Weisæth, L. (1989). A study of behavioural response to an industrial disaster. *Acta Psychiatrica Scandinavica, 80*, 13–24.

Wind, T. R., Rijkeboer, M., Andersson, G., & Riper, H. (2020). The COVID-19 pandemic: The 'black swan' for mental health care and a turning point for e-health. *Internet Interventions, 20.* https://doi.org/10.1016/j.invent.2020.100317

Wolfenstein, M. (2018). *Disaster: A psychological essay.* Routledge.

Young, A. (1997). *The harmony of illusions: Inventing post-traumatic stress disorder* (Vol. 11). Princeton University Press.

Jacquleen Joseph is Professor and Dean at the Jamsetji Tata School of Disaster Studies (JTSDS), Tata Institute of Social Sciences (TISS), Mumbai. She has a Masters' degree in Social Work, followed by an MPhil and a Ph.D. in Psychiatric Social Work from the National Institute of Mental Health and Neuro Sciences (NIMHANS), Bangalore. She has been associated with JTSDS since its inception. Her research, field action, and teaching centre around psychosocial care and support in disaster and humanitarian contexts starting with Tsunami 2004 to the most recent Balasore Train Disaster 2023. She has secured several competitive research and networking grants and has contributed to the emerging discipline of disaster studies through her numerous journal articles, book chapters and books.

Chapter 3
COVID-19 Pandemic and Mental Health and Psychosocial Interventions in India: Decoding Past and Informing Future

Aparna Joshi

Abstract COVID-19 pandemic, along with its devastating physical health threats, also contributed to distressing mental health and psychosocial (MHPS) consequences. Worldwide, health systems and voluntary sectors made efforts to respond to these impacts through a variety of interventions. Despite the large body of available literature on the mental health implications of and responses to the pandemic, the literature from low-income and middle-income countries (LMICs) where the majority of the global population lives, and where health resources have historically been marginal, remains scanty. India presents a prototypical example of problems faced by LMICs and yet stands as a pioneer with its mental health programmes and policies. Against this backdrop, the current chapter aimed to undertake a secondary literature review to document support measures and interventions undertaken to address the MHPS impact of the COVID-19 pandemic in India. Thematic analysis of the secondary literature showed that MHPS interventions during the COVID-19 pandemic in India largely originated from a diverse set of stakeholders from three sectors, namely Government, Non-governmental organizations (NGOs) and community-level initiatives. The interventions could be grouped into three thematic areas: (1) For those diagnosed with COVID-19, (2) For the general public and (3) For vulnerable groups. Interventions ranged from drafting guidelines, creating reliable information sources, telemental health and counselling services, providing relief measures to address basic needs, and providing protection services to awareness campaigns and advocacy efforts. These results offer valuable lessons for imagining and organizing mental health services in the future. They also include the need for foregrounding and prioritizing mental health and conceptualizing it through a psychosocial, inclusive and rights-based lens. The chapter ends by appealing for a coordinated and collaborative approach towards mental health service provision and response.

Keywords Psychosocial interventions for covid-19 · Psychosocial impact of pandemic

A. Joshi (✉)
Tata Institute of Social Sciences (TISS), Mumbai, India
e-mail: aparna.joshi@tiss.edu

U. Vindhya (ed.), *Psychosocial Interventions for Social Issues in Contemporary India*,
https://doi.org/10.1007/978-981-96-6553-2_3

Background

The World Health Organization (WHO) decleared 2019 Corona Virus Disease (COVID-19) as an international public health emergency on January 30, 2020. The pandemic, along with its devastating physical health threats, contributed to distressing mental health and psychosocial consequences. The pandemic and the subsequent lockdowns, caused disruption and disorder in the lives of millions worldwide. These were mainly detrimental for poor and vulnerable people in countries with pre-existing weak social support networks and economic resources to buffer against livelihoods that were lost (Kola et al., 2021). Worldwide, health systems and voluntary sectors initiated various interventions to respond to the mental health and Psychosocial (MHPS) impact of the pandemic (Moreno et al., 2020).

Despite the extant literature currently available on the mental health implications of COVID-19, work from low and middle-income countries (LMICs), where 83% of the global population lives and where health resources have historically been marginal (Liese et al., 2019) remains scanty (Kola et al., 2021). India presents a prototypical example of problems faced by LMICs in the form of its high burdens of mental health and low budgetary and human resources, further complicated by social factors such as poverty, rapid urbanization, internal migration alongside unequal economic and social structures (Rathod et al., 2017). At the same time, with its mental health programmes and policies, India stands as an exemplary forerunner in mental health initiatives among the LMICs (Suhas et al., 2023).

Against this backdrop, the current chapter aims to present a secondary literature review to document support measures and interventions to address the MHPS impact of the COVID-19 pandemic in India. This documentation serves to describe the key elements of these interventions and inform future directions.

Introduction

COVID-19: Mental Health and Psychosocial Impact and Interventions in the World

Early evidence of the mental health and psychosocial impact of the COVID-19 pandemic showed that people around the world were severely affected, including concerns of increased suicidal behaviour. In addition, the pandemic severely hindered access to mental health services (World Health Organisation, 2022).

A systematic review of the data on the global prevalence and burden of depressive and anxiety disorders in 204 countries and territories during the COVID-19 pandemic estimated an increase of 27.6% in depression and 25.6% in anxiety disorders in the general population due to the pandemic (COVID-19 Mental Disorders Collaborators, 2021). This increase resulted from the collective effects of the virus spread, containment measures such as lockdowns, closures of schools and businesses, public transport restrictions, and decreased social interactions and isolation. The prevalence of these disorders was most significantly increased in countries hit hardest by the pandemic (COVID-19 Mental Disorders Collaborators, 2021). Other mental health consequences of the pandemic were insomnia, posttraumatic stress disorder (PTSD) or posttraumatic stress syndrome (PTSS), eating disorders, obsessive–compulsive disorder (OCD), bipolar disorder, and further psychological effects (Agrawal et al., 2022).

Some of the economic and social problems caused by the pandemic involved disruption in student lives and educational activities, increased financial load on the family, reduced couple satisfaction and increase in disputes, disruption in social relationships, heavy economic burden and unemployment, exacerbation of segregation and poverty, and declining trends of social capital among communities (Alizadeh et al., 2023; Hosseinzadeh et al., 2022). Studies also showed that the most vulnerable groups faced adverse economic and psychological effects due to the physical distancing measures (Li et al., 2023). Resource diversion from other areas to COVID responses in many countries led to disproportionate effects on vulnerable groups, leaving them with unmet health and mental health service and social security needs (Moreno et al., 2020).

The massive mental health and psychosocial impact created by the pandemic was met with the MHPS response that ranged from traditional psychiatry and psychotherapy-based interventions to those adopting socioeconomic strategies. Worldwide, the available health and mental health infrastructure of the countries was leveraged to address the MHPS consequences of the pandemic. Given the severe mobility restrictions, mental health services largely shifted to online and digital modalities and included tele-mental health for detection and diagnosis, as well as medication and treatment management (Moreno et al., 2020). Psychotherapy interventions were informed mainly by cognitive-behavioural and mindfulness therapy approaches. These also included psychoeducational interventions to reduce symptoms of anxiety, depression, insomnia and stress (Ye et al., 2022).

Other psychosocial interventions majorly comprised measures such as the provision of reliable COVID-19 information for public health education, mental health prevention/promotion and treatment using technology-based interventions, use of physical activity for promoting individual mental health and awareness building around healthy coping strategies for reduction of COVID-19-related anxiety and stress (for example, spending time with family, seeking spiritual guidance, and talking with friends or partners online) (Safieh et al., 2022).

Psychosocial interventions from sectors other than health, such as education, employment, and social welfare, involved policy adaptations for short quarantine durations, dissemination of reliable COVID-19-related information, provision of essential supplies and suggestions for improved interpersonal communication and strategies to cope with boredom (Safieh et al., 2022). Economic actions included cash payments to vulnerable groups (such as workers), offering financial and nutritional grants and lending, subsidies and capital injection, reduction in debt amounts, relaxations in taxes, reimbursement of loans and special buying drives to help economically disadvantaged groups (Azmand et al., 2021). Other interventions included support from government and non-governmental organizations (NGOs) for domestic violence victims, provision of shelters and nutrition for refugees, migrants, homeless and support workers, and measures for older adults by providing goods and services. Some interventions also aimed to increase social support and connectedness, especially among vulnerable groups (Azmand et al., 2021).

Mental Health and Psychosocial Impact of COVID-19 Pandemic in India

India encompasses around 18% of the global population. It contributes significantly to the global burden of mental disorders, with one in seven Indians being affected by mental disorders, amounting to about 200 million people (Sagar et al., 2020).

The first case of COVID-19 in India was reported in January 2020. Subsequently, the Government of India declared the disease a national disaster on March 25, 2020, leading to lockdowns (extended three times) and further shutting down educational institutions, workspaces and modes of transport (Adhikari et al., 2020). The pandemic and the prolonged lockdown severely affected the health, economy, livelihood, and social and professional interactions of the masses (Gulat et al., 2023). The social and economic consequences of the pandemic were distressing, too (Gupta et al., 2022).

Similar to the global trends, studies from India showed the occurrence of mental health dysfunction, with anxiety, stress, and depression (Shukla & Singh, 2021). Studies specifically measuring pandemic's mental health impact as a function of gender, age, and income showed that loss of a job, death of the family's earning member or mishap in the family, and increased prices contributed to increased anxiety, with women showing more significant anxiety than men due to the increased burden of household chores and childcare responsibilities (Gulati et al., 2023). Reviews showed that certain groups were further vulnerable to the MHPS impacts of the pandemic, including those diagnosed with COVID-19 infection, frontline workers, migrants, women and children, elderly, LGBTQIA+ individuals and those with prior mental health problems (Joshi, 2021; Joshi et al., 2022; Roy et al., 2021).

History suggests that while infectious disease outbreaks or pandemics are known to bring significant mental health impacts, countries divert limited resources toward pandemic containment, leaving mental health concerns and treatments less attended (Roy et al., 2021). Similarly, in India, physical health and relief measures occupied centre stage in India's response to the pandemic, leaving mental health a late entrant in the list (Joshi, 2021). The massive MHPS impact created by the pandemic led to further struggles in India's already-flailing mental health systems.

Barring a few exceptions of early articles (e.g., Rangaswamy et al., 2022; Roy et al., 2021), there remains a paucity of comprehensive reviews documenting mental health and psychosocial interventions and support measures carried out during the COVID-19 pandemic in India. Such documentation is necessary for critically analyzing existing literature and providing recommendations for future directions.

Mental Health Interventions and Conceptual Frameworks

Several competing frameworks exist for conceptualizing mental health and psychosocial support (MHPSS) and interventions. These can be broadly grouped into two categories: Clinical and socio-environmental (Miller et al., 2021).

The clinical framework encompasses two approaches: The psychological approach (aimed at altering psychological variables such as emotional dysregulation, maladaptive cognitions and behaviour patterns and trauma-related phenomena) and the biological approach (diagnostic or psychiatric approach, informed by the biomedical viewpoint and involves categorizing people based on sets of symptoms they show) (Miller et al., 2021). These two sub-variants share an emphasis on the treatment of severe forms of distress and illness and predominantly focus on intrapersonal or individual-level factors as intermediaries of change. The focus is on psychological or pharmacological interventions traditionally offered by trained mental health practitioners in health and clinical settings. On the other hand, the social-environmental framework (akin to the psychosocial approach) prioritizes the contribution of environmental-level variables in the causation and maintenance of distress. It focuses on changing environment-level factors and mobilizing social resources for distress reduction and strengthening well-being and resilience. These interventions are carried out by varied actors and in various settings (Miller et al., 2021).

Despite the tensions and seeming contradictions between these two frameworks in terms of their causal analysis and response preferences, a call has been made in recent times for greater dialogue and multilevel interventions for a comprehensive response (Miller et al., 2021). The Inter-agency Standing Committee guidelines for humanitarian and emergency settings capture the complementarity and possible synergy between clinical and social-environmental frameworks (IASC, 2007). 'Mental health and psychosocial support' (MHPSS) is a broader term used to connote " Any type of local or outside support that aims to protect or promote psychosocial well-being and/or prevent or treat mental disorder" (IASC, 2007: 1). Recent international guidelines have confirmed that MHPSS is not confined to a single sector but requires a multi-sectoral approach with the involvement of partners in health, education and protection (including gender-based violence protection, child protection and community-based protection) (UNHCR, 2024). Definitions such as these acknowledge the real distress experienced by individuals and the need for effective treatment but also go beyond a mere diagnostic lens. They conceptualize mental health responses along the continuum and actively acknowledge the need to address symptoms and their social contexts and determinants.

Mental health and psychosocial interventions include interpersonal or informational activities, techniques, or strategies focusing on biological, emotional, cognitive, behavioural, interpersonal, social, or environmental factors for symptom reduction and improving functionality and well-being (Miller et al., 2021). These can be stand-alone activities or executed in combination with other interventions. These interventions are provided in a variety of settings (e.g., inpatient, outpatient or primary clinics, hospitals, private practitioners, educational institutions such as schools and colleges, community settings, and digital or online settings), modalities (psychotherapies, rehabilitation, community-based treatments, peer support services, and integrated care interventions) and formats (such as individual, family, group, digital) (Miller et al., 2021). They are provided by specialists (social workers, psychiatrists, and psychologists) and non-specialists (community volunteers and collectives, religious leaders and peer providers) (Institute of Medicine, 2015).

The COVID-19 pandemic, with its complex mental, psychological, interpersonal, social and economic impact, has meant that such a multifaceted framework is required to conceptualize mental health responses and interventions. This framework must acknowledge individual and interpersonal level factors and needs and their interplay with the larger socioeconomic and cultural influences (Joshi, 2021). A dialogical approach (between clinical and socio-environmental viewpoints) to MHPS interventions, described in the section above, is a befitting framework to understand and analyze India's response to its mental health and psychosocial needs. Hence, this approach has informed the secondary literature review conducted in the present chapter and the results analyzed.

Methods

Research Questions

The following research questions guided the secondary review of the literature:

1. What is the nature of mental health and psychosocial support strategies and interventions implemented to address the MHPS impact of the COVID-19 pandemic for the general public as well as vulnerable groups in India?
2. Who were the stakeholders involved, and what were the contexts or settings in which these interventions were carried out?
3. What insights from these interventions can guide the services for improving mental health in India?

Search Strategy and Analysis

A comprehensive search was undertaken over several databases to conduct a secondary review and identify pertinent literature published from January 2020–April 2024. The literature reviewed included academic articles published in peer-reviewed journals (empirical research from quantitative and qualitative studies, review articles and conceptual papers) and book chapters. Considering that many of the interventions carried out during the COVID-19 pandemic in India were documented in non-academic or semi-academic spaces, grey literature in the form of newspaper articles, opinion pieces, and articles published on websites was hand-picked and included in the review.

Key search terms involved 'novel coronavirus', 'COVID-19', 'mental health', 'psychosocial interventions', 'psychosocial support', 'psychotherapy', 'vulnerable groups' and 'India'. Different combinations of key terms, including the terms for vulnerable populations and specific MHPSS responses, were used to search relevant literature.

Interventions from a range of actors and settings addressing mental health concerns, as well as their determinants, were selected for the analysis. These interventions were situated at the population level or the level of specific groups and communities, including those belonging to vulnerable sections across different geographies in India. Interventions were located not only within health or clinical sectors but also in other sectors such as social, economic, educational, protection, etc. The evidence was synthesized using thematic analysis proposed by Braun and Clarke (2006).

Results

The COVID-19 pandemic caused significant disruptions in the already flailing mental health service system in India. Online surveys conducted to evaluate the impact of the lockdown and COVID-19 pandemic on mental health services in various medical institutions, training centres and the private sector showed the collapse of regular mental health services to a large extent and a reduction in revenue generation for the private sector (Grover et al., 2020a, 2020b).

A closer analysis of India's response to the pandemic shows that the two strands of health and relief measures continued to occupy centre stage in the early phases. Mental health response was a late entrant and was initiated by a diverse range of actors and stakeholders (Joshi, 2021). These responses were introduced by three major stakeholders, namely National and State Governments, Non-governmental and civil society organizations, and community-based groups (Rangaswamy et al., 2022). The following section presents themes derived from the literature review. The interventions have been grouped into three broad thematic areas: (1) MHPS interventions for individuals diagnosed with COVID-19 (2) MHPS interventions for general public (3) MHPS interventions for vulnerable and marginalized groups and been further organized into sub-themes. Each of these themes briefly describes the mental health impacts of the pandemic and MHPS interventions carried out in response to those impacts.

1. **MHPS interventions for COVID-19-diagnosed individuals**

Patients who were diagnosed with or suspected to have contracted COVID faced a range of stressors, including social stigma and discrimination (Nair et al., 2022). Quarantine, isolation, and struggles with the health system, coupled with financial and practical constraints, affected their mental health (Joshi, 2021).

Given the low levels of awareness and high risk posed by COVID-19, the Indian Government, with its reach and public health infrastructure, took a multi-pronged approach to tackle the onslaught caused by the pandemic and its psychosocial impacts. Saving lives, containing the transmission of the virus, preventing infection, and managing and minimizing impact on physical health, were priorities. It was also important to clarify misconceptions and stigma around the disease. This was attempted through strengthening of medical and healthcare infrastructure, provision of reliable information, creating awareness around preventive measures, provision of logistic and financial support to the states, undertaking vaccination drives, manufacturing of COVID-19 vaccines, and training and capacity building for healthcare professionals (PIB, 2021). The government initiated online capacity programmes to train health workers to provide psychosocial support to patients. The Indian Council of Medical Research drafted a Guidance document for psychosocial counselling for COVID-19 Positive Patients and their family members and a Guidance document for psychosocial support for healthcare workers (ICMR, 2021a).

Counseling support was made available by hospitals and organizations to those diagnosed with COVID-19 through helpline services. The UDHAVI helpline, initiated by a tertiary care medical institution in Vellore, was established to directly link emergency responders and the general population to address the public's perceptions and concerns, share accurate information regarding the disease and vaccination, and raise awareness about the current government guidelines. The helpline services were organized into four content areas: general information, medical advice, counselling, and logistics support and the services were provided by a multidisciplinary team (Sasidharan et al., 2023). In Jharkhand, COVID-related services were delivered through the existing 104 health information helpline (HIHL, established through a public–private partnership in 2014), and outbound calls were made by the staff to follow up with COVID-19 patients who were in home isolation (Nawaz et al., 2023). Similarly, tele-counseling interventions were initiated by Dharwad Institute of Mental Health and Neurosciences (DIMHANS), which was designated as a COVID testing center during the pandemic. These services were aimed at either infected persons receiving medical care at special COVID centers or under home quarantine. Counseling services included supportive counseling, sleep hygiene advice, general information on COVID, problem-solving strategies, relaxation techniques and mindful mediation, grief counseling, family counseling and stress management.

Medical institutions and training centres expanded their telemedicine services and integrated mental health responses within the same, with three-fourths of these centres, offering services to patients with COVID-19 infection. In most of the institutes, mental health professionals were involved at different levels in the COVID-19 responsibilities such as provision of helpline services to the general public, screening people in quarantine for mental health issues, providing clinical care to patients diagnosed with COVID-19, screening health care workers (HCWs) for mental health issues, and training of HCWs (Grover et al., 2020a, 2020b). In-person counseling services in the form of telepsychiatry outpatient services, consultation-liaison psychiatry for COVID-19 patients, group counseling, supportive counseling, and psychosocial counseling center for relatives were provided in Dedicated COVID-19 hospitals (Santre et al., 2021).

2. MHPS interventions for general public

2.1 Preventive measures and Guidelines

Realizing the enormous impact of COVID-19 on the mental health of the general people, the government, in collaboration with the National level Institutes, undertook several preventive initiatives. MOHFW-GOI web portal provided a list of videos, advisories and resource materials on coping with stress during COVID, yoga and meditation advice, taking care of the mental health of vulnerable groups, etc. (MoHFW|Home, 2020). Some of the early strategies included issuing guidelines/ advisories on managing mental health concerns. A few examples of these guidelines include 'Management of mental health issues for different segments of the society' and 'Minding our minds during COVID-19' by the Ministry of Health and Family Welfare (MoHFW), Government of India, and 'Mental Health in the times of COVID-19 Pandemic-Guidance for general Medical and Specialized Mental Health Care Settings' by the National Institute of Mental health and Neurosciences (NIMHANS) (Manjunatha, Kumar & Math, 2020). These National-level guidelines provided directions to the government's efforts to address mental health concerns of the communities in India.

2.2 Online and Digital Interventions

Against the backdrop of the mobility restrictions posed by the pandemic, the subsequent disruptions in the provision of face-to-face mental health services and a large treatment gap, technology-based mental health solutions emerged as an effective alternative (Carter et al., 2021). In the initial stages, the MoHFW, India launched a toll-free helpline number for 'Behavioural Health', for anyone needing mental health assistance during the COVID-19 pandemic. Community Mental-Health Digital platform MANAS, a comprehensive, scalable, and national digital well-being platform and an app, was launched to promote well-being across age groups (PIB, 2021). Other central and teaching medical and psychiatric institutions, too, set up online and telemedicine services during the initial stages of the pandemic. Several state governments also launched helpline-based and in-person initiatives (wherever possible) to address the mental well-being of populations and specific vulnerable groups (Roy et al., 2021). Some regional responses preceded national-level initiatives; for example, the Kerala State Government constituted a multidisciplinary team in February 2020 to initiate integrated efforts by several sectors and also established a state helpline (John et al., 2024).

National and state-level NGOs, regional psychology chapters, mental health organizations and academic institutions, too, initiated helplines. For example, iCALL, a national-level technology-assisted mental health and psychosocial counselling initiative of the Tata Institute of Social Sciences (TISS) (Functional since 2012), started additional helplines to address the mental health and psychosocial impact of the COVID-19 pandemic. Documentation of the helpline calls showed that the nature of concerns presented by the callers was often a mix of psychological, relational, social, economic and practical issues, further appealing for more expanded psychosocial conceptualizations of mental distress (Joshi, 2021; Joshi et al., 2021, 2022). Considering the adverse mental health impact of the pandemic on vulnerable groups in India, iCALL started an additional helpline for 13 Indian states in an attempt to meet the support and mental health needs of vulnerable populations (Gaur, 2020).

Helpline counsellors were at the forefront of addressing distress issues on an ongoing basis, making them vulnerable for secondary trauma and necessitating the need for structured and continuous training, supervision and support (Joshi et al., 2021). Rahbar, another field action project of TISS, provided online supervision to mental health practitioners and care workers, offering remote counselling and supporting children and individuals diagnosed with Covid-19 and the supervision was based on principles of social justice, trauma-informed, and strengths-based practice (Duggal et al., 2022). It involved helping supervisees recognize the impact of client stories on themselves, teaching them how to identify and manage indirect trauma including activities such as grounding and somatic exercises. Supervisees' knowledge and skills were strengthened, and the social justice lens highlighted the need for systemic and organizational responses and focused on strengthening client empowerment through rights-based and advocacy frameworks (Duggal et al., 2022).

Given the difficulties families and couples faced in India during the pandemic (Joshi, 2021), Sukoon, another field action project of TISS, initiated a five-session online psychoeducational support group for relational well-being among young adults. Results at the end showed that participating in the group helped its members gain greater awareness of their relational dynamics and identify strengths, areas for growth and strategies to navigate relational challenges created by the COVID-19 pandemic (Joshi et al., 2021).

The initiatives mentioned above were a part of TISS's COVID-19 Task Force that was constituted to support people, institutions, and processes in the ongoing efforts to mitigate the ill effects of the pandemic where faculty, students and alums across campuses joined hands to offer diverse services through field action and policy support to both national and state governments. The above-mentioned efforts indicate the role of National level academic institutes in responding to the psychosocial impacts of the pandemic.

3. MHPS interventions for vulnerable groups

3.1 Mental health and psychosocial interventions for migrants

Before the COVID-19 pandemic as well migrant workers in India suffered multiple stressful experiences in the form of economic difficulties and experiences of discrimination and marginalization. Initially meant for 21 days, the lockdown during COVID-19 was extended over the next two months, leaving the footloose migrant workers with the maximum brunt of this decision (Adhikari et al., 2020). The mishandling of migrant mobility and the scapegoating of migrants due to them being the most visible commuters during the pandemic generated a trust deficit among migrants (Adhikari et al., 2020). There were extensive reports of police aggression and maltreatment at the hands of officials (Adhikari et al., 2020; Rajan et al., 2020). Mental health and psychosocial impacts of these crises included emotional distress, reduced self-esteem, feelings of social disconnection and helplessness, depression and anxiety, self-harm and suicide and substance abuse (Singh, 2021).

In the early stages of the pandemic, the Ministry of Health and Family Welfare highlighted the need for treatment of dignity and respect to the migrants and information about available assistance from central as well as state governments (Adhikari et al., 2020; Ministry of Health & Family Welfare, 2020). The Ministry of Home Affairs also appealed to the state governments to provide for medical and psychological needs of the migrant workers along with food and shelter requirements (Tiwary, 2020). The national-level mental health helpline initiated by NIMHANS was extended to migrants as well.

Some of the psychosocial interventions for migrants during the pandemic focused on helping migrants who were temporarily sheltered at relief camps. For example, NIMHANS, upon the directives of the Supreme Court, assisted the State government (of Karnataka) in addressing mental health concerns of migrants in relief camps and shelter homes across the city of Bengaluru (Chander et al., 2021). A mental Health Professionals team comprising Psychiatrists, Clinical Psychologists and Psychiatric Social Workers visited migrants in these camps along with 11 Mobile Medical Units (MMU) and screened them for physical and mental health concerns. The intervention provided included emotional support, advice on COVID-related precautions to be implemented at the camps, brief counselling for those who showed signs of mental disorders and linkages with the nearby District Mental Health Programme (DMHP) team for medical interventions and also to the National COVID Psychosocial Helpline (Chander et al., 2021).

The Department of Psychiatry of Government Medical College and Hospital, Chandigarh, also carried out a similar psychosocial intervention with 61 migrant workers from various states lodged in a shelter home upon the directives of the Ministry of Health and Family Welfare, Government of India (Chavan et al., 2021). This 12-step intervention was informed by Maslow's theory of hierarchy of needs. It addressed a variety of needs such as including food and water supply, a comfortable and safe living environment, medical attention and contact with family and involved assurance of support from the government, attempts to improve migrants' self-esteem and sense of hope and psychosocial and counselling services by the DMHP teams (Chavan et al., 2021; Singh et al., 2020).

Some of the other psychosocial interventions for migrant workers included relief-work-based measures. For example, the Stranded Workers Action Network (SWAN) spontaneously initiated a relief effort after the first announcement of the lockdown (Adhikari et al., 2020). The relief efforts included a range of strategies such as appeals for funds and volunteers for relief work, proactive follow-up calls to distress messages from migrants on WhatsApp groups and other social media platforms, and connecting stranded workers with NGOs and with government rations. An amount worth 6 million was raised through crowdsourced funding and transferred directly to the workers' accounts between 27 March 2020 and 3 July 2020 (Adhikari et al., 2020).

Interventions were also carried out by National level academic institutions. For example, the Community-Led Action Learning and Partnership (CLAP) project initiated by TISS (an offshoot of an ongoing field action project called Transforming M-East Ward), worked closely with migrants and residents from the M-East, one of the poorest of the 24 wards of Mumbai, as far as human development indices are concerned. The project surveyed 26,000 households in 26 *bastis* of M East ward, to study the impact of the pandemic on various domains such as health, education, livelihood, housing and education (Shelar, 2021). Results showed that the impact of the loss of income meant that many people could not pay rent and buy groceries and basic medications. TISS was actively involved in relief work and community mobilization; and initiated a helpline for support in collaboration with the local health department (Shelar, 2021).

3.2 Child and Adolescent-focused Interventions

The COVID 19 pandemic posed many challenges for children, adolescents and young individuals. These included experiences of stress, anxiety, closure of educational institutions, disturbance in routines, mobility restrictions leading to home confinement with reduced interactions with peers and educators, increased family violence, restricted physical activity, worry about future and career etc., further affecting their mental health (Modi & Kalra, 2022; Patra & Patro, 2020).

Given the importance of schools in children's lives, some of the early interventions from the Government involved ensuring continuity of educational activities. Against the backdrop of the school closure, disruption in academic activities, and the digital divide in accessing online education among students, the Ministry of Human Resources Development (MHRD) promoted digital education through online platforms and TV and RADIO. Several online programs were developed by the Indian government to engage teachers, parents, and students through the dissemination of written and audio-visual educational material. To deal with the stress and anxiety around learning, exams, and evaluation, the MHRD took policy-level decisions related to public schools in terms of reduction in the syllabus, cancellation of exams, lenience in corrections, and promotion of students to higher grades etc. Several non-governmental organizations (for example, Sampark, operating in six Indian states, Pratham, Mumbai, Eklavya, Madhya Pradesh, Vidya, based in major cities and Think zone, Virtual all India presence) too stepped forward to ensure continuity of education by supporting students with educational aids as well as material (Chugh & Ravichandran, 2022a, 2022b).

Several government and NGO led responses were initiated to address the mental health impact of the pandemic on children and young individuals during the pandemic. The Ministry of Health and Family Welfare (MoFHW) along with NIMHANS released an advisory for 'taking care of Mental Health of children during COVID-19' which comprised simple strategies for stakeholders involved in the care of children (NIMHANS & MoFHW, n.d.). UNICEF in collaboration with the Childline India Foundation, launched a manual titled, 'Psychosocial Support for Children during COVID 19: A Manual for Parents and Caregivers'.

To address the mental health vulnerabilities of young students, the Ministry of Education started a programme called 'Manodarpan', offering psychosocial support by providing a toll-free helpline number and launching a website. A handbook on the life skills necessary to survive a health crisis was released, too (Ministry of Education, n.d.). The tele-mental health services were expanded to address mental health issues of children, adolescents and young individuals. Specific states, too, initiated measures for the well-being of children and young people. For example, Kerala state, as part of a larger programme called 'Our Responsibility to Children' (ORC), launched the first-of-its-kind peer-run helpline, 'Kutty desk' and also a Play hub: an infotainment program engaging children to help them get rid of the boredom and tension due to social isolation (Praveen, 2021).

Offline and online initiatives informed by specific psychotherapy models such as positive psychology and mindfulness-based interventions (Chhajer & Hira, 2024; Pal et al., 2023) were undertaken to address mental health and well-being of children and adolescents in school and community settings. The use of Arts-based therapies (Prakashan & Banerjee, 2024) and group-based interventions (Burhans, 2022) during the pandemic was also found to be effective in improving children's mental health and resilience.

While all children were at risk of adverse impacts during COVID-19 pandemic, children in vulnerable situations were further prone to adverse mental health and psychosocial impacts. Children in childcare institutions were one of the groups who experienced tremendous disruptions during the pandemic. During the pandemic, the Supreme Court of India's directives in April 2020 instructed the Child Welfare Committees, Juvenile Justice Boards, Child Care Institutions (CCI), and state governments to take measures to protect children in care institutions and settings. Unfortunately, some of these measures led to abrupt reunification with families that were psychologically and financially ill-prepared for their return. Children who had no families to return continued in residential care while the CCI staff struggled to execute the physical distancing measures, provide medical care, offer psychosocial support to children who were anxious and grieving, and ensure continuation of educational activities (CTWWC, 2022). The young Care Leavers (young individuals, on turning 18, leaving child care institutions) were stuck at CCIs and faced difficulties in various life domains (Modi & Kalra, 2022).

In response to these realities, measures to mitigate the harmful impacts of the pandemic on vulnerable children included designing legal frameworks as well as guidance tools by the National and State Governments, capacity enhancement and training of national and state-run institutions, academic institutions, and the child protection systems, vaccination drives, announcement of schemes to support of children who lost parents to COVID-19, provision of free rations and essentials to families and children, sanitization of CCIs and establishment of a national care leavers network and monetary support for care leavers (CTWWC, 2022). Non-governmental as well as UN organizations too undertook supportive measures such as expedited case management, development of a Package of Case Management and Virtual Monitoring Tools, organization of recreational activities for children in CCIs, follow-up with those who were with families, provision of life skills programmes and counselling services virtually, facilitating access to education (CTWWC, 2022) and designing of aftercare outreach programme (Modi & Kalra, 2022). There were also attempts by the government to take action against the increased incidents of child trafficking and child labour by promoting and publicizing the dedicated central helpline number for children, 1098 (Chug & Ravichandran, 2022a).

Several initiatives were started to build the capacities of stakeholders and enhance the well-being of children and young people. Support, Advocacy & Mental health interventions for children in Vulnerable circumstances and Distress (SAMVAD), a national initiative under the deployment of the National Institute of Mental Health and Neuro Sciences (NIMHANS), worked in the areas of child protection and mental health of children in challenging situations by training child protection functionaries as well as helping professionals in India (NIMHANS, n.d.).

Other academic institutions, too, undertook initiatives to build capacities of functionaries and stakeholders working with children and youth in vulnerable situations. iCALL a field action project of the Tata Institute of Social Sciences (TISS) in collaboration with UNICEF and the Department of Women and Child Development (DWCD) Maharashtra, designed a unique curriculum and executed a capacity-building initiative aimed to equip child protection functionaries, NGOs and service providers to offer psychosocial support to children and adolescents in vulnerable situations. The initiative involved a needs assessment study and the development and delivery of a 15-session statewide online programme on mental health and psychosocial well-being of children in childcare institutions and other vulnerable situations (iCALL, n.d). Another field action project of TISS, School Initiative for Mental Health Advocacy (SIMHA), leveraging its existing school networks, launched a webinar series and other training initiatives to build the capacities of teachers and counsellors (Duggal & Bagarswala, 2020).

3.3 MHPS Interventions for women survivors of gender-based violence (GBV)

Similar to the global trends, India too witnessed a spurt in domestic violence during COVID-19, leading to a shadow pandemic. The extended lockdowns and the resultant forced house-boundedness led to an increase in women's unpaid household work, disruption in work-life balance and isolation from social and economic support as well as access to protection and health services (and additionally, these were diverted towards addressing disease prevention). Loss of jobs and financial insecurities caused by the pandemic, accompanied by substance abuse in many cases, further contributed to men exercising more control over their partners, making women further vulnerable to violence (Markan et al., 2022; Mittal & Singh, 2020).

Gender-based violence programming during COVID-19 in India adopted strategies in three key domains- public/government, non-governmental and digital space.

In the public sector, the Ministry of Women and Child Development attempted to increase coordination between One-Stop centers providing legal and psychosocial support to survivors of gender-based violence and local medical teams, police, shelter homes, working women's hostels and mental health facilities (Markan et al., 2022). The National Commission for Women launched a WhatsApp number for reporting emergency cases of domestic violence. It formed a special team for the speedy redressal of complaints and facilitation of support and security with the help of state police and administration (*Deccan Herald*, 2020). The government also disseminated information about its helplines for rescue and support of abused women during the lockdown. State governments (in some cases in collaboration with non-governmental organizations) initiated campaigns towards non-tolerance of violence against women, as well as helplines and emergency helpdesks for support (Markan et al., 2022). The family counselling centres (FCC) started providing help over WhatsApp messages and phone calls. The counsellors worked closely with the local police, civil society organizations and village committees to reach out to women even within their constrained realities (Mahapatro et al., 2022).

In the digital spaces, the NGOs leveraged social media influencers' support to create awareness about GBV and encourage women to seek assistance. NGOs rallied towards mobilizing focused social media campaigns to fight against online and offline GBV. This was an attempt to reach out to women who were otherwise finding it difficult to voice their concerns and access help (Markan et al., 2022). Online mediums were not only used for direct support and service provision but also for disseminating information about existing resources and building capacities of stakeholders who worked with issues of gender-based violence. For example, iCALL, a leading national level technology assisted mental health and psychosocial counselling initiative and a field action project of the TISS, in collaboration with the United Nations Population Fund (UNFPA), proactively assessed the functioning of existing women's helplines in the country and released a list of these helplines during the first few months of the lockdown (iCALL, 2020). Akshara Centre, a women's rights organization from Mumbai in collaboration with TISS- RCI-VAW (A field action project of TISS addressing issues of violence against women and children), and the Department of Women and Child (Government of Maharashtra) started an app called "Stand-up against violence". This app collated mobile numbers of State agencies, NGOs, service providers, and women's groups working on GBV issues across Maharashtra, thus making it easier for women survivors and supporters to seek help (Stand up against violence- WebApp. Akshara-empowering women and girls) (Markan et al., 2022). A Campaign titled, '#LockdownonDomesticViolence' was launched under this collaboration which received 3.5 million views in the first week of its launch. Special Cell for women and children, a field action project of the Tata Institute of Social Sciences, launched a helpline 'Mala Bolaincha Aahe (I want to talk)' to address concerns of violence against women.

3.4 Mental health and psychosocial interventions with healthcare providers

Health workers, especially those working in the frontline and primary healthcare, were among the most affected communities worldwide and in India during the pandemic. They were confronted with deficient infection control measures, a dearth of personal protection equipment, inadequate training and surveillance, and a shortage of human resources (Behera et al., 2020). Many experienced an increase in their work volume and intensity, additional responsibilities, and adaptations to new protocols. Being at the front lines of the care duties, they were vulnerable to both physical risk as well as mental health and psychosocial impacts of the pandemic. Multisite studies from India reported signs of psychological distress and burnout (Menon et al., 2022); and review articles noted higher levels of depression, anxiety, and stress among healthcare workers and professionals during the early phase of the COVID 19 pandemic in India (Sharma et al., 2023).

The Health Ministry, during the early phases of the pandemic, undertook several measures to enable training and capacity building for healthcare professionals (PIB, 2021). The Ministry and Indian hospitals took measures such as provision of personal protective equipment, enforcement of physical distancing recommendations, sanitization, trainings and measures for staff well-being in the form of provision of food and beverages, transportation facilities, on-time payment of salaries, clear guidelines and seeking feedback from the healthcare providers (Joseph et al., 2022).

In order to address the stress and mental health consequences of the pandemic for healthcare providers, NIMHANS in collaboration with the Department of Health and Family Welfare, Government of Karnataka, released a document titled, 'Caring for healthcare warriors- Mental health support during COVID-19'. This guidance document provided a framework for addressing mental health needs of healthcare personnel and for self-care and care of colleagues in distress (Manjunatha & TS, 2020). Indian Council of Medical Research (ICMR) too released a Guidance Document for the 'Psychosocial Support for Health Care Workers during COVID-19 pandemic' aimed at ensuring the optimal mental health of healthcare workers dealing with COVID-19 patients (ICMR, 2021b). iCALL, a field action project of TISS in collaboration with the United Nations Population Fund (UNFPA), initiated a national helpline called Swasthi and a web page to provide psychosocial support and resources for health and mental healthcare providers and also for frontline workers. The helpline received more than 500 calls from healthcare providers and frontline workers from different parts of India.

3.5 **Interventions with LGBTQIA+ Individuals**

As India continued to reel from the pandemic, the LGBTQIA+ community faced myriad problems. Queer individuals encountered heightened levels of distress and aggravation of pre-existing socioeconomic inequalities, discrimination, job losses and violations due to prior vulnerabilities that were adversely triggered by the lockdown (Sengupta, 2021). Many queer individuals were cut off from their preferred social support systems and forced to cohabit with unaccepting families, which in turn led to invisibalization of their gender and sexuality expressions and experiences of violations and violence (Joshi, 2021). There were cases of forced marriages of lesbians and trans men during lockdowns. And if they resisted, they were either evicted or forced to flee home (Sengupta, 2021).

Given the immediate healthcare and relief needs of the queer community, a list of NGOs providing immediate relief resources (food, medical, livelihood and shelter assistance) was compiled by the Pink List India (The Pink list India, n.d.). Special funding drives were started to support relief work for LGBTQIA+ individuals. Peer-led online interventions were undertaken to increase COVID-19 knowledge and protective behaviours and reduce psychological distress among queer individuals

(Newman et al., 2021). Queer collectives further intensified their efforts to provide support through existing helplines. Organizations such as Sappho For Equality (a Kolkata-based feminist organization that works for the rights of sexually marginalized women and trans men), Y'all (a queer collective based in Manipur) and Nazaria (A Queer Feminist Resource Group), reported receiving large number of crisis calls as soon as the pandemic hit India (Nazaria, 2020; Sengupta, 2021). A list of health and mental health care resources was compiled by the Mariwala Health Initiative (MHI, n.d.). Efforts were also made to provide support through counselling services, virtual hangouts, social media conversations, documentation of safety and self-care measures for LGBT*QIA + people and financial assistance (Nazaria, 2020). Additionally, there were instances of specific provisions made by states for trans persons in the form of healthcare facility reservations and food and medicine provisions and financial assistance.

3.6 **Interventions for individuals with a prior history of mental illness and the older adults**

Past studies have shown that there is often worsening of symptoms among people with pre-existing mental health conditions during pandemics, and the same was the case with COVID-19. Some of the risk factors worsening existing mental health symptoms during the pandemic included anxiety and uncertainty around the changing nature of the disease, information and quarantine practices, social isolation, disruptions in routine, overall increase in stress levels, sleep problems and struggles in accessing support, mental health services and medication (Chatterjee et al., 2020; Rangaswamy et al., 2022). Guidelines, drafted by NIMHANS, were issued for mental health care settings on behalf of the health ministry in April 2020. These guidelines focused on care and community support through existing community outreach programs, such as the District Mental Health Program for patients diagnosed with severe mental disorders and staying at home (NIMHANS, 2020).

The pandemic also adversely impacted older adults in India due to the physical threats posed by the disease, loneliness and isolation, reduced flexibility in adjusting to new situations, travel restrictions, challenges in using smartphones and communication technology, etc. (Mukku & Sivakumar, 2020). Hence, NIMHANS, in 2021, issued guidelines for addressing mental health concerns of older people. National-level organizations such as HelpAge India undertook several measures to assist and support local administrations in facilitating the government's vaccination drive and providing relief and rations to disadvantaged elders and their communities through its various program interventions.

Discussion

The extensive mental health and psychosocial impact caused by the COVID-19 pandemic in India warranted a comprehensive response, and yet mental health interventions were late to enter the list of responses (Joshi, 2021) as also seen during past disasters (Roy et al., 2021). MHPS interventions primarily originated from three sectors: Government, Non-governmental organizations and community-level initiatives during the pandemic.

The early stages of the pandemic saw MHPS responses predominantly introduced by the National and State Governments (in collaboration with National level teaching Institutes in some cases) alongside health initiatives for infection control. These responses included the development of guidance documents and capacity-building initiatives for care professionals and providers working in the health and mental health sectors aimed at early detection of signs of distress and providing psychological first aid and mental health treatment. Some of these guidance documents also directed national-level plans for organizing health and mental health services (NIMHANS, 2020). Responses also involved designing and disseminating information and advisories to the general public and vulnerable groups for self-help, stress management, and helping others in distress. These initiatives are similar to many others undertaken in low- and middle-income countries during the COVID-19 pandemic, aimed at crisis intervention, mitigation of COVID-19 stressors, management of distress and promotion of mental health (Kola et al., 2021).

Before the pandemic, mental health services in India were largely delivered in face-to-face settings. Given the mobility restrictions and severe service disruptions caused by the pandemic, mental health and support initiatives had to shift to online and digital modalities. Telepsychiatry, Helplines, online digital platforms, websites, awareness campaigns etc. were initiated to detect early signs of distress, disseminate COVID-related information, provide mental health care, support and psychological first aid, and conduct psychotherapeutic interventions. These were started by a range of stakeholders, including National and state-level Governments, teaching Institutes and professional bodies, as well as NGOs, volunteers and peer supporters. In some cases, these were targeted to help larger populations, while in others, to support specific vulnerable groups and contexts. Worldwide, remote mental health services have become a reality post-pandemic. Mental health services, informed mainly by existing diagnostic, psychotherapeutic or psychoeducational approaches, have largely shifted to synchronous or asynchronous digital and online formats during the COVID-19 pandemic due to their wide reach, accessibility, cost-effectiveness and scalability (Li, 2023; Witteveen et al., 2022). There is growing evidence of short-term and long-term advantages, especially in low and middle-income countries (Moreno et al., 2020).

The role of NGOs, community-based organizations, and the voluntary sector has always been important in India's mental health response prior to the pandemic, and it has continued to emerge as significant during the pandemic (Thara & Patel, 2010). During the pandemic, NGOs were involved in preparedness, response, service delivery, awareness creation, and advocacy efforts to mitigate the consequences of the pandemic, particularly amongst the poor and vulnerable groups. Given their proximity and connection with the communities and field-level realities, their presence in geographies that were unreachable during COVID due to mobility restrictions and their commitment to the cause, the volunteer sector and NGOs were seen to mobilize relief-related work as well as health and mental health support at the grassroots levels (Challagalla, 2021; Choudhary & Subr, 2023). In many situations, NGOs and the voluntary sector played a role in highlighting gaps, inequities and injustices in existing responses and demonstrating innovative and rights-based solutions.

The COVID-19 pandemic, while an equalizer in India at one level, also disproportionately affected poor and vulnerable populations such as migrants, poor, women, children, elderly, LGBTQIA+ individuals, people with pre-existing conditions, and others. Prior to the pandemic itself, there were socioeconomic and cultural inequalities in India that contributed to the vulnerabilities of the marginalized sections. The pandemic further aggravated these. Resultant stress could not be merely conceptualized through the limiting lens of mental health symptoms. In a similar vein, traditional mental health responses such as diagnosis, medication and counselling were not always appropriate and adequate in responding to issues of structural inequalities and social injustice (Burgess, 2020). These required multisectoral response (Moreno et al., 2020). The Inter-Agency Standing Committee, which coordinates responses to humanitarian emergencies in its first briefing notes with MHPSS recommendations in February 2020, highlighted the need to address vulnerabilities of specific populations such as older people, children, front-line workers, and individuals in quarantine, as well as guidance on combating stigma (IASC, 2020). The present review of MHPS interventions in India also showed the responses (especially from NGOs and the voluntary sector) addressing specific vulnerabilities and resultant distress among marginalized groups. While the traditional mental health framing still informed some of these interventions, others went beyond the health sector (social, community, economic, education, protection and welfare) in addressing the needs of the vulnerable groups.

The COVID-19 pandemic required all countries to launch and implement diverse programmes addressing population level and individual needs. The pandemic highlighted the necessity for not only addressing distress symptoms but also ensuring basic needs, equity, non-violence and human rights (Kola et al., 2021), requiring dialogue and coordinated response across sectors (including the voluntary sector and communities) and departments (Moreno et al., 2020). The MHPS response in India during the pandemic also witnessed cross-sector efforts occasionally. This was particularly the case in addressing the MHPS needs of vulnerable groups such as migrants, survivors of violence and children and young people, where social determinants and pre-existing inequalities contributed largely to distress generation.

Lessons from the past and directions for the future

The efforts made to respond to the Mental health and psychosocial impacts of the COVID-19 pandemic in India, while heartwarming at one level, also point towards glaring inadequacies of the mental health systems in India at another. These inadequacies and gaps pertain to the largescale treatment gaps and the conceptualization and framing of mental health responses. Based on the insights gained from the present review and lessons learned, the following section provides recommendations for organizing and reimagining mental health services and support in India.

Foregrounding and prioritizing mental health

The pandemic, with its largescale impact, has highlighted the importance of mental health. Post-pandemic times have seen greater awareness and vocabulary around issues of mental health. The pandemic needs to be treated as a wake-up call for prioritizing and foregrounding mental health by investing in mental health financing, human resources, training, implementation, and research. There is also a need for an equitable distribution of mental health services and for services to be available, affordable and of quality.

Reconceptualizing and redefining mental health

The pandemic has clearly underlined the need for conceptualizing mental health beyond the restricted biomedical and diagnostic understanding and for expanding it to cognize the role of social, economic and cultural factors in shaping people's mental health. Mental health also needs to be conceptualized beyond the discrete model of the presence or absence of symptoms and instead thought of as a continuum reflecting the diversity and complexity of the mental health needs of individuals and communities. Given the progressive policy (National Mental Health Policy, 2014, National Suicide Prevention Strategy, 2022) and legislative measures (The Mental Health Care Act, 2017, Rights of Persons with Disabilities Act, 2016) within the mental health sector in India in recent times, mental health also needs to be conceptualized as a Rights issue.

Integrating mental health into public health and development initiatives

This revised understanding and conceptualization of mental health has significant implications for mental health service delivery. The National Mental Health Programme and its subsequent implementation arm, the District Mental Health Programme, are fundamentally based on integrating mental health services into the existing public health infrastructure to make these services accessible to the masses. Despite their stated aims and continued expansion, the programmes have been severely criticized for their uneven coverage across geographies, constraints in human and financial resources, inadequate training for the team involved, less emphasis on preventive and promotive aspects and near absence of community participation (Gupta & Sagar, 2018). The most critical criticism pertains to its bio-medical framing of mental health issues and almost singular dependence on pharmaceutical solutions to psychosocial problems (Jain & Jadhav, 2009).

The pandemic has highlighted the need for full integration of mental health in plans for universal health coverage (Rangaswamy et al., 2022) and for services that are not merely diagnostic, pharmacological and/or mental health-institution-based. It is essential to make accessible and culturally sensitive psychosocial services available to individuals and communities. These will include various options such as counselling and psychotherapy, peer support, community-based interventions, shelter homes, protection services, legal aid, financial aid and livelihood opportunities. These services should target not only the curative aspects of mental health but also the promotive and preventive aspects (Joshi, 2021). Community-based and community-led initiatives need to be acknowledged and strengthened. This review of MHPS initiatives in India has also highlighted the impressive efforts made by NGOs and civil society organizations and the role of peer support, thus underscoring the need for financing and supporting these initiatives.

Online treatment and therapy options have seen accelerated growth during the COVID-19 pandemic and, therefore, need to be leveraged to make mental health services accessible and affordable to the common public. However, it is also vital to remember the challenges and drawbacks associated with using remote therapies. These include concerns of unequal access to technology, digital divide and literacy issues, Data privacy and confidentiality issues, ethics and regulations, etc. Given India's diverse cultural and socioeconomic realities, Telehealth and digital services can't be conceptualized as replacing face-to-face mental health services but as ways of augmenting or complementing them.

Apart from effectively incorporating mental health services into public health infrastructure, integration here also refers to a conscious attempt to emphasize mental health and psychosocial support in development, social welfare, and social protection measures. Mental health is as much a development issue as a health agenda. There is a reciprocal relationship between developmental contexts and mental health, with each affecting the other. It is, therefore, essential that development agendas and initiatives in various sectors such as housing, education, employment, workplace, social protection, social welfare, criminal justice and legal systems, humanitarian initiatives etc., make conscious efforts to integrate issues of MHPS in their fold.

Collaborating for mental health

Mental distress and well-being are affected by a range of factors situated at different levels of ecology and an interplay among them. This necessitates that mental health promotion and interventions are carried out by a diverse set of stakeholders and not just specialists. These include help and care providers, community workers, teachers, communities, families of people, local leaders, traditional and religious healers etc. Public policies and developmental efforts must protect mental health; and Leadership must initiate inter-sectoral collaboration to involve a wide range of stakeholders within and beyond the health sector (Patel et al., 2018). Mental health interventions need to come out of the silos and initiate dialogues and collaborations across actors and settings.

Inclusive and rights based mental health

The COVID-19 pandemic has effectively brought forth stark realities of disproportionate impact on the mental health on vulnerable groups in India. It is, therefore, essential to recognize the adverse socioeconomic realities confronted by these groups, along with issues of unequal access to support and welfare structures and unique mental health service needs that arise from the same. 'One fit for all approach' that ignores these realities and excludes vulnerable groups from service nets, will need to be urgently changed.

Inclusion also refers to active efforts to centre and learn from the experiences of service users and communities. The role of people with lived experience of mental ill health, their families and caregivers and other vulnerable groups needs to expand beyond nominal participation. Instead, it should be considered as experts by experience, leading to meaningful engagement and further facilitation of policy and programmatic planning (Kola et al., 2021). Alongside, barriers and threats to mental health, as well as issues of stigma and discrimination, must be addressed (Patel et al., 2018). Similarly, the role of communities and peer-led initiatives must also be urgently acknowledged.

Conclusion

It has taken a pandemic to remind all of us of the importance of mental health and psychosocial well-being. The suffering caused by the pandemic and efforts undertaken in response, provide valuable insights in assessing strengths and gaps in the existing mental health services in India. The impressive endeavours made by diverse stakeholders during the pandemic have brought optimism for imagining a new future. The pandemic has highlighted an urgent need for reconceptualizing mental health beyond the diagnostic lens and for expanding mental health responses to diverse sectors and stakeholders. It has also underscored linkages between the psychological and socioeconomic realities, necessitating a collaborative and comprehensive response. It is hoped that the reminders given by the pandemic will continue to inform and shape future mental health perspectives and services in India.

References

Adhikari, A., Goregaonkar, N., Narayanan, R., Panicker, N., & Ramamoorthy, N. (2020). Manufactured Maladies: Lives and livelihoods of migrant workers during COVID-19 lockdown in India. *The Indian Journal of Labour Economics, 63*(4), 969–997. https://doi.org/10.1007/s41027-020-00282-x

Agrawal, S., Dayama, S., & Galhotra, A. (2022). COVID-19 mental health challenges: A scoping review. *Journal of Education Health Promotion, 26*(11), 375. https://doi.org/10.4103/jehp.jehp_426_22.PMID:36618463;PMCID:PMC9818617

Alizadeh, H., Sharifi, A., Damanbagh, S., Nazarnia, H., & Nazarnia M. (2023). Impacts of the COVID-19 pandemic on the social sphere and lessons for crisis management: A literature review. *Nat Hazards (Dordr),10*,1–26. https://doi.org/10.1007/s11069-023-05959-2. Epub ahead of print. PMID: 37360799; PMCID: PMC10088618.

Azmand, S., Joulaei, H., & Fatemi, M. (2021). *Non-medical interventions to reduce burden of Psychosocial and economic impacts of COVID-19 pandemic: A scope review* (in press). https://doi.org/10.5812/semj.118177

Behera, D., Praveen, D., & Behera, M. R. (2020). Protecting Indian health workforce during the COVID-19 pandemic. *Journal of Family Medicine and Primary Care, 9*, 4541–4546. https://doi.org/10.4103/jfmpc.jfmpc_925_20

Braun, V., & Clarke, V. (2006). Using thematic analysis in psychology. *Qualitative Research in Psychology, 3*(2), 77–101. https://doi.org/10.1191/1478088706qp063oa

Burgess, R. (2020). COVID-19 mental-health responses neglect social realities. *Nature.* https://doi.org/doi.org/10.1038/d41586-020-01313-9

Burhans. (2022). *Implementing Nae Disha, a youth resilience intervention, in urban North India during the COVID-19 pandemic*. https://aii.unimelb.edu.au/wp-content/uploads/2022/03/Nae-Disha-in-pandemics-Report.pdf. Accessed on March 1, 2024.

Carter, H., Araya, R., Anjur, K., Deng, D., & Naslund, J. A. (2021). The emergence of digital mental health in low-income and middle-income countries: A review of recent advances and implications for the treatment and prevention of mental disorders. *Journal of Psychiatric Research, 133*, 223–246. https://doi.org/10.1016/j.jpsychires.2020.12.016. Epub 2020 December 13.

Challagalla, S. (2021, July 1). *Dealing with the pandemic: Contributions of the NGOs*. https://indiafoundation.in/articles-and-commentaries/dealing-with-the-pandemic-contribution-of-ngos/GOs. Accessed on January 15, 2024.

Chander, R., Murugesan, M., Ritish, D., Damodharan, D., Arunachalam, V., Parthasarathy, R., Raj, A., Sharma, M. K., Manjunatha, N., Bada, M. S., & Kumar, C. N. (2021). Addressing the mental health concerns of migrant workers during the COVID-19 pandemic: An experiential account. *International Journal of Social Psychiatry, 67*(7), 826–829. https://doi.org/10.1177/0020764020937736

Changing the way we care (CTWWC). (2022). *The impact of COVID-19 on children's care: India*. https://bettercarenetwork.org/sites/default/files/2022-10/case_sudy_india_covid19_final.pdf. Accessed on March 2, 2024.

Chatterjee, S. S., Barikar, C. M., & Mukherjee, A. (2020). Impact of COVID-19 pandemic on pre-existing mental health problems. *Asian Journal of Psychiatry, 51*, Article 102071. https://doi.org/10.1016/j.ajp.2020.102071

Chavan, B. S., Arun, P., & Singh, G. P. (2021). Psychosocial intervention model for migrant workers during extended lockdown: The Chandigarh model. *Indian Journal of Psychiatry, 63*(2), 175–178. https://doi.org/10.4103/psychiatry.IndianJPsychiatry_542_20

Chhajer, R., & Hira, N. (2024). Exploring positive psychology intervention and mindfulness-based intervention in nature: Impact on well-being of school students in India. *Frontiers in Public Health, 12*, 1297610. https://doi.org/10.3389/fpubh.2024.1297610

Choudhary, A., & Subr, B. (2023). *Role of community based organizations in the pandemic opportunities for growth challenges to survival.*

Chugh, L., & Ravichandran, R. (2022). Issues that affected the mental health of children in India during COVID-19 and efforts taken by the Indian Government to address them. *Global Journal of Medicine and Public Health, 11*, 4. https://nicpd.ac.in/ojs-/index.php/gjmedph/article/view/3802

Chugh, L., & Ravichandran, R. (2022). *Small hands-big battles: Challenges encountered by Indian children and the approaches implemented by the Indian government to alleviate them during COVID-19 pandemic*. https://doi.org/10.20944/preprints202205.0339.v1

COVID-19 Mental Disorders Collaborators. (2021). Global prevalence and burden of depressive and anxiety disorders in 204 countries and territories in 2020 due to the COVID-19 pandemic. *The Lancet, 398*(10312), 1700–1712.

Department of Psychiatry, NIMHANS. (2020). *Mental health in the times of COVID-19 pandemic—Guidance for general medical and specialized mental health care settings*. https://nimhans.ac.in/wp-content/uploads/2020/04/MentalHealthIssuesCOVID-19NIMHANS.pdf

Duggal, C., & Bagarswala, L. (2020). Promoting well-being and resilience of young people during COVID-19: An initiative with schools. In L. S. S. Manickam (Ed.), *COVID-19 pandemic: Challenges and responses of psychologists from India* (pp.63–75). The Editor.

Duggal, C., Dua, B., & Kothari, A. (2022). Holding space for those who heal: Reflections from the Rahbar Supportive Supervision Programme during the Covid 19 pandemic. *The Clinical Supervisor, 41*(2), 127–148. https://doi.org/10.1080/07325223.2022.2111624

Gaur, V. (2020, December 14). UNDP, TISS to launch tech-assisted counselling for those battling mental distress during pandemic. *The Economic Times*. https://economictimes.indiatimes.com/news/politics-and-nation/undp-tiss-to-launch-tech-assisted-counselling-for-those-battling-mental-distress-during-pandemic/articleshow/79726477.cms?from=mdr. Accessed on February 27, 2024.

Grover, S., Dua, D., Sahoo, S., & Chakrabarti, S. (2020a). Profile of patients availing psychiatry emergency services pre and post lockdown at a tertiary care center of North India. *Asian J Psychiatry, 54*, Article 102448. https://doi.org/10.1016/j.ajp.2020

Grover, S., Mehra, A., Sahoo, S., Avasthi, A., Tripathi, A., D'Souza, A., Saha, G., Jagadhisha, A., Gowda, M., Vaishnav, M., Singh, O., Dalal, P. K., & Kumar, P. (2020b). State of mental health services in various training centers in India during the lockdown and COVID-19 pandemic. *Indian J Psychiatry, 62*(4), 363–369. https://doi.org/10.4103/psychiatry.IndianJPsychiatry_567_20

Gulati, N., Nanda, C., & Hora, R. K. (2023). COVID-19 and its impact on mental health as a function of gender, age, and income. *Discover Mental Health, 3*(1), 4. https://doi.org/10.1007/s44192-022-00025-y

Gupta, S., & Sagar, R. (2018). National mental health programme-optimism and caution: A narrative review. *Indian Journal of Psychological Medicine, 40*(6), 509–516. https://journals.sagepub.com/doi/10.4103/IJPSYM.IJPSYM_191_18

Gupta, V., Santosh, K. C., Arora, R., Ciano, T., Kalid, K. S., & Mohan, S. (2022). Socioeconomic impact due to COVID-19: An empirical assessment. *Information Processing & Management, 59*(2), Article 102810. https://doi.org/10.1016/j.ipm.2021.102810

Hosseinzadeh, P., Zareipour, M., Baljani, E., & Moradali, M. R. (2022). Social consequences of the COVID-19 pandemic. A systematic review. *Invest Education Enferm, 40*(1), Article e10. https://doi.org/10.17533/udea.iee.v40n1e10.PMID:35485623;PMCID:PMC9052715

iCALL. (2020). A Directory of Helplines for Women and Girls in Distress. https://icallhelpline.org/wpcontent/uploads/2020/10/helpline-directory.pdf

iCALL|Home. (2024a). https://icallhelpline.org/about-the-program-unicef/. Accessed on February 15, 2024.

iCALL|Home. (2024b). https://icallhelpline.org/strengthening-response-to-violence-against-women-and-girls/. Accessed on February 15, 2024.

Indian Council of Medical Research (ICMR). (2021). *Guidance document for the psychosocial support for healthcare workers*. Downloaded from https://www.icmr.gov.in/pdf/covid/techdoc/Guidance_Psychosocial_counselling_HCW.pdf. Accessed on March 20, 2024.

Inter Agency Standing Committee. (2007). *IASC guidelines on mental health and psychosocial support in emergency settings*. World Health Organization. https://doi.org/10.1037/e518422011-002

IOM (Institute of Medicine). (2015). *Psychosocial interventions for mental and substance use disorders: A framework for establishing evidence-based standards*. The National Academies Press.

Jain, S., & Jadhav, S. (2009). Pills that swallow policy: Clinical ethnography of a community mental health program in northern India. *Transcultural Psychiatry, 46*(1), 60–85.

John, C. E., Gunasekaran, I., & Maria, R. N. (2024, March 1). *COVID-19: Taking heed from Kerala's mental health interventions*. The Wire. https://science.thewire.in/health/covid-19-kerala-mental-health/

Joseph, L., Agarwal, V., Patel, P. J., Majumder, J., & Jayalakshmi, J. (2022). Measures taken by Indian hospitals toward healthcare worker and workplace safety during COVID-19 pandemic. *QAI J Healthc Qual Patient Saf, 2022*(3), 21–27.

Joshi, A. (2021). COVID-19 pandemic in India: Through psychosocial lens. *Journal of Social and Economic Development, 23*(Suppl 2), 414–437. https://doi.org/10.1007/s40847-020-00136-8

Joshi, A., Joshi, A., Chatterjee, I., Kantak, C., & Puntambekar, A. (2021). Facilitator lessons from online psychoeducational group for relational well-being in India during COVID-19 pandemic. *Journal of Family Therapy, 43*(2), 314–328. https://doi.org/10.1111/1467-6427.12337

Joshi, A., Tamanna, S., Babare, T., & Auti, N. (2022). Caller concerns and mental distress during COVID-19: Findings from a counselling helpline in India. *Indian Journal of Social Work, 83*(1). https://journals.tiss.ac.in/ijsw/index.php/ijsw/article/view/749

Joshi, A., Tammana, S., Babre, T., & Kallianpur, R. (2021). Psychosocial response to COVID-19 pandemic in India: Helpline counsellors' experiences and perspectives. *Counselling & Psychotherapy Research, 21*(1), 19–30. https://doi.org/10.1002/capr.12378

Kashish supports LGBTQIA+ community organizations with funds for COVID-19 relief. (2020, November 3). *Times of India*. https://timesofindia.indiatimes.com/city/mumbai/kashish-mumbai-supports-lgbtqia-community-organizations-with-funds-for-covid-19-relief/articleshow/79024495.cms

Kola, L., Kohrt, B. A., Hanlon, C., Naslund, J. A., Sikander, S., Balaji, M., Benjet, C., Cheung, E. Y. L., Eaton, J., Gonsalves, P., Hailemariam, M., Luitel, N. P., Machado, D. B., Misganaw, E., Omigbodun, O., Roberts, T., Salisbury, T. T., Shidhaye, R., Sunkel, C., & Patel, V. (2021). "COVID-19 mental health impact and responses in low-income and middle income countries: Reimagining global mental health": Correction. *The Lancet Psychiatry, 8*(5), Article e13. https://doi.org/10.1016/S2215-0366(21)00090-0

Li, J. (2023). Digital technologies for mental health improvements in the COVID-19 pandemic: A scoping review. *BMC Public Health, 23*, 413. https://doi.org/10.1186/s12889-023-15302-w

Li, L., Taeihagh, A., & Tan, S. Y. (2023). A scoping review of the impacts of COVID-19 physical distancing measures on vulnerable population groups. *Nature Communications, 14*, 599. https://doi.org/10.1038/s41467-023-36267-9

Liese, B., & Gribble, R., & Wickremsinhe, M. (2019). International funding for mental health: A review of the last decade. *International health, 11*(10),1093. https://doi.org/10.1093/inthealth/ihz040

Mahapatro, M., Prasad, M. M., & Singh, S. P. (2022). Domestic violence and Covid-19: Policy and pattern analysis of reported cases at the family counseling center (FCC) in Alwar, India. . *Sex Resarch and Social Policy, 28*, 1–9. https://doi.org/10.1007/s13178-022-00782-z

Manikappa, S., Shetty, K. V., Ashalatha, K., Bamney, U., & Sachetha, G. M. (2024). Tele-counseling services for COVID-19 patients: Experiences from a state mental health institute in South India. *Journal of Education and Health Promotion, 13*(1), 505. https://doi.org/10.4103/jehp.jehp_292_23

Manjunatha, N., & Jaisoorya, T. S. (2020). *Care for health care warriors—Mental health support during COVID-19*. https://www.researchgate.net/publication/342672227_Care_for_Health_Care_Warriors_-_MentalHealthSupport_During_COVID-19

Manjunatha, N., Kumar, C. N., & Math, S. B. (2020). *Mental health in the times of COVID-19 pandemic guidelines for general medical and specialised mental health care settings.*

Mariwala Health Initiative. (n.d.) *Resources for LGBTQI community during COVID*. https://mhi.org.in/voice/details/resources-lgbtqi-community-during-covid/. Accessed on February 20, 2024.

Markan, M., Dhingra, R., Segan, M., Dabla, V., Sagar, M., Neogi, S., Dey, S., & Chakravarty, N. (2002). Gender-based violence programming in times of COVID-19: Challenges, strategies and recommendations. *Front in Global Womens Health, 6*(3), 952688. https://doi.org/10.3389/fgwh.2022.952688

Menon, G. R., Yadav, J., Aggarwal, S., Singh, R., Kaur, S., Chakma, T., Periyasamy, M., Venkateswaran, C., Singh, P. K., Balachandar, R., Kulkarni, R., Grover, A., Mishra, B. K., Viray, M., Devi, K. R., Singh, K. H. J., Saha, K. B., Barde, P. V., Thomas, B., … Panda, S. (2022). Psychological distress and burnout among healthcare worker during COVID-19 pandemic in India-A cross-sectional study. *PLoS One, 10*(3), e0264956. https://doi.org/10.1371/journal.pone.0264956

Miller, K. E., Jordans, M. J. D., Tol, W. A., & Galappatti, A. (2021). A call for greater conceptual clarity in the field of mental health and psychosocial support in humanitarian settings. *Epidemiology and Psychiatric Sciences, 30*, Article e5. https://doi.org/10.1017/S2045796020001110.

Ministry of Education|Home. https://manodarpan.education.gov.in/. Retrieved March 6, 2024, from https://www.mohfw.gov.in/

Ministry of Health and Family Welfare. (2020). *Psychosocial issues among migrants during COVID-19*. Government of India. https://covid19dashboard.mohfw.gov.in/pdf/RevisedPsychosocialissuesofmigrantsCOVID19.pdf. Accessed on March 1, 2024.

Mittal, S., & Singh, T. (2020). Gender-based violence during COVID-19 pandemic: A mini-review. *Front Glob Womens Health, 8*(1), 4. https://doi.org/10.3389/fgwh.2020.00004

Modi, K., & Kalra, G. K. (2022). Assessing the impact of COVID-19 and the support provided to youth leaving care in India. *Youth, 2*, 53–66. https://doi.org/10.3390/youth2010005

MoHFW|Home. (2020). Retrieved April 6, 2020, from https://www.mohfw.gov.in/

Moreno, C., Wykes, T., Galderisi, S., Nordentoft, M., Crossley, N., Jones, N., Cannon, M., Correll, C. U., Byrne, L., Carr, S., Chen, E. Y. H., Gorwood, P., Johnson, S., Kärkkäinen, H., Krystal, J. H., Lee, J., Lieberman, J., López-Jaramillo, C., Männikkö, M., & Arango, C. (2020). How mental health care should change as a consequence of the COVID-19 pandemic": Correction. *The Lancet Psychiatry, 8*(7), Article e16. https://doi.org/10.1016/S2215-0366(21)00216-9

Mukku, S. S. R., & Sivakumar, P. T. T. (2020). Mental health care of older adults during coronavirus disease (COVID-19) pandemic: Challenges and way ahead in India. Indian Journal of Psychological Medicine, *42*(5), 495–496. https://doi.org/10.1177/0253717620944824

Nair, S., Joshi, A., Aggarwal, S., Adhikari, T., Mahajan, N., Diwan, V., Stephen, A., Devi, K. R., Mishra, B.K., Yadav, G. K., Kohli, R., Sahu, D., Gulati, B.K., Sharma, S., Yadav, J., Ovung, S., Duggal, C., Sharma, M., … Vardhana Rao M. V. (2022, January). Development & validation of scales to assess stigma related to COVID-19 in India. *Indian Journal of Medical, 155*(1), 156–164. https://doi.org/10.4103/ijmr.ijmr_2455_21. PMID: 35859441; PMCID: PMC9552373.

National Commission for Women launches WhatsApp number to report domestic violence during coronavirus lockdown. (2020, April 10). *Deccan Herald*. https://www.deccanherald.com/india/national-commission-for-women-launches-whatsapp-number-to-report-domestic-violence-during-coronavirus-lockdown-823726.html

National Institute of Mental Health and Neurosciences & Ministry of Health and Family Welfare. (2022). Taking care of mental health of children during COVID-19' which comprised simple strategies for stakeholders involved in the care of children. https://www.mohfw.gov.in/pdf/mentalhealthchildrean.pdf

National Institute of Mental Health and Neurosciences, SAMVAD|Home. https://nimhanschildprotect.in/reports/. Accessed on February 15, 2024.

National Mental Health Policy. (2014). Ministry of Health and Family Welfare, Government of India. *National Health Mission*. https://nhm.gov.in/images/pdf/National_Health_Mental_Policy.pdf

National Suicide Prevention Strategy. (2022). Ministry of Health & Family Welfare. https://main.mohfw.gov.in/sites/default/files/National%20Suicide%20Prevention%20Strategy.pdf

Nazaria. (2020). *The impact of COVID-19 on the human rights of LGBT persons, communities and/or populations Submitted by Nazaria to OHCHR*. https://www.ohchr.org/sites/default/files/ImpactCOVID19LGBTpersons.pdf. Accessed on February 21, 2024.

Nawaz, A., Singh, B., Singh, A., Mukherjee, C., Rathnam, N., & Hegde, S. (2023). Leveraging health information helpline to sustain healthcare delivery during the COVID pandemic: Experiences from a state in Eastern India. *Indian Journal of Public Health, 67*(1), 28–34. https://doi.org/10.4103/ijph.ijph_604_22

Newman, P. A., Chakrapani, V., Williams, C., Massaquoi, N., Tepjan, S., Roungprakhon, S., Akkakanjanasupar, P., Logie, C., & Rawat, S. (2021). An eHealth intervention for promoting COVID-19 knowledge and protective behaviors and reducing pandemic distress among sexual and gender minorities: Protocol for a randomized controlled trial (#SafeHandsSafeHearts). *JMIR Research Protocols, 10*(12), e34381. https://doi.org/10.2196/34381

Pal, A., Mukhopadhyay, P., & Pal, N. (2023). An online mindfulness-based intervention influences the health-related quality of life of Indian children and adolescent during COVID-19 pandemic: A randomized controlled trial. *International Journal of Contemporary Pediatrics, 10*, 887–893. https://doi.org/10.18203/2349-3291.ijcp20231495

Patel, V., Saxena, S., Lund, C., Thornicroft, G., Baingana, F., Bolton, P., & UnÜtzer, J. Ü. (2018). The Lancet Commission on global mental health and sustainable development. *Lancet, 392*(10157), 1553–1598. https://doi.org/10.1016/S0140-6736(18)31612-X

Patra, S., & Patro, B. K. (2020). COVID-19 and adolescent mental health in India. *Lancet Psychiatry, 7*(12), 1015. https://doi.org/10.1016/S2215-0366(20)30461-2

Prakashan, N., & Banerjee, B. (2024). Expressing through creativity: An intervention for the mental health of children living at child care institutions in Goa, India. *Residential Treatment for Children & Youth, 1–28*. https://doi.org/10.1080/0886571X.2024.2319741

Praveen, M. P. (2021, July 21). In Kerala, a help desk by the children for the children. *The Hindu*. https://www.thehindu.com/news/national/kerala/in-kerala-a-help-desk-by-the-children-for-the-children/article35439575.ece.

Press Information Buearu (PIB), Community Mental-Health Digital platform MANAS launched by the Principal Scientific Adviser. Downloaded from https://pib.gov.in/PressReleaseIframePage.aspx?PRID=1711860. Accessed on March 20, 2024.

Press Information Bureau, Ministry of Information and Broadcasting, Government of India. (2021). *Effective response in the face of a pandemic: Measures adopted by the government of India to combat COVID-19 (Ministry of Health and Family Welfare)*. Downloaded from https://static.pib.gov.in/WriteReadData/specificdocs/documents/2021/dec/doc2021122421.pdf. Accessed on March 28, 2024.

Rajan, I., Sivakumar, P., & Srinivasan, A. (2020). The COVID-19 pandemic and internal labour migration in India: A 'crisis of mobility.' *The Indian Journal of Labour Economics, 63*(4), 1021–1039. https://doi.org/10.1007/s41027-020-00293-8

Rangaswamy, T., Grover, S., Tyagi, V., & Bhan, A. (2022). How did the mental health care system in India respond to COVID 19 pandemic? *Schizophr Bull Open, 3*(1), sgac043. https://doi.org/10.1093/schizbullopen/sgac043

Rathod, S., Pinninti, N., Irfan, M., Gorczynski, P., Rathod, P., Gega, L., & Naeem, F. (2017). Mental health service provision in low- and middle-income countries. *Health Serv Insights., 28*(10), 1178632917694350. https://doi.org/10.1177/1178632917694350.PMID:28469456;PMCID:PMC5398308

Rights of Persons with Disabilities Act. (2016). The Ministry of Social Justice and Empowerment. https://www.indiacode.nic.in/handle/123456789/2155

Roy, A., Singh, A. K., Mishra, S., Chinnadurai, A., Mitra, A., & Bakshi, O. (2021). Mental health implications of COVID-19 pandemic and its response in India. *International Journal of Social Psychiatry, 67*(5), 587–600. https://doi.org/10.1177/0020764020950769

Safieh, J., Broughan, J., McCombe, G., McCarthy, N., Frawley, T., Guerandel, A., Lambert, J. S., & Cullen, W. (2022). Interventions to optimise mental health outcomes during the COVID-19 pandemic: A scoping review. *International Journal of Mental Health and Addiction, 20*(5), 2934–2955. https://doi.org/10.1007/s11469-021-00558-3. Epub 2021 June 15. PMID: 34149329; PMCID: PMC8204922.

Santre, M., Panse, S., Wadgaonkar, G., & Haritha, S. (2021). Counseling patients with COVID-19: An experience at dedicated COVID-19 hospital. *Industrial Psychiatry Journal, 30*(Suppl 1), S285–S287. https://doi.org/10.4103/0972-6748.328831

Sagar, R., Gururaj, G., Dhaliwal, R. S., Singh, A., & Ferrari, A. (2020). The burden of mental disorders across the states of India: The global burden of disease study 1990–2017. *Lancet Psychiatry, 1*, 148–161. https://doi.org/10.1016/S2215-0366(19)30475-4. Epub 2019 Dec 23. PMID: 31879245; PMCID: PMC7029418.

Sasidharan, B. K., James, R. I., Sathyendra, S., Harsh, R., Jeba Sundararaj, J., Ravindran, V., Thomas, H., H.,Ashok, N., Thirunavukkarasu, M. M., Punitha, J. V., George, T. K., Isaac, B. T. J., Zechariah, A. J., David, S. N. J., Yesupatham, D. P., Irodi, A., Aruldas, V., Keshava, S. N., Zachariah, A., … Mammen, J. J. (2023). UDHAVI community support during India's SECOND COVID-19 wave: A descriptive study on a tertiary care center's pandemic response helpline. *Glob Health Sci Pract, 11*(5), e2200315. https://doi.org/10.9745/GHSP-D-22-00315

Sengupta, S. (2021, October 7). *Family prejudice, lack of safe spaces: What the pandemic has meant for India's LGBTQI community*. The Wire. https://thewire.in/lgbtqia/lgbtqi-community-pandemic-family-support-groups

Sharma, S. K., Joseph, J., Dhandapani, M., Varghese, A., Radha, K., Das, K., Jangra, N., Rozha, P., Varkey, B. P., & Rachel, R. (2023). The psychological morbidity among health care workers during the early phase of Covid-19 pandemic in India: A systematic review and meta-analysis. *Indian Journal of Community Medicine 48*(1), 12–23. https://doi.org/10.4103/ijcm.ijcm_159_22

Shelar, J. (2021, July 18). The epidemic to follow the Covid-19 pandemic. *Hindustan Times*. https://www.hindustantimes.com/cities/mumbai-news/the-epidemic-to-follow-the-covid-19-pandemic-101626589322875.html

Shukla, J., & Singh, R. M. (2021). Psychological health amidst COVID-19: A review of existing literature in the Indian context. *Clinical Epidemiology and Global Health, 11*, Article 100736. https://doi.org/10.1016/j.cegh.2021

Singh, G. P. (2021). Psychosocial and mental health issues of the migrants amidst COVID-19 pandemic in India: A narrative review. *Indian Journal of Psychological Medicine, 43*(6), 473–478. https://doi.org/10.1177/02537176211044802

Singh, G. P., Arun, P., & Chavan, B. S. (2020). Migrant workers' needs and perceptions while lodged in a shelter home in India during the COVID-19 pandemic. *Primary Care Companion CNS Disorder, 22*(6), 20m02753. https://doi.org/10.4088/PCC.20m02753

Suhas, S., Arvind, B., Sukumar, G., Banandur, P., Nirisha, L., Kumar, C., Benegal, V., Rao, G., Varghese, M., Gururaj, G., NMHS National Collaborators Group. (2023). A bird's eye view of the mental health systems in India. *Indian Journal of Psychiatry, 65*(12), 1214–1222. https://doi.org/10.4103/indianjpsychiatry.indianjpsychiatry_845_23

Thara, R., & Patel, V. (2010). Role of non-governmental organizations in mental health in India. *Indian Journal Psychiatry, 52*(Suppl 1), S389–S395. https://doi.org/10.4103/0019-5545.69276

The Inter Agency Standing Committee (IASC)|Home. (2020, June 25). *IASC guidance on operational considerations for multisectoral mental health and psychosocial support programmes during the COVID-19 pandemic.* https://interagencystandingcommittee.org/iasc-reference-group-mental-health-and-psychosocial-support-emergency-settings/iasc-guidance-operational-considerations-multisectoral-mental-health-and-psychosocial-support

The Mental Healthcare Act. (2017). The Ministry of Law and Justice. https://www.indiacode.nic.in/bitstream/123456789/2249/1/A2017-10.pdf

The PinkList India|Home. (2024). https://www.pinklistindia.com/queerelief. Accessed on February 25, 2024.

Tiwary, D. (2020). Provide counselling to migrants: Centre to states. *Indian Express*. https://indianexpress.com/article/india/coronavirus-india-lockdown-provide-counselling-to-migrants-centre-to-states-6359601/. Accessed on March 1, 2024.

UNHCR (2024). *Mental health and psychosocial support (MHPSS): Emergency handbook.*

Witteveen, A. B., Young, S., Cuijpers, P., Ayuso-Mateos, J. L., Barbui, C., Bertolini, F., Cabello, M., Cadorin, C., Downes, N., Franzoi, D., Gasior, M., John, A., Melchior, M., McDaid, D., Palantza, C., Purgato, M., Van der Waerden, J., Wang, S., & Sijbrandij, M. (2022). Remote mental health care interventions during the COVID-19 pandemic: An umbrella review. *Behaviour Research and Therapy, 159*, Article 104226. https://doi.org/10.1016/j.brat.2022.104226

World Health Organisation (WHO). (2022, March 2). *Mental health and COVID-19: Early evidence of the pandemic's impact: Scientific brief*. https://www.who.int/publications/i/item/WHO-2019-nCoV-Sci_Brief-Mental_health-2022.1. Accessed on January 22, 2024.

Ye, Z., Li, W., Zhu, R. (2022, November 1). Online psychosocial interventions for improving mental health in people during the COVID-19 pandemic: A systematic review and meta-analysis. *Journal of Affective Disorders, 316*, 120–131. https://doi.org/10.1016/j.jad.2022.08.023.

Aparna Joshi is an Assistant Professor, School of Human Ecology, Tata Institute of Social Sciences (TISS), Mumbai, India. She is a trained psychologist and has completed her PhD from TISS Mumbai. She has over 25 years of experience as an academician, researcher, interventionist and practitioner. Her research interests include mental health and psychosocial well-being and interventions, couple and family therapy, gender, violence against women, and youth mental health. Currently, she leads two field action projects at TISS, namely iCALL, a national-level technology-assisted mental health and psychosocial well-being initiative and Sukoon, an initiative addressing couple and family well-being.

Chapter 4
Feminist Psychosocial Intervention Approaches to Respond to Domestic Violence Against Women: Evolution and Emerging Evidence from India

Sangeeta Rege and Padma Bhate-Deosthali

Abstract Using a feminist lens, this chapter focuses on psychosocial services for mitigating domestic violence (DV) faced by women in India. It traces the evolution of such services, beginning with the campaigns by the autonomous women's movement in India in the 1970s, and subsequently by non-governmental organizations (NGOs) to highlight DV, with the primary focus in the early years being on demanding the state for legal reform, and for establishment of services for those affected by DV. The first section of this chapter describes the evolution of approaches of several such organisations engaged in feminist counselling to respond to DV, although the term 'feminist counselling' was not specifically used then to describe the nature of support they provided to the survivors. The second section presents a conceptualisation of DV as a public health issue and elaborates on the development of a feminist counselling model by CEHAT, a Mumbai-based NGO, with which the authors have a long-standing association. This section also offers evidence related to the impact of feminist counselling based on perspectives of women survivors accessing the services. The chapter concludes by presenting a recent initiative led by CEHAT in collaboration with different NGOs to conceptualise outcome indicators for understanding successful and effective outcomes of feminist counselling.

Keyword Autonomous women's groups · Feminist counselling · Domestic violence · Outcome indicators

S. Rege (✉)
CEHAT, Mumbai, Maharashtra, India
e-mail: sangeetavrege@gmail.com

P. Bhate-Deosthali
ICRW, New Delhi, India

U. Vindhya (ed.), *Psychosocial Interventions for Social Issues in Contemporary India*,
https://doi.org/10.1007/978-981-96-6553-2_4

Introduction

The issue of Violence against women (VAW) was brought onto the public domain by autonomous women's groups in India in the late 1970s (Agnihotri & Mazumdar, 1995; Kannabiran & Menon, 2007). By taking up and publicising individual cases of violence—of dowry deaths and custodial rape in particular—and demanding action against the perpetrators, they questioned the social, cultural and economic context of power relations that sanctioned VAW, and highlighted the need for a range of services and support, anchored in feminist principles, that those affected by such violence needed. This chapter focuses on the role of the autonomous women's groups and subsequently of non-governmental organizations (NGOs) in conceptualising and implementing a framework of psychosocial support for survivors of domestic violence (DV), grounded in feminist principles and strategies. In particular, the chapter draws on the efforts by the Centre for Enquiry into Health and Allied Themes (CEHAT), a Mumbai-based non-governmental research organisation to conceptualize DV as a public health issue, to develop a feminist counselling model in the setting of a public hospital-based crisis centre to respond to DV, and to provide evidence on the impact of such counselling on women's lives and well-being and their perception of such services. Finally, the chapter presents a recent initiative led by CEHAT in collaboration with different NGOs across the country to develop outcome indicators for defining outcomes of feminist psychosocial interventions in the arena of DV.

Evolution of Psychosocial Interventions to Address DV in India

Instances of different forms of VAW were foundational to the emergence and spread of the movement led by autonomous women's groups in the 1970s (Gandhi & Shah, 1992; Ray, 2002). Gender-specific forms of violence were seen as rooted in unequal power relations and as violations of constitutional rights to life, liberty, and dignity (Shirwadkar, 2009). Challenging the notion that VAW and DV in particular was a 'private' affair within the family, the autonomous women's movement, attempted to make violence visible, through their campaign strategies ranging from street play performances, distribution of pamphlets, and staging protests in public spaces (Desai, 1985; Phadke, 2003). Women's groups in Delhi such as Saheli and Stree Sangharsh were some of the earliest groups protesting against DV and the movement slowly spread to other parts of the country (Kumar, 1998). The early years of the movement focused on bringing legal reforms to redress the issue of dowry harassment and custodial rape (Agnihotri & Mazumdar, 1995; Gandhi & Shah, 1992; Katzenstein, 1989). The decade of 1980s thus saw formation of several autonomous women's groups across different states of India drawing attention to the patriarchal biases and seeking to create awareness about forms and types of VAW both outside and within the homes. The first national autonomous women's group conference by Mumbai based group Forum Against Oppression Of Women (FAOW) in 1980 had ambitious agenda. The conference deliberated on concerns with regards to role of state agencies such as police, courts and health system and its apathy to VAW; but what is of significant interest is that even then, despite the fact that the movement largely represented middle class, upper caste and urban women, they were critical of the fact that the movement was dominated by middle class and upper caste women. The conference deliberations included the urgency to reflect on the lack of representation of Dalit and tribal women from India. Similarly, they reflected on lack of representation of women from the minority communities and their participation (Desai, 1985). Members discussed about the need for cross movement solidarity to ensure that their voices were stronger and to ensure representation of women from different communities. They decided to engage with other movements in India such as trade unionists, health activists and development professionals to embed the issue of VAW in their respective campaigns. The conference ended with a resolve to ensure furthering of the different agenda points deliberated and develop stronger campaigns to demand state accountability to redress VAW (Burte, 2013).

As the campaign started to gain momentum, women started speaking out and seeking support from women's groups. The nature of support offered by women's groups was not formalised however, as 'psychosocial intervention'. Volunteers from the movement created spaces in their own homes, if women were thrown out of their homes, provided much needed emotional support, and also discussed legal options to deal with domestic violence (Burte, 2013).

By the 1980s the campaign of women's groups against DV had gathered momentum. Women's groups had to multi-task on several aspects related to DV; providing individual support for women, appearing in the courts on their behalf, taking up litigation and fund raising for campaigns. The thrust of the campaign during the early period was primarily on legal reforms and demanding the state to take punitive action against the perpetrators of DV. These campaigns led to fruition in terms of law and policy such as the criminalisation of domestic violence by introduction of Section 498A in the Indian Penal Code in 1983; the introduction of 'dying declaration' for women reporting with severe burn injuries, the setting up of family counselling centres, family courts, and shelter homes for women affected by domestic violence; and eventually the enactment of the Protection of Women from Domestic Violence Act in 2005, a rights-based civil law that provided a definition of domestic violence for the first time in Indian law, and several civil remedies to protect women from DV (Agnes, 1999; Jaising, 2009).

Autonomous women's groups such as the Women's Centre, and Majlis in Mumbai, Jagori and Saheli in Delhi, Vimochana in Bengaluru and Sakhi in Kerala sought to structure their support services to women and girls facing domestic violence. They developed unique strategies of bringing women together for sharing their lived experiences of domestic violence. The structure of these gatherings started with individual women speaking about the violence faced by them, followed by guided discussions by volunteers. In this process volunteers encouraged women to discard feelings of shame, and provided perspectives about the larger context in which oppression against women was systematically allowed. Women coming to the centres were exposed to films, songs and group readings to discuss domestic violence (Mitra, 2001). These activities helped to bring issues such as domestic violence, hitherto regarded as 'personal' into the public arena, and to articulate violence as rooted in patriarchal structures of unequal power relations and also as violations of constitutional rights to liberty and dignity. Such discussions enabled women to discover myriad ways in which patriarchy operated in their everyday lives and took form of control over their reproduction, labour and sexuality, disallowing them from having property and inheritance to their names (Gupte, 2013). Women's groups felt that such methods would not only help women heal from the domestic violence they faced but also create support for other women and in turn create a solidarity amongst women (Burte, 2013).

Having carried out support activities with women for almost a decade, some voluntary groups began to reflect upon the outcomes of support offered. Most women facing domestic violence wanted to reconcile and continue their matrimonial relationship. Not many women sought to join the movement which was contrary to the view of activists who believed that their on-going discussions about power imbalances in relationships would change women's world view and assist them to confront violence (Mitra, 2001). By the 1990s, women's groups were also stretched for resources as all support activities were volunteer based. Some of them arrived at the decision to gradually restrict the individual support work with women. For instance, Saheli, one of the autonomous Delhi- based groups, in an article "Case work debate in Saheli" raised several critical aspects about case work practice. Women of different classes came for support but very few eventually volunteered for offering support to other women. After providing support to individual women for more than a decade, the organization felt it was at a cross roads about whether to continue "servicing" women or to engage with the state-led initiative called Family counselling centres to redress the issue of domestic violence against women. To quote from the article, *"Some of us in Saheli felt that the very nature of casework is inherently curative, rather than preventive. Unless it is accompanied by active efforts to organize for social and structural change, casework can only provide symptomatic relief to a few individual women. Yet casework, by becoming a primary activity of Saheli, consumed the energies of volunteers so completely that campaigns on issues emerging from the casework did not receive enough attention"* (Saheli Women's Resource Centre, 1995).

Despite a long history of voluntarism in India, the decades of 1980s and 1990s witnessed a "veritable mushrooming" of NGOs (Sheth & Sethi, 1991, p. 49). Their genesis in post-independence India, however, can be traced to the first five-year plan and setting up of the Central Social Welfare Board (Asian Development Bank [ADB], 2009; Sharma, 2011). The Board sought to provide financial and technical support to the setting up of NGOs especially in the arena of development for women and children. The seventh five-year plan particularly lay emphasis on role of NGOs for two interrelated activities: delivery of services to those in need; and public campaigns in the pursuit of social transformation and securing social justice in development related issues of the country. With funding from domestic, government and international donors, the NGOs began to get involved in the arena of DV against women. They started evolving pragmatic methods of responding to DV by way of setting up crisis centres in the community, provision of legal aid, engaging with community structures to change gender norms, creating women's collectives amongst others (Rege & Chandrasekhar, 2013). Some of these organisations were spearheaded by the erstwhile autonomous women's groups and feminist principles such as "personal is political", "sisterhood is powerful" and "we have a right over our bodies" continued to be the guiding principles for DV response and prevention work (Gupte, 2013).

The decade of 1990s witnessed a structured response by NGOs to violence against women in general and to DV in particular. The activities ranged from gender awareness trainings, setting up of counselling centres, helpline services, creating micro-credit committees, initiating self-defence classes for girls, amongst others (Haksar, 1986; Santhya & Jejeebhoy, 2017; Suneetha & Nagraj, 2006). The terms 'feminist counselling' or 'feminist psychosocial support' had not yet, however, entered the lexicon or practice of these organizations. Despite formal training of psychologists in counselling, counsellors from the field of mainstream psychology did not actively respond to DV, perhaps because mainstream psychology has been rather slow to critically engage, from a feminist perspective, with issues of gender-based inequities and power differentials in the aetiology of violence in particular (Vindhya, 2013). Even though the decade of 2000 began to witness a small number of mental health professionals provide counselling services from a feminist perspective to women facing domestic violence, adaptation of theoretical orientations with feminist values, skills and principles continues to be sparse (Joshi, 2019).

Furthermore, while efforts to provide feminist counselling to women have emerged from different contexts in the last two decades or so, limited documentation is available with regards to the approach and methods for implementing them on ground. An early effort, made almost a decade ago, sought to document implementation of a feminist perspective in counselling as well as the diversity of interventions by NGOs in dealing with DV survivors (Rege & Chandrasekhar, 2013). These initiatives emphasized the critical need to embed feminist principles such as 'personal is political', 'validating women's experiences', 'avoiding victim-blaming', and 'right to bodily autonomy' while dealing with DV survivors. These principles in interventions help to illumine to women that acts of violence are rooted in imbalances in power relations between men and women (Vindhya, 2013). Feminist principles thus encourage discussions related to control over women's bodies, reproductive abilities, mobility and sexuality (Rege, 2008).

One of the first and key principles of support highlighted by women's groups in 1980s comprised offering a *non-judgemental space* for women to speak about the violence. This not only enabled active listening to the women's concerns, but sent the message that the domestic violence they were facing in their lives is not just a personal issue but a political one. At one level, individual support to them continued and on the other, groups developed innovative ways of breaking silence on the issue of domestic violence. There was a constant link made between individual support and the socio-political context in which violence against women occurred. Vimochana and Women's centre were one of the first formalised counselling groups creating monthly meeting forums for women to participate in learning about economic and legal rights and to also learn from each other's stories of violence and resilience. Early activists recognised that married women facing violence received no support from their parental families thus pushing them to continue living in abusive relations. They started raising important questions about parental responsibilities and support for their daughters living in abuse. Breaking the silence around violence was encouraged by encouraging them to disclose DV to friends, neighbours as well as members at work place to create a network of support for themselves (Rege & Chandrasekhar, 2013).

Autonomous groups of the 1980s such as Sahiyar, Saheli and Jagori created a non-threatening space to bring those perpetrating violence at the table and negotiate ways to stop violence. Such negotiations ensured that women's interests were at the centre and that no violence could be justified. Women who did not want to continue the relationship were supported by reaching out to legal aid committees. *Ensuring access to legal aid* was thus the second key principle in psychosocial support provided to the survivors. While some of the organisations had lawyers who volunteered their time, others did not. Groups like Vimochana and Saheli developed the concept of "out of court settlements". Innovative techniques such as people's committees comprising of respected members from the community to discuss concerns of women and ways of reaching an amicable settlement with women's interests at the core. While responding to individual women facing violence continued, it was also important to draw community support for women and for the community to stand with women facing domestic violence. *Improving access to social and community resources* was thus another key principle of feminist psychosocial intervention (Vindhya & Lingam, 2019). Groups such as Swadhar and Stree Mukti Sanghatana (2013) were at the helm of community awareness and mobilisation through street plays and awareness drives (Rege & Chandrasekhar, 2013).

Although the term 'intersectionality perspective' had not come into specific use, the expanse and scope of activities of several organizations demonstrated their recognition of overlapping layers of disadvantage stemming from the intersections of gender with caste, class, religion, region and so on. For instance, organisations such as Masum (Gupte & More, 2007) and Vanagana created unique strategies for responding to domestic violence faced by women in rural areas. At the outset, they recognised that caste was an important axis of discrimination and linked closely to the issue of violence against Dalit communities and more so against women from these communities. The methodology adopted to work within the community was that of building local leadership was by creating teams of rural Dalit women. These teams received training to support women facing DV. As local leadership started to gather momentum, issues of employment for women, skilling to set up small scale business and increasing women's participation in decision making at the level of their communities started to take pace. Many of the rural team members engaged in providing counselling, enabling women to record police complaints as well as encouraging them to take steps to stop violence. Some of the survivors of domestic violence joined the organisational teams to support other women to deal with the violence they faced (Rege & Chandrasekhar, 2013).

Similarly, the Women's Action and Research group (WRAG) (K.K. et al., 2014) was set up in the context of increased communalisation and its impact on the minority community in general and women in particular (Burte, 2013). Initiated as a research initiative to respond to the aftermath of communal violence in Mumbai in 1992, WRAG documented Muslim women's socio-economic concerns in the aftermath of communal riots. It was in this course of work that several women expressed the need to have a space to be able to discuss their deep concerns related to a range of issues including domestic violence. Members of WRAG responded to the felt need of women by equipping existing resources—Mahila Mandals in communities to respond to domestic violence. Members of the Mahila Mandal went through elaborate training workshops to equip them with information about a range of issues such as schemes and policies for women, skills to respond to domestic violence, negotiation with perpetrators of violence, meetings with police and community members. This trajectory was also echoed by "Shaheen women's centre" in Andhra Pradesh that was set up in aftermath of communal riots. Their efforts assisted members of the minority community to build their lives with the help of skills-based trainings for women and girls. As women started to develop comfort and speak with members of the group, they decided to set up a counselling centre for women facing DV. Many of the women and girls who enrolled in their training centres were themselves survivors of DV and eventually became support workers for women dealing with DV. The efforts mentioned above signify ways in which feminists sought to engage and organise women on a variety of issues that impacted their lives- be it caste-based oppression, effects of communalism on women. Their response to violence against women in general and domestic violence in particular was informed of the intersectional issues of marginalisation (Rege & Chandrasekhar, 2013). The participation of several women's groups in the Beijing conference on women's empowerment, organized by the United Nations in 1995 provided further impetus to discuss impact of communalism on minority community in general and women in particular.

The decade of 2000 saw the formalisation of psychosocial counselling practices by organisations such as Susamvad, Swayam, Olakh and Humsafar. Susamvad and Swayam primarily worked with DV survivors with trained in social workers as well as psychologist. Olakh and Humsafar provided legal services as well as psychosocial support as a part of their activities. Their lawyers were trained in feminist perspective that shaped their ideologies in litigation against DV (Rege & Chandrasekhar, 2013).

Box 1: Centering principles: personal is political', 'validating women's experiences', 'avoiding victim-blaming', and 'right to bodily autonomy'

The 1980s –

- Autonomous women's groups bring VAW both both outside and within the homes into public domain.
- Genesis of support services to women and girls facing domestic violence

The 90s-

- NGOs providing VAW services with a feminist and intersectional lens focusing on gender awareness trainings, setting up of counselling centres, helpline services, creating micro-credit committees, initiating self-defence classes for girls
- Groups for responding to Muslim women post-communal riots

The 2000s-

- NGOs focusing on psychosocial interventions with a feminist perspective
- Small number of mental health professionals provide counselling services from a feminist perspective

The 2010s

- OSCs, Helplines
- Upscaling of Dilaasa, Special Cell for women and children

One of the earliest efforts to respond to DV survivors facing mental health problems was by Bapu Trust, a Pune-based organization (Modi, 2007). Their counselling methodology enabled an understanding of the cyclical nature of domestic violence and mental ill health. They brought forth the issue of victimisation of DV survivors due to mental illness and their treatment by family members as well as the state. They stressed the need for prioritising the need to deal with mental illnesses faced by DV survivors and subsequently focus on social support (Modi, 2007).

Lastly, it is important to recognise that the disciplines of psychology and psychiatry largely remained on the periphery and hardly engaged with the autonomous women's movement or with the issue of violence largely because of their predominant focus on the individual and intrapsychic explanations for violence. The feminist emphasis on the other hand, has been on societal norms that create and structure imbalances in power and access and control over resources (Davar, 1999, 2001; Vindhya, 2005, 2013). Although feminist psychological scholarship is very limited in India, and it is beyond the scope of this chapter to go into the tension between feminist discourse and mainstream psychology, it has critiqued the discipline of psychology for victim-blaming of women facing domestic violence and attributing psychopathology to offenders of domestic violence, thereby absolving them from any responsibility for their acts and behaviours, and thereby denying justice to women (Vindhya, 2005).

Redressing Domestic Violence as a Public Health Issue: Conceptualising Feminist Counselling for Women

The autonomous women's movement in India has critiqued the health system on a range of issues, beginning with the feminist demand for bodily autonomy (Ram, 1998). Some of the objections raised for instance, have been on imposition of contraceptives on women in the name of family planning; mechanical use of amniocentesis for sex determination; unscientific medical tests on rape survivors; and sub optimal care by health professionals for women succumbing or surviving burns due to DV (Bhate-Deosthali & Lingam, 2016; Qadeer & Viswanathan, 2004; Ram, 2001; Ramasubban & Jejheebhoy, 2000; Ravindran, 1995; Sarojini, 2006; Unnithan & Pigg, 2014). However, a direct engagement by health systems to bring about a change in response to VAW has largely been missing, although it is clear that the health system has a crucial role in responding to women survivors of violence (Deosthali- Bhate et al., 2018). The public health system is an important and often the first facility that receives women suffering from psychological and physical health consequences as a result of violence; and therefore, has the legal responsibility of collecting medical and forensic evidence as well as providing expert witness account in the court of law (Bhate-Deosthali & Duggal, 2013). Recognising the importance of a health systems response to VAW, the Centre for Enquiry into Health and Allied Themes (CEHAT)—a research centre of Anusandhan trust embarked in collaboration with the public health system in Mumbai and established Dilaasa—a hospital-based crisis centre in 2001 (CEHAT, 2001). The centre was conceptualised as a counselling outpatient department of a public hospital in Mumbai to provide psychosocial counselling to women facing violence. This was the first initiative in India to collaborate with a public hospital in creating services for women facing DV (Deosthali- Bhate et al., 2012).

The team relied on the feminist principles developed by the autonomous women's groups of the 1980s and 1990s in India. Further, given the paucity of literature on feminist methods and practices related to counselling in India, the team also studied specific literature on feminist therapies developed by western feminist psychologists (Deosthali et al., 2005; Enns, 2004; Worell & Remer, 2003).

The Dilaasa feminist counselling model emerged from these different learnings. A unique aspect of counselling in a public hospital is that women may be "referred" by Health professionals to the Dilaasa centre as against women voluntarily seeking support from community counselling centres This necessitated explaining services of the centre and seeking consent before initiating counselling. Given the context of a public hospitals, women often came with grievous injuries and would be in pain due to the health consequence of violence (fractures, burns, injuries, tears, contusions, lacerations etc.) and therefore the first point of contact with them would be in a hospital ward. This again required seeking out private space even in a busy ward to assure women of privacy and confidentiality. A crucial element of counselling was discussing the impact of violence on health, explaining effects of self-harming behaviours on physical and psychological well-being and encouraging them to think of self-valuing behaviours. Recognising the serious effects of violence on health, the team developed a set of questions so that counsellors could assess the safety of women and in accordance develop a safety plan in collaboration with the survivors (Rege, 2008). 'Accidental' poisoning was a crucial aspect with which several women and girls were admitted to the hospital. Speaking with them, the team realized that most of them had tried to end their lives due to unbearable domestic violence. This close association of DV with suicide attempts often led to a dilemma whether the issue of suicide attempts should be dealt with by the counsellors or should they be referred to a psychiatrist. Given that psychiatrists in a public health facility in particular, do not offer counselling, it was crucial that counsellors/social workers of Dilaasa be trained to respond to mental health consequences arising out of DV, in order to fill the gap in current health response to DV. This required the team to devise a distinct counselling strategy for women and girls so that they disclose the violence, and develop strategies to deal with it, and help to prevent recurrence of attempt to end their life.

Based on the experiences of crisis counselling at the Dilaasa centre, the team evolved the primary *goals* of counselling as validating the women's feelings and experiences, supporting their decisions, respecting autonomy, and mitigating feelings of inferiority, powerlessness, and disrespect in order to enhance their agency (Rege, 2008). The key feminist *principles* underlying the counselling include (a) *avoidance of victim-blaming* and instead, recognizing that every woman who pursues formal redress is essentially challenging the structures and power of patriarchy; (b) understanding of the intersectional nature of social inequities organized by caste, class, religion, ethnicity etc. with DV and that DV cannot be dealt with in isolation; and (c) social justice for social change cannot be achieved if violence against women is ignored or overlooked (Rege et al., 2010).

The team felt the need to document the Dilaasa approach to feminist counselling because, as mentioned earlier, it was the first such initiative in a public health system to respond to DV. Similarly, this was the only intervention that sought to equip social workers to respond to mental health consequences of DV and provide counselling. Such documentation was expected to assist new counsellors working with the health system to respond to DV (Burte et al., 2005). The team also documented ethical dilemmas arising in the course of counselling (Rege et al., 2010). These different learnings enabled the team to develop a concrete training program for new counsellors in the public health field. The table below shows the scope of activities of Dilaasa in the year 2021–2023 (Table 4.1).[1]

Table 4.1 Persons reached through Dilaasa Mumbai

Sr. No	Activities	Number
1.	No. of DV survivors receiving psychosocial care	2546
2.	No. of Counsellors trained in Feminist Counselling	150
3.	No. of Health Professionals trained to respond to DV	2016

[1] Healthprofessionals comprise doctors and nurses working in 11 public hospitals.

Assessing the Impact of Counselling

Most of the studies pertaining to "effectiveness" or "efficacy" of psychosocial counselling for domestic violence have emerged from high income countries (Micklitz et al, 2023; Ogbe et al, 2020; Trabold et al, 2020). Available global evidence discusses mental health interventions using cognitive behaviour therapy, empowerment counselling and interpersonal psychotherapeutic interventions offered to women subjected to DV (Craven et al., 2023; Hackett et al., 2016; Worell & Remer, 2003). However, no studies are specifically available on impact/ efficacy of these interventions on women facing DV in the Indian context.

Additionally, a bulk of research has focused on the epidemiology of violence—its prevalence, severity, nature, and detrimental effects on the physical and mental health of victims and survivors; and on building evidence on what works to prevent violence against women (Ellsberg et al, 2015; Morrison et al, 2007). But as noted by Ellsberg et al. (2015), there is limited evidence on the impact of counselling/advocacy interventions on the health and well-being of victims and survivors. There remains a significant debate regarding appropriate measures and indicators for evaluating DV interventions with some working in the field being averse to using indicators, such as re-abuse/stop abuse, as women have no control over whether they are abused again by their violent intimate partners or ex-partners. Many critics are advocating for the use of outcome measures that are determined and defined by victims and survivors themselves.

CEHAT endeavoured to build an evidence-based model and therefore from the very inception, there was a commitment to regularly analyse all program data to improve the interventions and also conceptualise research studies to understand experiences of women users of psychosocial services and assess impact of counselling related to domestic violence. The following section synthesizes findings of three different studies that endeavoured to understand the role of feminist psychosocial counselling in mitigating domestic violence experienced by women. The first study relates to women survivors' perceptions about Dilaasa and its location; the second study refers to the impact of counselling intervention offered to women survivors seeking antenatal services in two hospitals; and the third section highlights counsellors' perspectives on providing women-centred care as a part of review of the upscaling of Dilaasa centres across public hospitals in Mumbai (Arora et al., 2018, 2021; CEHAT, 2004).

Women Survivors' Perceptions About Dilaasa Counselling Centre in a Public Hospital

The objective of this study was to understand the relevance of hospital-based crisis centre- Dilaasa for women facing domestic violence. During the study research participants were asked to share how they perceived the accessibility of Dilaasa's services and counsellors, the location of the Centre (within a government hospital), the timings, and the range of services offered. They were also asked to share their opinions about both the advantages and disadvantages of the Centre's structure and set-up. The study comprised of speaking to women who were former clients, those who were currently seeking services and those that did not return for counselling after their first visit. This was done to ensure that the team documents responses across the spectrum of clients seeking services.

The following aspects of counselling were found to be useful:

- Validation of women's feelings and experiences by counsellors
- Feeling that Dilaasa is a safe, comfortable, unthreatening, and confidential space for women
- Awareness about linkages between the violence she is experiencing and her physical and mental health status.
- Increased belief that women are not to blame for the violence in their lives (reduction in feelings of self-blame) and that there is no excuse or valid reason for this abuse.

Women reported that the location of Dilaasa in a hospital was of particular significance for emergency cases as well as for women who needed to access immediate treatment as well as counselling services. Its location in a public hospital made it more accessible as it offered privacy and anonymity for women who faced extreme restrictions on their mobility or suspicion from their abuser/s and families. They also said that counsellors made themselves available even on days when there was a large number of women awaiting services and that they were always treated with respect and were provided full attention. Women particularly found specific aspects of counselling useful. These were validation of their feelings and experiences by counsellors. They noted that counsellors helped them become aware of the impact of violence on their physical as well as psychological health. Despite being a counselling centre in a public hospital, all women found Dilaasa as a safe, comfortable, unthreatening, and confidential space for women. Women recalled that counsellors helped them to increase belief in self by discussing violence in their lives as a result of power inequities in relationships and that there was no excuse for domestic violence. This study was of significance as there had been concerns and fears that women survivors' privacy and confidentially would be compromised due to Dilaasa's location in a public hospital. Dilaasa was able to demonstrate that a feminist counselling intervention can be established in a public hospital (Deosthali-Bhate et al., 2012).

Evaluating Psychosocial Intervention for Responding to DV Against Pregnant Women

Given the dearth of evidence on efficacy of feminist counselling intervention in India, CEHAT conducted a study in two public hospitals in Mumbai, India. Over a period of six months; 2778 women coming for Ante natal check-up (ANC) were asked about experiences of violence, 2515 women consented to being asked about domestic violence. Of these 442 (16%) of women reported experiencing violence. women were offered counselling services and were also provided at least one in person follow up and one telephonic counselling. They were followed up post-delivery to understand the impact of psychosocial counselling on their health and well-being in relation to the domestic violence. The study was able to capture the changes in understanding of the phenomenon of violence among women. These changes are critical as the shift in mindset propels women to take action against ongoing violence. As per our knowledge, this is the only study that has identified qualitative outcomes of impact of counselling intervention.

The most common change among women as a result of the intervention was an understanding of the intrinsic relationship between violence and their health. The other important changes were recognising violence as an issue of power and the need to raise their voice against violence. The results of the study indicate positive impacts of intervention on coping and safety behaviour of women. There was a significant number of women who acted against violence with the support of informal (family, friends, neighbours) and formal systems (police, counselling centre, helpline) as a result of the counselling intervention. All women felt equipped to use at least one safety strategy in the event of an episode of violence, while some women also did it to ensure future safety. The effects of the intervention were also reflected in the health outcomes of the women at six weeks after delivery, where 84 per cent of women reported better health status. The findings of the study are summarised below (Arora et al., 2018).

Increased knowledge, skills and critical consciousness: Women often perceive that they are responsible for the violence they are facing and tend to normalize it because of gender role socialization. Raising critical consciousness forms an essential element of empowerment counselling (Sullivan, 2018). Dilaasa counselling addresses woman's mindsets related to violence such as normalizing violence, considering violence as her fault, not involving natal family due to perceptions of burdening them etc.

Recognizing violence as an issue of power: A large majority of survivors reported that they recognised violence as an issue of power, recognised the impact of violence on health and the need to raise voice against violence. According to the feminist counselling principles, violence is perpetrated by an abuser in order to stay in a powerful position which is ascribed by the rigid gender roles of our society (Rege, 2008). Women are able to see that the abuser does not inflict violence because of illness, stress or addiction, neither does he inflict abuse because of the "other woman" in case of extra- marital relationship, or because someone instigates him/ her (marital family).

Recognizing the impact of violence on health: Many women participating in the study reported that they were able to recognize how violence was impacting their health. They described it as; "not eating properly", "always thinking about abuse" and not being able to seek healthcare because of violence. One such example is that of a 24-year woman who was a post graduate and not employed stated; "When I talked to counsellor I realized how violence from husband is making me sick. It (the counselling intervention) has actually positively affected my health as I started eating properly."

Recognising the need to confront voice against violence: Several women said that the counselling intervention helped them to understand that violence is not acceptable and there is a need to raise one's voice against it. The women were able to articulate that they had to do something about the abuse to change their situation. They discussed steps taken by at an individual level to address the violence. These ranged from taking up a job, moving out of the house, raising voice against the abuser, joining a livelihood programme, undergoing MTP and even arriving at a decision to giving their child up for adoption. Findings of the study indicated that almost half the women in the study (51%) women adopted an action at the individual level. action to safeguard their well-being after receiving counselling intervention.

Mitigating feelings of self-blame and guilt: Social conditioning of women results in the acceptance of violence as a part of domestic lives. Mitigating feelings of self-blame and guilt has been defined as the ability of women to realize that the violence they are facing is not their fault Women often try to locate the fault in themselves, such as not being able to cook or take care of the household or husband's needs or marital family. 67 per cent reported on their ability to comprehend that violence had an impact on their health. Post counselling intervention, 24% women said that discussions with counsellor helped them build a positive self-image because the message that violence was not their fault stayed with them.

Safety of women: Domestic violence affects not only the physical but the emotional safety of women as well. There is evidence from the various intervention research studies carried out in Western countries that safety planning activity with women greatly improves their situation (Ramsay et al., 2009; Tirado-Muñoz et al., 2014). These activities help women build their capacity to engage in activities that can promote their safety and well-being (Ford-Gilboe et al., 2017). Another element to be emphasized during such intervention is the psychological safety of women. This is a key component of safety planning as women facing violence experience a lot of emotional health consequences, including suicidal ideation (Alhusen et al., 2015).

During, post-intervention assessment, women were asked about the safety measures adopted by them. These strategies were documented both in response to an immediate episode of violence as well as those that were implemented by women to ensure safety in future. 62 per cent of women recalled a safety measure at the time of the post-intervention assessment and asserted that they would adopt it in future. These women shared the preferred safety measures that they were planning to use. 37 per cent of the women filed a non-cognizable complaint against the abuser in which the police record the statement of women about violence but do not take any action against the abuser. This complaint plays a significant role as evidence of documentation of violence faced by women in case they want to take legal action against the abuser in future The other most common (35 per cent) safety related strategy adopted by women was keeping their valuables in a safe place. Women narrated being more aware of keeping important documents, and belongings in a safe space so that if the violence escalates and she has to leave her documents are not damaged/confiscated by the abuser. These include Aadhar cards, marriage certificates, birth certificates of children, property papers, ATM card, jewellery and bank account details.

Change in violence faced by women: Women participating in the study were followed *up* at two points of time. One was before their delivery and the other was at six weeks post-delivery. There was no sexual violence reported before the delivery and at six weeks after delivery by women. Emotional violence was the most common form of violence reported by women before delivery as well as six weeks after delivery. Women's narrative indicated that it had reduced to 2.5 times at six weeks post-delivery. Similarly, there was substantial decrease reported by women in financial violence.

Physical and emotional health: To measure the health status of women at six weeks post-delivery, women were asked about the change in their health status in the form of "better, worsen and remained same". The women who shared that their health improved were nearly 84 per cent, while for remaining the health status remained the same. The women who reported no improvement in their health status were significantly less likely to act at the informal and formal level.

Counsellors' Perspectives on Women-Centred Care for Survivors of Violence

Dilaasa centres have been upscaled to 11 public hospitals in the city of Mumbai since 2016. A review of the implementation of Dilaasa was carried out by CEHAT to identify the facilitators, barriers, inputs and processes for scale-up of VAW interventions. As part of this study, counsellors were interviewed to understand their interface with the health system, provision of crisis intervention services, and challenges faced by them in providing services to survivors (Arora et al., 2021).

Counsellors articulated how they addressed survivors' guilt or blame by validating their experience and sending an unequivocal message that violence was not her fault. Counsellors also receive survivors who are on a gender spectrum as well as women and girls in same sex relationship. They usually get admitted to hospital following an assault and/or attempted suicide after which they are referred to Dilaasa. Interviews with counsellors showed that counsellor reiterated to gender and sexually diverse people that they should not feel shame about their identity and that the law recognises their identity. Most importantly counsellors were able to provide an alternate perspective to survivors by explaining the phenomenon of VAW as an issue of power and control which is rooted in gendered power relations, that this is not just directed at an individual woman but is experienced by many women in a patriarchal society. The feminist principle of respecting women's autonomy was practised by counsellors by respecting survivors' wish to not disclose all details in the first counselling interview, respecting their decisions about continuing to live with abuser and focusing on a safety plan so that women can priortise their safety and have a backup plan in case they decided to leave the abusive home.

Counsellors reported that they focused on recognising the impact of violence on health. From direct and indirect health consequences to recognising how certain health conditions can trigger violence in women's lives. Being in a health system, safety assessment forms a crucial aspect of crisis counselling. Counsellors ask several questions to assess the severity and frequency of violence, change in the nature of violence over time, and women's perception of their safety at home. Based on all this, the safety plan is prepared. Each woman's situation is unique, depending on whether she is going back to the abusive home or leaving it. Safety assessments of survivors include enquiries about suicidal thoughts. When women endure violence over long periods can get frustrated and angry and may express thoughts of suicide to the counsellor. The counsellors encourage them to overcome thoughts of suicide, consequences of attempted suicides. The counsellors explained that women ask counsellors to conduct meetings with those perpetrating them and sometimes counsellors also feel the need for such meetings. In such situations, they explained having a woman centred approach to joint meetings with abusers and their families. But counsellors also explain the limitations of such meetings because the perpetrators may not agree to change their behaviour, and sometimes violence may also escalate. Before conducting it, they prepare women on how to speak and approach the issues in the meeting and counsellors act as a facilitator by encouraging her to speak out and agree to stop violence. It was evident that a feminist perspective and strategies were integrated in the upscaled Dilaasa crisis intervention departments.

Conceptualising Outcome Indicators for Psychosocial Counselling with a Feminist Perspective

Most knowledge about feminist strategies to mitigate DV in India continues to be in the form of oral histories of organisations. There is a lack of dialogue on commonly agreed upon strategies in psychosocial interventions to respond to DV. This could be one of the reasons for the poor uptake of feminist counselling practices by the mainstream counselling centres established by the Government of India (GOI). One Stop Centres is one such recent flagship program of the GOI, started in 2016 and currently there are 769 OSCs operational across India (Ministry of Women and Child Development, 2024). One of the many challenges experienced by OSCs relates to lack of awareness of feminist perspective and its integration in counselling for the survivors (Suresh, 2023). It is in this context of the critical need for collectivising an understanding on "what works to respond to DV", SAHAJ, a Vadodara-based organization in collaboration with CEHAT decided to embark on initiating a dialogue with collectives and organisations specifically engaged on responding to DV. CEHAT's counselling model at Dilaasa as well as evidence backed studies put the team in the unique position of initiating such a dialogue. SAHAJ has been engaged in state and national level advocacy campaigns to address gender inequities and has engaged with national networks in India in addressing violence against women. Both organisations convened to bring together those engaged in responding to DV and specifically providing psychosocial counselling with a feminist orientation (CEHAT & Sahaj, 2021). What emerged at the consultation was that almost all organisations focused on two forms of survivors-centred approaches, one being case work and the other joint meetings with the abuser (Box 2).

Box 2: Indicators of Success that emerged from the discussions

Intrapersonal

- Improvement in survivor's mental health
- Reduction in stress/depression/anxiety
- Increase in confidence & self-esteem- Improvement in Decision-making skills
- Improvement in social skills/networking ability
- Improved ability to make and maintain friendships
- Increase in responsibility towards oneself
- Increase in self-care
- Increase in understanding of oneself
- Taking legal steps to address violence (police/court)
- Taking steps to/ Becoming economically independent
- Increased independent mobility

Interpersonal

- Reduction in violence/moving out of violent relationships
- Improvement in support from Natal Family/community members
- Reduction in isolation- increased social networks within/outside family
- Improvement in Inter-personal relationships (with family members, friends, children, colleagues etc)
- Increase in responsibility towards family (natal)- Women supporting other survivors in similar situations
- Survivors engaging with the larger women's movement and becoming agents of change themselves

Source (CEHAT & Sahaj, 2021)

These indicators include intrapersonal and interpersonal markers of immediate and long-term outcomes. From keeping herself safe, improving her well-being, taking a stand against violence to taking steps towards becoming independent are some examples of immediate outcomes. The long-term outcomes are related to centring self-care, questioning violence against herself and seeing it as a structural issue, building relationships with children to alleviate consequences on them and their relationship, and becoming a change agent herself.

These outcomes are context-specific and vary per woman. Women's mindsets vary as their internalisation of gender roles, justification of domestic violence, stigma associated with 'breaking" a marriage, and support from parental /natal families, are factors that facilitate or inhibit women's struggle to take a stand and stop violence in their lives.

Joint Meetings. A joint meeting is a meeting organised to facilitate negotiation / mediate for nonviolent behaviour from the abusive partner or other perpetrators from the family. This is an opportunity to work with men, educate them and stop violence.

Box 3: Indicators of Success Indicators of Success of Joint Meetings

- The goal of a joint meeting was achieved: an agreement was reached based on what the woman wanted, upholding her right to live in a home without violence.
- Principles of joint meeting followed: Non-acceptability of violence communicated to the perpetrator
- Clear definition of non-negotiables in a signed agreement
- Adherence to an agreement resulting in the elimination of violence

Source (CEHAT & Sahaj, 2021)

Joint meetings are facilitated by most organisations and the approach to it varies based on their location—police, health facility or community. The role of a counsellor is to create a safe space where the woman can clearly state what she wants such as living separately from the abuser, stopping violence, maintenance, access to employment/education, custody of children, amongst others. These negotiations may not yield results in one meeting but may require multiple meetings and therefore the process becomes critical as mentioned in the above box. The principles of joint meeting and the non-negotiables are most important as it may take the abuser some time to take a decision. In this process, the safety of the woman becomes paramount. The non-negotiables refer to conditions agreed to in the agreement at the end of each meeting. Instead of mentioning conditions such as 'the woman will not call/visit her natal family', 'she will behave herself', where the onus is on changing the woman's behaviour, there should be a clear agreement to stop "violence of any form."

As counselling can be done only if the person is willing or admits that the person needs help, it becomes difficult for a crisis intervention centre/counselling centre to insist on counselling the 'perpetrator'. But as a feminist practice, joint meetings as mentioned above are an opportunity to talk to and educate the male perpetrators.

Some of the conditions that led to successful outcomes of counselling were parental family support, support from friends, neighbours as well as colleagues at work place as well as women's economic independence. Some of the barriers experienced were lack of support from law enforcement agencies such as police, courts that discourage women from accessing formal redressal mechanisms.

Conclusion

To conclude, the autonomous women's movement in India had initially drawn attention to the issue of Domestic Violence against women in India in the 1970s. The task before the movement was to raise issues of several forms of oppression against women starting with dowry demands and dowry deaths to other forms of domestic violence as well as sexual violence. Consistent campaigns by them helped women to speak out about the violence faced by them. This led volunteers from the movement to create support structures for women disclosing violence. Although the autonomous women's movement did not use the term 'intersectionality', it is evident from the above account that they did critically examine social dimensions such as caste, class, religion and their intersections to violence against women, while engaging with the issue. This enabled the women's groups and organisations in subsequent years to integrate critical feminist intersectional thought in the development of their counselling practices. As is evident from the chapter, the effectiveness of feminist counselling practices for violence against women lies in examination of VAW with intersections of women's personal, social and political identities. The Dilaasa hospital-based crisis centre is an example of building on feminist principles contributed by the autonomous women's movement and their adaptation in a public hospital setting. Despite the integration of feminist perspectives in counselling for DV, such an approach in counselling has however, not been adequately mainstreamed either in research and practice of psychology or social sciences in India. While the paper provides only a glimpse of the importance of embedding a feminist perspective in counselling, it is important to add to the evidence base related to implementation of feminist counselling in domestic violence redressals in India. Similarly, it is crucial to influence mainstream practice of government counselling centres to integrate feminist principles in their efforts to respond to DV.

Lastly, the authors are cognisant of recent efforts by structurally excluded groups that have questioned the ableist, casteist and homophobic attitudes of mainstream counsellors (Ranade et al., 2023). They find the feminist practices that do adopt a gender and intersectional lens inadequate and limited in their ability to understand structural exclusion based on caste, sexual and gender identity and disability (Daruwalla et al., 2013). Queer and Dalit activists are therefore currently vocal about the need for mental health interventions that recognise the intersections of sexual and gender identity with caste and disability and the experience of violence by socially excluded groups within homes and outside.

References

Agnihotri, I., & Mazumdar, V. (1995). Changing terms of political discourse: Women's movement in India, 1970s–1990s. *Economic and Political Weekly, 30*(29), 1869–1878.

ADB Nongovernment Organization and Civil Society Center. (2009). *Overview of civil society organizations in India*. https://www.adb.org/sites/default/files/publication/28966/csb-ind.pdf

Agnes, F. (1999). *Law and gender inequality in India: The politics of women's rights in India.* Oxford University Press.

Alhusen, J. L., Ray, E., Sharps, P., & Bullock, L. (2015). Intimate partner violence during pregnancy: Maternal and neonatal outcomes. *Journal of Women's Health, 24*(1), 100–106. https://doi.org/10.1089/jwh.2014.4872

Arora, S., Bhate-Deosthali, P., & Rege, S. (2018). *Responding to domestic violence for improving maternal health outcomes: An evaluation of a counselling intervention for pregnant women in Mumbai.* Centre for Enquiry into Health and Allied Themes and Municipal Corporation of Greater Mumbai. https://www.cehat.org/uploads/files/Responding%20to%20Domestic%20Violence%20in%20Pregnancy.pdf

Arora, S., Thomas, D., Bhate-Deosthali, P., Baxi, A., & Rege, S. (2021). *Scaling up the health-systems response to violence against women: A review of the implementation of Dilaasa crisis centres in 11 public hospitals of Mumbai.* Centre for Enquiry into Health and Allied Themes. https://www.cehat.org/uploads/files/SVRI_report_Scaling_up.pdf

Bhate-Deosthali, P., & Duggal, R. (2013). Rethinking gender-based violence and public health policies in India. In K. Nakray (Ed.), *Gender-based violence and public health: International perspectives on budgets and policies* (pp. 184–196). Routledge.

Bhate-Deosthali, P., & Lingam, L. (2016). Gendered pattern of burn injuries in India: A neglected health issue. *Reproductive Health Matters, 24*(47), 96–103. https://doi.org/10.1016/j.rhm.2016.05.004

Burte, A. (2013). The spirit of resistance. In P. Bhate-Deosthali, S. Rege & P. Prakash (Eds.), *Feminist counselling and domestic violence in India* (pp. 19–47). Routledge—Taylor & Francis Group.

Burte, A., Rege, S., & Deosthali, P. (2005). *Choosing to live: Guidelines for suicide prevention counselling in domestic violence.* Centre for Enquiry into Health and Allied Themes. https://www.cehat.org/uploads/files/sucide%282%29.pdf

Craven, L. C., Fields, A. M., Carlson, R. G., Combs, E. M., & Howe, E. S. (2023). Counselling interventions for victims of intimate partner violence: A systematic review. *Journal of Counselling & Development, 101*(3), 346–358. https://doi.org/10.1002/jcad.12478

Centre for Enquiry into Health and Allied Themes. (2001). *Working towards right to health and health care: Nine years of Anusandhan trust: Six years of Centre for Enquiry into Health and Allied Themes (CEHAT).* https://www.cehat.org/reportPdfs/17012444072812.pdf

Centre for Enquiry into Health and Allied Themes. (2004). *Counselling impact study.* [Unpublished research report].

Centre for Enquiry into Health and Allied Themes & SAHAJ. (2021). *Assessing progress in interventions addressing domestic violence against women report of a national consultation.* CEHAT & SAHAJ. https://www.cehat.org/uploads/files/Convening%20report%20draft.pdf

Daruwalla, N., Chakravarty, S., Chatterji, S., Shah More, N., Alcock, G., Hawkes, S., & Osrin, D. (2013). Violence against women with disability in Mumbai, India: A qualitative study. *Sage Open, 3*(3). https://doi.org/10.1177/2158244013499144

Davar, B. V. (1999). *Mental health of Indian women: A feminist agenda.* Sage Publications India.

Davar, B. V. (Ed.). (2001). *Mental health from a gender perspective.* Sage.

Deosthali-Bhate, P., Maghnani, P., & Malik, S. (2005). *Establishing Dilaasa: Documenting the challenges.* Dilaasa and Centre for Enquiry into Health and Allied Themes.

Deosthali-Bhate, P., Ravindran, T. K. S., & Vindhya, U. (2012, April 28). Addressing domestic violence within health care settings. *Economic and Political Weekly, 47(17),* 66–75.

Deosthali-Bhate, P., Rege, S., Pal, P., Nandi, S., Bhatla, N., & Kashyap, A. (2018). *Role of the health sector in addressing intimate partner violence in India: A synthesis report.* International Center for Research on Women.

Desai, A. R. (1985). Women's movement in India: An assessment. *Economic and Political Weekly, 20*(23), 992–995.

Ellsberg, M., Arango, D. J., Morton, M., Gennari, F., Kiplesund, S., Contreras, M., & Watts, C. (2015). Prevention of violence against women and girls: What does the evidence say? *The Lancet, 385*(9977), 1555–1566. https://doi.org/10.1016/S0140-6736(14)61703-7

Enns, C. Z. (2004). *Feminist theories and feminist psychotherapies: Origins, themes and diversity* (2nd ed.). The Haworth Press.

Ford-Gilboe, M., Varcoe, C., Scott-Storey, K., Wuest, J., Case, J., Currie, L. M., Glass, N., Hodgins, M., MacMillan, H., Perrin, N., & Wathen, C. N. (2017). A tailored online safety and health intervention for women experiencing intimate partner violence: The iCAN plan 4 safety randomized controlled trial protocol. *BMC Public Health, 17*(273), 1–12. https://doi.org/10.1186/s12889-017-4143-9

Gandhi, N., & Shah, N. (1992). *The issues at stake: Theory and practice in the contemporary women's movement in India.* Kali For Women.

Gupte, M., & More, A. (2007). *Chakrabhed: Kautumbik hinseche dushtachakra and surksha niyojan* [Marathi Publication]. MASUM.

Gupte, M. (2013). Why feminism should inform our routine interventions in domestic violence. In P. Bhate-Deosthali, S. Rege, & P. Prakash (Eds.), *Feminist counselling and domestic violence in India* (pp. 48–89). Routledge.

Hackett, S., McWhirter, P. T., & Lesher, S. (2016). The therapeutic efficacy of domestic violence victim interventions. *Trauma, Violence, & Abuse, 17*(2), 123–132. https://doi.org/10.1177/1524838014566720

Haksar, N. (1986). Women and violence. *Economic and Political Weekly, 21*(49), 2126–2127.

Jaising, I. (2009). *Handbook of law on domestic violence.* Lexis Nexis.

Joshi, A. (2019). *Counsellors' journeys of working with domestic violence issues* (Doctoral Thesis, Tata Institute of Social Sciences). School of Social Science, Tata Institute of Social Sciences. http://hdl.handle.net/10603/256474

K.K., L., Umashankar, S., Nainar, V., & Patel, V. A. (2014, May 21). *Women's Research and Action Network (WRAG): Report of activities 2010–2014* [PowerPoint Slides). SlidesShare. https://papers.ssrn.com/sol3/papers.cfm?abstract_id=3182465

Kannabiran, K., & Menon, R. (Ed.). (2007). *From Mathura to Manorama: Resisting violence against women in India.* Kali for Women.

Katzenstein, M. F. (1989). Organizing against violence: Strategies of the Indian women's movement. *Pacific Affairs, 62*(1), 53–71.

Kumar, R. (1998). *History of doing: An illustrated account of movements for women's rights and feminism in India 1800–1990.* Kali for Women.

Micklitz, H. M., Glass, C. M., Bengel, J., & Sander, L. B. (2023). Efficacy of psychosocial interventions for survivors of intimate partner violence: A systematic review and meta-analysis. *Trauma, Violence, & Abuse, 25*(2), 1000–1017. https://doi.org/10.1177/15248380231169481

Mitra, N. (2001). Community based initiatives in the struggle against domestic violence. *The Indian Journal of Social Work, 62*(3), 414–429.

Modi, P. (2007). Consultation of users and survivors: YMCA, 26th September 2007. *Aaina: A mental health advocacy newsletter, 7*(3), 18–21. Pune, Bapu Trust for research on mind and discourse, https://baputrust.com/wp-content/uploads/2020/02/aaina-nov-2007.pdf

Morrison, A., Ellsberg, M., & Bott, S. (2007). Addressing gender-based violence: A critical review of interventions. *World Bank Research Observer, 22*, 25–51.

Ogbe, E., Hermon, S., Van den Bergh, R., & Deyomme, O. (2020). A systematic review of intimate partner violence interventions focused on improving social support and/mental health outcomes of survivors. *PLoS ONE, 15*(6), Article e0235177.

Phadke, S. (2003). Thirty years on: Women's studies reflects on the women's movement. *Economic and Political Weekly, 38*(43), 4567–4576.

Qadeer, I., & Viswanathan, R. (2004). How healthy are health and population policies? The Indian experience. In A. Castro & M. Singer (Eds.), *Unhealthy health policies: A critical anthropological examination* (pp. 145–163). Altamira Press.

Ram, K. (1998). *Na shariram nadhi,* my body is mine: The urban women's health movement in India and its negotiation of modernity. *Women's Studies International Forum, 21*(6), 617–631. https://doi.org/10.1016/S0277-5395(98)00076-4

Ram, K. (2001). Rationalising fecund bodies: Family planning policy and the modern Indian nation state. In M. Jolly and K. Ram (Eds.), *Borders of being: Citizenship, fertility and sexuality in Asia and the Pacific.* University of Michigan Press.

Ramsay, J., Carter, Y., Davidson, L., Eldridge, S., Hegarty, K., Rivas, C., Taft, A., Warburton, A., Dunne, D., & Feder, G. (2009). Protocol: Advocacy interventions to reduce or eliminate violence and promote the physical and psychosocial well-being of women who experience intimate partner abuse. *Campbell Systematic Reviews, 5*(1), 1–31. https://doi.org/10.1002/CL2.57

Ramasubban, S., & Jejheebhoy, S. (2000). *Women's reproductive health in India.* Rawat Publications.

Ranade, K., Kumar, N., Raju, M. S., Somaiya, A., Pai, P., Roychowdhuri, I., & Singh, A. (2023). *Trans affirmative mental health care guidelines: Results of a mixed-method inquiry in three cities of India.* Tata Institute of Social Science. https://tiss.edu/uploads/files/Trans_Affirmative_Mental_Health_Care_Guidelines.pdf

Ravindran, T. K. S. (1995). Women's health policies: Organizing for change. *Reproductive Health Matters, 3*(6), 7–11.

Ray, R. (2002). *Fields of protest: Women's movement in India.* Zubaan Publishers.

Rege, S., Deosthali, P., & Contractor, Q. (2010). *Challenges in domestic violence counselling: A casebook.* Centre for Enquiry into Health and Allied Themes.

Rege, S., & Chandrasekhar, A. (2013). Feminist domestic violence interventions in India. In P. Bhate-Deosthali, S. Rege, & P. Prakash (Eds.), *Feminist counselling and domestic violence in India* (pp. 126–175). Routledge.

Rege, S. (2008). *Guidelines for counselling: Women facing violence.* Centre for Enquiry into Health and Allied Themes and Dilaasa.

Saheli Women's Resource Centre. (1995). *The "Casework" debate in Saheli: Souvenir 1995.* https://sites.google.com/site/saheliorgsite/other-issues/the-casework-debate-in-saheli

Santhya, K.G., & Jejeebhoy, S.J. (2017). *Acceptability and effectiveness of helpline services: Perspectives of women in distress and service providers: Policy brief.* Population Council. https://doi.org/10.31899/pgy8.1000

Sarojini, N. B. (2006). *Women's right to health.* National Human Rights Commission.

Sheth, D. L., & Sethi, H. (1991). The NGO sector in India: Historical context and current discourse. *Voluntas: International Journal of Voluntary and Nonprofit Organizations, 2*, 49–68. https://doi.org/10.1007/BF01398670

Sharma, G. (2011). NGOs in India: Historical roots, meanings, characteristics and types—A narrative and conceptual account. In *Non-governmental organisations and empowerment of women: A study on some selected NGOs of Darjeeling district of West Bengal* (pp. 44–74) (Doctoral Thesis, University of North Bengal). Department of Political Science, University of North Bengal. https://ir.nbu.ac.in/handle/123456789/1393

Shirwadkar, S. (Ed.). (2009). *Family violence in India: Human rights, issues, actions and international comparisons.* Rawat Publications.

Sullivan, C. M. (2018). Understanding how domestic violence support services promote survivor well-being: A conceptual model. *Journal of Family Violence, 33*(2), 123–131. https://doi.org/10.1007/s10896-017-9931-6

Suneetha, A., & Nagaraj, V. (2006). A difficult match: Women's actions and legal institutions in the face of domestic violence. *Economic and Political Weekly, 41*(41), 4355–4362.

Suresh, N. (2023, May 5). One stop, many challenges: Sakhi centres struggle to support women survivors of violence [Blog post]. *India Spend.* https://www.indiaspend.com/governance/one-stop-many-challenges-sakhi-centres-struggle-to-support-women-survivors-of-violence-861666

Stree Mukti Sanghatana. (2013). *Stree Mukti Sanghatana: Annual report: January to December 2013*. https://streemuktisanghatana.org/wp-content/uploads/2018/04/Annual-report-2013-final.pdf

Tirado-Muñoz, J., Gilchrist, G., Farré, M., Hegarty, K., & Torrens, M. (2014). The efficacy of cognitive behavioural therapy and advocacy interventions for women who have experienced intimate partner violence: A systematic review and meta-analysis. *Annals of Medicine, 46*(8), 567–586. https://doi.org/10.3109/07853890.2014.941918

Trabold, N., McMahon, J., Alsobrooks, S., Whitney, S., & Mittal, M. (2020). A systematic review of intimate partner violence interventions: State of the field and implications for practitioners. *Trauma, Violence & Abuse, 21*, 311–325. https://doi.org/10.1177/1524838018767934

Unnithan, M., & Pigg, S. L. (2014). Sexual and reproductive health rights and justice: Tracking the relationship. *Culture, Health and Sexuality, 16*(10), 1181–1187. https://doi.org/10.1080/13691058.2014.945774

Vindhya, U. (2005). Battered conjugality: The psychology of domestic violence. In K. Kannabiran (Ed.), *The violence of normal times: Essays on women's lived realities* (pp. 197–223). Women Unlimited.

Vindhya, U. (2013). Feminist counselling for domestic violence: Some issues of theory and practice. In In P. Bhate-Deosthali, S. Rege & P. Prakash (Eds.), *Feminist counselling and domestic violence in India* (pp. 93–125). Routledge.

Vindhya, U., & Lingam, L. (2019). Social action committees: Community intervention to reduce gender-based violence. *Indian Journal of Gender Studies, 26*(3), 263–287.

Worell, J. W., & Remer, P. (2003). *Feminist perspectives in therapy; Empowering diverse women* (2nd ed.). John Wiley & Sons.

Sangeeta Rege is a Consultant at CEHAT, Mumbai. Her areas of interest include the interface of gender with health, gender-based violence, medical education and ethics in health care. She is engaged in research, training and advocacy on health as a human right. She led CEHAT's public interest litigation seeking right to health care for rape survivors that paved the way for development of a health sector protocol for rape care in India.

Padma Bhate-Deosthali Ph.D has experience in research, training, and policy advocacy in the areas of gender-based violence, gender in medical education, health policy research, regulation of private health sector, and women and work, with a focus on health and human rights. She was a member of the Steering Group of the GDG-WHO for developing policy and clinical practice guidelines for responding to VAW and also member of the National Committee under the MoHFW for drafting the "Guidelines and Protocols for medico-legal care for victims/survivors of sexual violence". She coordinated the setting up of Dilaasa, a public hospital-based crisis centre on domestic violence in Mumbai. She currently works at ICRW.

Chapter 5
Psychosocial Interventions with Communities to Prevent Violence Against Women and Girls in Complex Urban Informal Settings

Nayreen Daruwalla, Sharanya Gautam, Gargi Khandekar, Vanessa D'Souza, Shanti Pantvaidya, and David Osrin

Abstract Violence against women and girls is a complex and multifaceted issue that is engrained in social and cultural realities, while impacting both the mental health and social wellbeing of survivors. The issue becomes even more challenging in the context of urban informal communities in cities like Mumbai where settlements are characterised by overcrowding, insubstantial housing, insufficient water and sanitation, lack of tenure, and hazardous locations. Psychosocial approaches to prevent and respond to violence against women and girls target a range of factors—behavioural, cognitive, emotional, interpersonal, social and environmental—with the aim of improving the health and wellbeing of women and girls. SNEHA's experience suggests that an interdisciplinary approach of interventions delivered by a range of professionals, including social workers and mental health practitioners, will help in formulating a more comprehensive and pragmatic theory of social change. This chapter explores the conceptualisation, evolution and evaluation of a theory-driven, community-led psychosocial approach to violence prevention that emphasizes locally relevant and scalable solutions.

Keyword Prevention strategies for violence against women · Theory of change · Community-led approaches to violence prevention

The chapter is grounded in the work of the Society for Nutrition, Education, and Health Action (SNEHA), a Mumbai-based NGO with over 23 years of experience addressing health and violence against women and children in the city's informal settlements, which host 41% of the city's households. It outlines the development of

N. Daruwalla (✉) · S. Gautam · G. Khandekar · V. D'Souza · S. Pantvaidya
Society for Nutrition, Education and Health Action, Mumbai, India
e-mail: nayreen@snehamumbai.org

D. Osrin
Wellcome Trust Fellow at University College London, London, England

U. Vindhya (ed.), *Psychosocial Interventions for Social Issues in Contemporary India*,
https://doi.org/10.1007/978-981-96-6553-2_5

SNEHA's community-driven violence prevention program, and argues that interventions for prevention of violence against women and girls in complex urban settings elicit greater participation and commitment from community members if delivered through psychosocial support.

SNEHA's community-led intervention program employs a socio-ecologic model as a framework for action at multiple levels, from the individual to society, to prevent violence. The program addresses the interplay between these levels and intersectional factors through primary, secondary, and tertiary prevention strategies. This comprehensive approach is more effective than any single intervention, fostering social change by leveraging community mobilization, participation, and behaviour change to prevent violence against women and girls.

In SNEHA's program, Primary prevention involves campaigns and group education to encourage individual voluntarism in identifying, responding to, and referring cases of violence. Secondary prevention includes comprehensive services like counselling, crisis intervention, coordination with public health facilities, police, legal aid, home visits, and mental health counselling. Tertiary interventions provide extended counselling, psycho-education, couple and family counselling, and legal support to empower survivors in making decisions about their situations.

Finally, the chapter discusses the development and evaluation of a theory of change for this program model, that also acknowledges the intervention functions of the behaviour change wheel developed by Michie and colleagues: increasing capability, opportunity and motivation in communities through training, education, enablement and modelling to build critical consciousness on the issue and understand the importance of participation. In conclusion, it discusses challenges, strategies and further directions for the design, implementation and evaluation of community-based psychosocial interventions to prevent violence against women and girls.

Introduction

Violence against women and girls is a complex phenomenon that is intricately linked to both the socio-cultural context in which violence occurs and the mental health of both survivors and those who commit it. This chapter discusses a theory-driven, multifaceted, community-led approach to violence prevention that is grounded in the social realities of the community, and based on locally relevant and scalable ways of preventing and addressing violence. It is based on the work of the Society for Nutrition, Education and Health Action (SNEHA) over the last 23 years in the complex urban informal settings of Mumbai, and describes the development of their community-driven violence against women and girl's prevention programme, outlining its inception, evolution, formulation of its theory of change, and the processes involved in its evaluation. Finally, it outlines the challenges in designing, implementing and evaluating psychosocial interventions to prevent violence against women and girls in community settings and suggests strategies to mitigate those challenges.

Background

Psychosocial Determinants of Violence Against Women and Girls: A Double Burden on Mental Health

Violence against women and girls is common and ubiquitous, with visible and hidden forms. Globally, 30% of women have ever experienced physical or sexual violence by an intimate partner, or sexual violence by a non-partner (World Health Organisation, 2024). The latest National Family Health Survey (NFHS-4) suggests that 21% of ever-married women in Maharashtra state—the location of SNEHA's work—have experienced intimate partner violence (International Institute for Population Sciences (IIPS) and ICF, 2017). SNEHA's monitoring data from its community-based programs over the years indicates that approximately 80% of cases related to violence against women and girls are domestic violence (DV) and intimate partner violence (IPV). Natal family violence accounts for 15%, sexual violence constitutes 3%, and the remainder is child sexual violence. Consequently, this chapter primarily focuses on the prevention of DV and IPV, while acknowledging the need to prevent other types of violence within community settings.

SNEHA's experience of working in community settings shows that violence against women and girls cuts across class, caste and cultures, and its reasons and manifestations are complex and interconnected. The experience of violence significantly affects women's mental health. At the same time, the relational, hierarchical, and historically ingrained aspects of gender amplify stressors on women's mental well-being, while also acting as pivotal determinants of domestic and intimate partner violence. Socially constructed gender norms, roles, and responsibilities frequently confine women to situations where they wield limited control over crucial life decisions. Patriarchal family structures often dictate the extent of a woman's autonomy and the choices available to her. Non-compliance with traditional social norms or neglecting domestic duties often subjects women to criticism, social ostracism, and even violence. The pressure to conform to patriarchal expectations and the lack of social support in managing domestic responsibilities contribute significantly to heightened stress levels, severely impacting women's mental well-being.

In 2019, SNEHA conducted a retrospective study of counselling records from the urban informal settlements of Dharavi and Govandi in Mumbai to understand the range of responses that a service for survivors of violence against women should provide (Daruwalla et al., 2024). A total of 2278 women accessed the counselling centres, of whom 75% were aged between 20 and 39, 65% were married, 15% were involved in informal labour and around 80% lived in *zopadpatti* (informal settlements) or *chawls* (housing built for industry workers). Clients described intimate partner violence (37%), domestic violence by a family member other than their partner (22%), or both (27%). Common forms of violence reported were emotional (88%), economic (73%), and physical (71%); 68% of clients reported episodes of neglect, 59% of coercive control, and 36% of sexual violence, while 77% had survived three or more forms of violence (Daruwalla et al., 2024). An analysis of these counselling records found that among the issues that survivors reasoned were at the root of their problems were difficulties in either their adaptation to their expected roles in the marital family or the failure of their partner to live up to theirs. 29% of clients said that their marital family neglected their needs and 26% that the family exerted too much control over them. The majority of clients (83%) were screened for depressive symptoms using the nine-item Patient Health Questionnaire (PHQ-9) and for anxiety using the Generalised Anxiety Disorder (GAD-7) scale. Screening suggested moderate or severe depressive symptoms in 39% and moderate anxiety symptoms in 35% (Daruwalla et al., 2024).

Psychosocial Approaches to Preventing Violence Against Women and Girls

Research points to the complex and interconnected ways in which violence impacts different facets of women's lives. Psychosocial approaches to violence prevention aim to address both psychological and social factors affecting an individual's well-being—acknowledging both the psychological and social determinants of violence and mental health. For example, Paphitis et al.'s (2022) review of psychosocial interventions to improve the mental health of women intimate partner violence survivors highlights that survivors experience multiple and competing negative psychosocial concerns, including the protection and care of children, physical health concerns, safety concerns, financial instability, legal proceedings, feelings of isolation and lack of social support, low self-esteem and feelings of grief, and managing ongoing threats from and relations with abusers, as well as ongoing trauma and psychological symptoms—without addressing which survivors may not receive the full support they need for recovery.

In community settings, psychosocial interventions comprise biological, behavioural, cognitive, emotional, interpersonal, social, or environmental level interventions with the aim of improving the survivor's health functioning and well-being. This is usually done through interpersonal or informational activities, techniques, or strategies. The success of interventions for survivors depends on careful design and delivery that considers cultural relevance, feasibility, and comprehensive support. Interventions are likely to be most effective when they are considered feasible by practitioners and survivors, and are culturally-relevant, trauma-informed, individually adapted and supported by communities and institutions (Paphitis et al., 2022). Therefore, both survivors and providers should be carefully considered and involved during the development and implementation of violence prevention interventions. Ensuring that service providers are supported in their roles will improve their acceptance and delivery of interventions, and therefore improve survivor outcomes (Paphitis et al., 2022). This aligns with the World Health Organization's (WHO) emphasis on the critical role of healthcare providers, particularly physicians and health professionals, as key stakeholders in identifying and intervening in cases of intimate partner violence, sexual violence, or suicidal behaviour. The WHO underscores the need for comprehensive care and psychosocial support to address the far-reaching consequences of gender-based violence (Harbishettar & Math, 2014). Further, meta-analyses (Alsina et al., 2024; Bacchus et al., 2018; Micklitz et al., 2023; Muluneh et al., 2021; White et al., 2024) and realist reviews (Paphitis et al., 2022; Rivas et al., 2019) have shown that interdisciplinary approaches and comprehensive strategies are more effective than individual actions when it comes to violence prevention. In this scenario, health care institutions emerge as key players, not only in providing care for survivors but also in recognizing the impact of violence on reproductive and mental health.

In their meta-analysis of randomised controlled trials studying psychosocial interventions for intimate partner violence in low- and middle-income countries, Turner et al. (2020) advocate for region-specific and integrated interventions, calling for collaborative efforts to combat the entrenched structural causes of violence against women and children. Such a comprehensive, intersectional strategy is imperative for creating a society where human rights are upheld and violence is unequivocally deemed unacceptable. Psychosocial interventions involve collaboration among mental health professionals, social workers, and community members, offering counselling, therapy, support groups, behavioural interventions, skills training, and psychoeducation to enhance both psychological functioning and social integration. Such multi-layered interventions—which cut across a range of underlying problems—can lead to gains across multiple outcomes alongside enhancing service accessibility for women facing multiple and complex needs, including complex mental health issues (Paphitis et al., 2022). Engaging approaches that cultivate community partnerships and employ participatory methods to generate community-wide solutions not only improve the likelihood of survivors seeking help but also ensure programme sustainability. Additionally, they decrease the risk of violence and survivor distress by empowering communities to support survivors and address the root causes of violence (Paphitis et al., 2022).

The Challenge of Urban Informal Settlements

Urban India is home to over 377 million people (Central Bureau of Health Intelligence, 2015; Ministry of Home Affairs, 2011). Informal settlements (slums) are features of urbanisation in India and have been described in two-thirds of cities and towns (Chandramouli, 2011). These settlements are characterised by overcrowding, insubstantial housing, insufficient water and sanitation, lack of tenure, and hazardous location (Ministry of Housing & Urban Poverty Alleviation, 2010; UN Habitat, 2003). Chandramouli (2011) estimates that 41% of Mumbai's households are in such settlements. Along with population density and stressful living conditions, risk factors for physical and sexual violence converge in Mumbai's urban informal settlements, driving the incidence of violence. These risk factors include poverty, exposure to parental violence, childhood maltreatment, limited education, unemployment, young adulthood, mental disorder, substance use, individual acceptance of violence, weak community and legal sanctions, and gender and social norms supportive of violence (Abramsky et al., 2011). In addition, women and girls in these communities lack both financial and social resources and an understanding of the possibility of relief from endemic violence.

SNEHA's Approach to Community-Based Violence Prevention

Overview of SNEHA

The Society for Nutrition, Education and Health Action (SNEHA) is a Mumbai-based non-government organisation addressing the health needs of women and children in the context of urban informal settlements in India. SNEHA was founded in 1998 by a group of leading neonatologists, headed by Dr. Armida Fernandez, former Dean of one of Mumbai's leading public hospitals. SNEHA aims to improve the health, nutrition and safety of women and children living in the most vulnerable urban informal settlements and works across the public health areas of maternal and child health, adolescent health, prevention of violence against women and children, and health systems strengthening.

SNEHA takes an integrated life-cycle approach that seeks to break the intergenerational cycle of poor health, a major by-product of poverty and deprivation. Its continuum of care approach intervenes at critical junctures: preconception, pregnancy, childbirth, postnatal, early childhood and adolescence, to bring about improvements in health and nutrition of women and children. SNEHA's interventions work with both vulnerable communities to improve health-seeking behaviour and awareness of health services and public health systems and health-care providers to improve service delivery through training, capacity building, data sharing and advocacy. During the years 2016–2023, SNEHA worked directly with over 406,000 women, children and healthcare workers, and indirectly reached a population of over 1.68 million in the Mumbai Metropolitan Region.

SNEHA's Programme on Prevention of Violence against Women and Children approaches the issue as a public health priority. It adopts an intersectoral approach focused on working with the survivor and her community as well as with public systems like the police, health care and legal systems which are vital in providing services to survivors of violence. The programme prioritises developing high-impact strategies for primary prevention, ensuring survivors' access to protection and justice, empowering women to claim their rights, mobilising communities around 'zero tolerance for violence,' and responding to the needs and rights of excluded and neglected groups. At the same time, it foregrounds enhanced coordination of the state response to crimes against women through a convergence approach that works with government and public systems to reinforce their roles in assuring basic social, civil and economic security.

Evolution of SNEHA's Violence Prevention Programme

SNEHA's work on prevention of violence against women and children started with a counselling centre in an extension of a large public hospital. The counselling centre opened in response to the experiences of health workers at Lokmanya Tilak Municipal General Hospital (LTMGH), Mumbai's largest public hospital. Women and children survivors of violence accessing hospital services had minimal interaction with doctors and nurses which tended to stop at treatment for injuries. Engaging with the wider issues—emotional, psychiatric, social, and legal—requires confidence, time, training, protocols and resources, all of which were in short supply. The centre was conceived as a means to address this gap through a partnership with the Municipal Corporation. Founded in 2000 at a municipal health facility in Dharavi, which at the time was one of the world's largest informal urban settlements, the Centre's location enabled access to the communities.

Reviewing our experiences, we think that three issues particularly influenced the centre's development: the relative invisibility of the problems with which we were trying to deal, women's desire to meet normative expectations and to keep the family together, and a spiralling need to connect with other service providers, families, and communities. While the counselling centre primarily assisted women experiencing domestic and intimate partner violence, including instances of sexual violence by non-intimate partners, cases involving homicide and suicide necessitated interventions extending beyond the scope of counselling and crisis interventions. These incidents posed challenges to providing justice to the survivor and her family as redressal meant liaising with many stakeholders and managing the community's expectations. We understood the criticality of two major interventions in the design and delivery of the programme: providing a range of resources to reduce distress and trauma from environmental factors, and providing access to counselling and mental health services to support reasoning through holistic, trauma-informed, and individualised interventions. These interventions were grounded in culture and context, honouring the complexity of each individual's situation, but at the same time interplayed with factors at the interpersonal and community level. These factors needed to be addressed at the community level as rehabilitation of survivors often required community support and solutions provided by community members were more plausible and sustainable.

An imperative need emerged to work on interpersonal and informational activities in communities to target biological, behavioural, cognitive, emotional, interpersonal, social or environmental factors to support survivors of violence and bring about a shift in community perspectives on the issue. A significant development was a gradual shift in emphasis from institutional support to community response and action and running programmes with other stakeholders like the police, public health doctors and state legal services to respond to violence against women and girls. The strategies were a mix of psychosocial interventions for prevention of violence against women and girls. The combined use of psychological interventions, aimed at motivating and persuading individuals to address violence, with various social interventions providing community-based opportunities to contest violence against women and children, and enhancing the skills of community members and service providers, led to the development of SNEHA's programme on prevention of violence against women and girls and its adoption of an ecological approach—emphasising the interconnectedness of individual, social, and environmental factors. The programme established a strong foundation for primary prevention by forming groups of women, adolescents, and men, as well as recruiting volunteers from these groups. These volunteers actively identified and intervened in cases of violence against women and girls. Secondary intervention was strengthened through building a coordinated response between counsellors and volunteers to provide crisis intervention and an extended response to survivors. We used technology to train our volunteers through the Little Sister online platform to map, identify and respond to survivors of violence in the community. Little Sister is a crowd-sourced notification system for domestic violence. It works in communities with the people residing there and gives real time, accurate mapped data on violence against women and children which makes giving appropriate support to survivors easier. *Sanginis* (Community Volunteers) were trained to form a surveillance team and equipped with smartphones and protocols for monitoring and responding to domestic violence incidents. An extended response to help survivors with legal provisions and restore their mental health was strengthened through consolidation of legal and mental health services.

Adapting a Socioecological Approach to Violence Prevention

As the programme's intervention consolidated organically, we recognised that it follows a socio-ecological model developed by Heise after the work of Bronfenbrenner (Bronfenbrenner, 1979; Heise, 1998). Heise's socio-ecological approach to violence against women conceptualises it as a multifaceted phenomenon grounded in the interactions among personal, situational and socio-cultural factors. It also establishes the factors that emerge as predictive of abuse at each level of the social ecology, with an understanding that prevention efforts need to address the determinants of violence at a range of levels—within families, communities, and societies.

The model recognises that supporting survivors of domestic violence should address a complex system of nested socioecological levels (the individual, her family, her community, and society) (Heise, 1998; Rege & Deosthali, 2010), and a range of needs that vary in intensity, duration, and outcome (Fulu et al., 2014). SNEHA's model for the Prevention of Violence Against Women and Children responds to the complex interplay of these individual, interpersonal, organisational, community, and public policy-related factors. The approach considers risk factors for violence, protective measures against it, and contributors to perpetration. Further, it highlights the necessity of implementing intervention strategies at multiple levels simultaneously, ensuring survivors receive comprehensive and holistic support (as described in Box 1):

Box 1: Socio-Ecological Approach to Prevention of Violence against Women and Girls

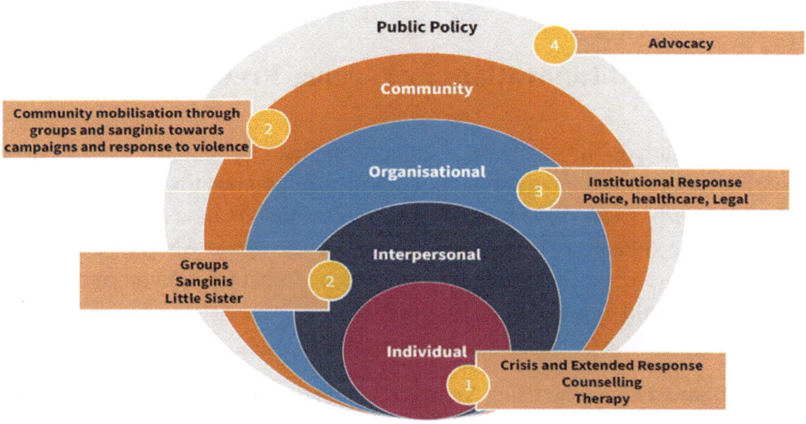

The programme addressed the interplay of factors that influence violence against women and children and gave us insights into the complex links between individual, relationship, community, institutional, and societal factors that put women at risk of experiencing or perpetrating violence.

The **individual** includes crisis and extended response, incorporating counselling and therapy. Prevention at the individual level with survivors and their abusers includes promoting attitudes, beliefs and behaviours that prevent violence.

The **interpersonal** includes our work at the relationship level and incorporates groups and *Sanginis* (women volunteers), who form relationships with women in communities, build awareness and connect individuals to SNEHA services. Prevention strategies at the relationship level include family focused interventions, fostering problem solving skills and promoting healthy relationships.

The **organisational** level includes interventions with the public systems including the police, healthcare and legal systems, including capacity building and training for police personnel and healthcare workers.

The **community level** interventions include community mobilisation work. Awareness building campaigns, pop-up information sessions, and women's, men's and adolescent groups are all part of community level interventions.

The **societal level** includes prevention strategies such as policy changing work as well as community mobilisation geared towards altering fixed beliefs and cultural norms that perpetuate violence.

Using a socio-ecologic model as a framework for action at different levels to prevent violence, from the individual to the home to the community to society, the programme tackles the interplay between levels and intersectional factors through primary, secondary and tertiary prevention strategies. Primary prevention seeks to stop domestic violence before it occurs. Secondary prevention seeks to prevent violence from continuing or escalating and respond to mental health needs. Tertiary prevention seeks to minimise the impact of violence and restore safety, mental health and wellbeing.

Community-Led Innovations in Violence Prevention

SNEHA's initiatives in furthering comprehensive, community-based violence prevention programmes have resulted in innovative methods towards fostering safer and healthier urban environments. Two examples, the Dharavi Biennale and Little Sister initiative (elaborated in Boxes 2 and 3), showcase SNEHA's innovations in addressing the complex challenges of violence against women and children's interventions within vulnerable communities.

Box 2: Dharavi Biennale: Using Art as a Medium to Expand Community Engagement

The Dharavi Biennale brought together art and science to address pressing urban health issues with the aim of highlighting Dharavi's significance in the cityscape while tackling themes like sanitation, women's safety, and mental health. This was done through innovative 'Artboxes'—art installations on various public health concepts including sanitation, women's safety, mental health, and violence.

Over a two-year span from February 2013, 23 Artboxes were created, showcasing artworks across three galleries, spanning from murals to films and theatre, highlighting diverse creative expressions. Additional events were organized to broaden participation in the lead-up to the main exhibition— the Alley Galli Biennale —encouraging community engagement and drawing attendees from across Mumbai.

The Biennale hosted participation from 41 Mentor Artists, 450 Participant Artists, and 14 Health Specialists in over 17 events, attracting 9000 visitors to the exhibition and 3340 attendees to ancillary programme events.

Data collected from 53 interviewees, including participants, mentor artists, volunteers, visitors, local artists, and Biennale team members, over eight months revealed insights into the impact of the event. Interviews with participants underscored their engagement in SNEHA's youth group programmes following involvement in workshops and events, indicating the effectiveness of community outreach efforts in challenging harmful beliefs. Since the Biennale, there has been a growing recognition among the residents of Dharavi of SNEHA's multifaceted approach beyond addressing violence against women and girls, extending to mental health, child nutrition, and sexual and reproductive health. http://www.dharavibiennale.com/

Box 3: Little Sister: Revolutionizing Violence Prevention with Simple Technology
Little Sister is a smartphone given to women volunteers (Sanginis) with a simple platform that focuses on enhancing surveillance, identifying violence, and providing immediate assistance in the realm of violence prevention. Operating as a notification system specifically designed for domestic violence in Dharavi, the app engages directly with the community and offers real-time, accurate data on incidents of domestic violence—facilitating the provision of appropriate support to survivors.

Little Sister has implemented a comprehensive strategy that involves training Sanginis (volunteers) to form a dedicated surveillance team equipped with smartphones and specific protocols. This team is responsible for monitoring and responding to domestic violence incidents promptly. Surveys have proven inadequate in capturing the severity and long-term nature of domestic violence incidents. In the context of domestic violence, where the issue often remains hidden, recurrent, and unspoken, Little Sister confronts the challenges associated with gathering data by moving beyond traditional survey methods and hospital records.

Developing the Programme's Theory of Change

The multi-layered, ecological approach of SNEHA's intervention to prevent violence against women and children presented some challenges to measuring its impact. It was crucial to understand what change meant to all our stakeholders, and that the concepts and principles involved in the intervention were well-defined to measure change. Five major components were considered in developing a theory of change:

1. **Programme goals:** the goals of the programme needed to be defined.
2. **Resource needs:** resources required to carry out psychosocial interventions were listed.
3. **Assumptions:** critical assumptions were defined. These included assumptions around the functionality and accessibility of counselling services, and the facilitation of core interventions (training, enablement and modelling) by community teams that motivate group members to volunteer to take action against violence against women and girls.
4. **Pathways to change:** pathways to change were mapped by examining early, intermediate and distal outcomes.
5. **Ceiling of accountability:** basic benchmarks were established to assess the success of the programme within the bounds of possible effects.

The theory of change developed in 2016 (Daruwalla et al., 2019) promoted a common understanding of the programme's purpose, emphasised the process of change, facilitated communication of the programme's design, clarified what aspects should be measured, enhanced engagement with existing evidence, and highlighted gaps in current service provision. The development of the theory was informed by existing theories around social norms, networks, and behaviour change (Davidoff et al., 2015; Michie et al., 2011), combined with tacit theory based on experience (Birckmayer & Weiss, 2000; Chen & Rossi, 1980; Mason & Barnes, 2007; Weiss, 1997).

Drawing from the theory of change, we focused on two aspects: what stimulates pro-social action and bystander intervention and identification, support and stopping of violence in survivor's lives. The theory of change focuses on a feedback loop of connections between primary and secondary prevention. Community members feel motivated and confident to identify and refer cases to support centres and resolution of cases throudh institutional actors increases their confidence in their own actions. Community activism is promoted through group discussions, reflections, wider campaigns which is linked ot providing cousnelling and legal support to survivors (Daruwalla et al, 2019) (Fig. 1).

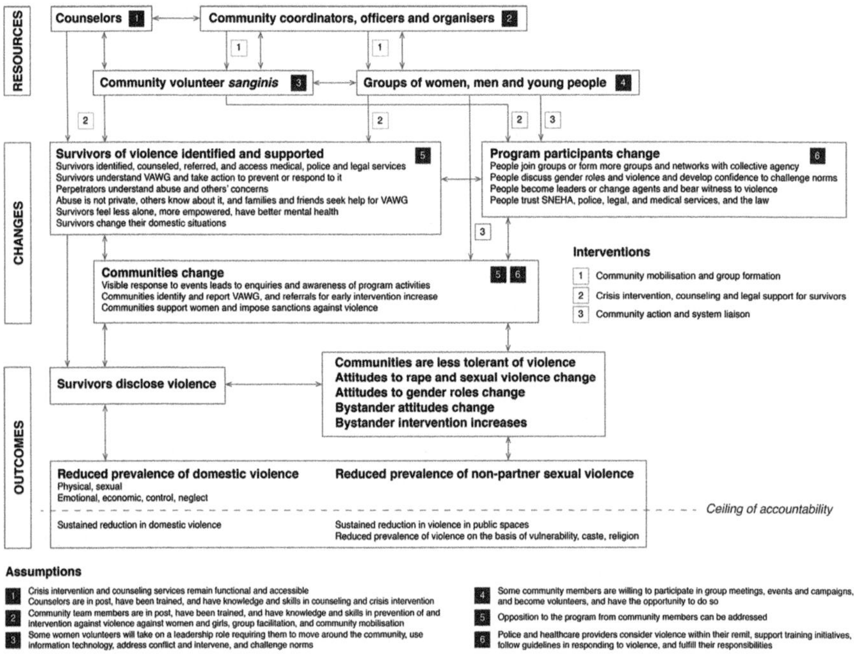

Fig. 1 Theory of Change for Community Mobilisation

(Daruwalla et al., 2019) Integrating a Behaviour Change Model (Michie et al., 2011) to Study the Mechanisms of Action

SNEHA's theory of change mentions immediate, intermediate and distal outcomes. While the distal outcomes such as reduced prevalence of violence could be evaluated using cross-sectional surveys, it was challenging to measure the immediate and intermediate outcomes and explain any change in behaviour at these levels. We were particularly interested in a framework that would explain phenomena, draw connections and make predictions of behaviour change through community mobilisation on the issue of violence against women and children: besides concentrating on changing social norms, how do communities challenge the broader social and institutional structures that undermine collective efforts to prevent violence?

We addressed this question by integrating the Capability, Opportunity, and Motivation model (COM-B) Model (Michie et al., 2011) within the Theory of Change. This model involves three essential conditions—capability, opportunity, and motivation—which form the hub of a 'behaviour change wheel' (BCW). It is based on a comprehensive causal analysis of behaviour and starts with the question: 'What conditions internal to individuals and in their social and physical environment need to be in place for a specified behavioural target to be achieved?' Capability refers to an individual's psychological and physical capacity to engage in an activity, and includes necessary knowledge and skills. Motivation encompasses thinking processes energizing and directing behaviour, including habitual processes, emotional responses, and analytical decision making. Opportunity comprises external factors enabling or prompting behaviour. Further, the behaviour change wheel specifies nine functions by which an intervention might stimulate change: education, persuasion, incentivisation, coercion, training, restriction, environmental restructuring, modelling, and enablement. Around them are placed seven categories of policy that could enable interventions to occur.

The process of development of SNEHA's theory of change pointed to interventions that involved education (awareness of the problem of violence and potential approaches to addressing it); training (workshops and training programmes); persuasion (of either perpetrators or community bodies); coercion (primarily of perpetrators, and often through linkages with the police); enablement (enabling group members and volunteers to carry out individual and collective actions against violence against women and girls; modelling (of exemplary successful actions by individuals and groups) as prominent functions and environmental restructuring (by helping group members and volunteers interface with police, health care and public systems) to ensure a coordinated response for survivors of violence. This has helped us think about structuring the psychosocial interventions for the programme in a systematic way.

Implementing the Community-Based Violence Prevention Model

SNEHA's intervention includes activities at the primary, secondary and tertiary levels of prevention. Conducting campaigns at the community level, group education with women, men and adolescent groups and building capacity of individual volunteers to identify, respond and refer are carried out under primary prevention. Secondary prevention is delivered through comprehensive services of counselling, psychoeducation, crisis intervention and coordination with health facilities, police, legal aid and home visits. Tertiary interventions include counselling and mental health assessments to help survivors manage distress, anxiety, depression and trauma along with role education, couple and family counselling and legal aid.

Our prevention activities involve two kinds of community outreach: group education and enablement and individual voluntarism. Meetings are conducted with women, men and adolescent groups to raise understanding and perspective on violence against women and girls, knowledge of rights and help-seeking provisions and encouraging them to take individual and collective actions. Individual action entails identification, response and referral support to survivors of violence and facilitate health and police measures. The three-year intervention is based on 'Aware, Act and Lead' to address and prevent violence in communities. This leads to agency building of group members and sanginis, improved digital literacy, prospects for employability and supportive social networks (Daruwalla et al., 2019).

Through this intervention, we aim to help people understand the gendered nature of violence, so that survivors make decisions, potential perpetrators think again, and others believe that action is possible. As a result of this, people will stand up against violence, individually and collectively, and community members will act to help survivors, will stop accepting violence, and will strengthen community structures that support a conviction that it is unacceptable. Our hypotheses are that women and girls will be more likely to disclose violence, that communities will become less tolerant of it, and that the prevalences of intimate partner and domestic violence will diminish. Supported by public engagement and advocacy, our ultimate goal is to establish a replicable community-led intervention model aimed at addressing the public health challenge posed by violence against women and girls.

Evaluating the Programme Model

Evaluations are underdeveloped given that endemic violence affects one-third of the world's women. It remains relatively invisible, stigmatised, and avoided by clinicians and public institutions. Although reviews recommend community mobilisation to address violence, evidence is limited. SNEHA's intervention was developed over 16 years of programmatic experience and two years of formative research and SNEHA's understanding of its effects is encapsulated in our theory of change. Following this, the organisation was interested in testing the effects of SNEHA's community mobilisation interventions through groups and volunteers to prevent violence against women and girls in Mumbai's slums through a randomised controlled trial. The trial—designed and conducted by SNEHA in collaboration with University College London—began in 2018 and compared 24 areas that received support services, engaged in community group activities, and utilised volunteer programmes, with 24 areas that solely received support services (Daruwalla et al., 2019). As of May 2024, SNEHA is conducting the final evaluation of trial data, after completing the three-year trial intervention and endline survey.

The trial aimed to determine the change in the prevalence of intimate partner violence and domestic violence after three years of community mobilisation. It also used a mix of data sources to examine reporting of violence to support services, community attitudes to violence, bystander intervention, gender equality, and the prevalence of non-partner sexual violence (Daruwalla et al., 2019). Broadly, the trial was designed to test the following hypotheses:

1. Community mobilisation for three years through group work and individual voluntarism along with support available for counselling and extended response will reduce the prevalence of domestic violence or sexual violence, and of domestic emotional or economic violence, control, or neglect.
2. A three-year community mobilisation intervention delivered along with the availability of support services will increase the disclosure of intimate partner or domestic violence to these services.

In terms of resources or inputs, the community mobilisation programme under evaluation covered a population of around 60,000 in 24 clusters of 500 homes in four large informal settlement areas of the city between 2018 and 2023. The outcomes expected and information collected at various levels of socioecology are described below:

- At the level of individuals, an intermediate outcome was that survivors of violence should disclose and receive support. One way to assess this was to use records of group activities and consultations with support services. As a result of community mobilisation, 4122 women disclosed concerns to a group member, of whom 3201 disclosed domestic or intimate partner violence. These are very large numbers, supported by the finding that 3795 women subsequently met with a counsellor.
- At the level of groups, the evaluation collected monitoring information on how often they met, how many people attended, what actions they took, and whether group members emerged as local volunteer activists. The reach of the programme over three years was broad and deep. Three women's groups with comprising 15–20 women in each group were established in each of 24 clusters of 500 homes—72 women's groups in all—and each group met about 20 times annually. Around 2340 women joined a group, over 2000 attended a meeting in any year, and an average 14 women attended each group meeting. Women from the 72 groups undertook 1916 individual actions to help survivors of violence and 1248 actions in concert with others

- At the level of organisation, the evaluation documented emerging institutional linkages, engagement with law enforcement and legal practitioners, the uptake of legal aid and the stories of women who engaged with them.
- At the level of communities, the evaluation documented the emergence of community change-agents and the number of survivors of violence accessing support services and resources facilitated by the community.

Challenges and Strategies

Psychosocial interventions and their evaluations face several challenges, particularly within the unique contexts of urban informal settlements. These settings present socio-culturally complex and sensitive issues that require careful understanding and response. Our programme, along with its evaluation, involves intervention and data collection on sensitive subjects from women, some of whom are survivors of violence. This raises critical issues such as consent, confidentiality, privacy, and the potential for causing further harm. Additionally, data collection can lead to recounting experiences of violence, causing psychological distress for participants and concerns about interviewer behaviour and data sharing.

The response to intervention activities may also follow 'dark logic', as elaborated in our theory of change. A woman's disclosure of violence may lead to reprisals and a short-term increase in abuse. Our activities might trigger vigilantism, leading to demands that we support perpetrators rather than survivors, punishment of the wrong person, changes in the type of abuse, or restrictive measures on women's mobility. There is also a small but significant risk of threats to team members and potential hostility from family or community members. For example, interview questions around the experience of violence, especially sexual violence, could be considered intrusive in a community setting and derail the evaluation process, as elaborated through an example in Box 4. When it comes to data collection and evaluation, we have identified issues including duty of care after disclosure, breach of confidentiality, veiling of interview content, and perpetration. Duty of care is an issue that has not been sufficiently addressed in previous research and trials. However, it is a crucial issue as an interviewee who discloses experience of violence—physical, sexual, emotional, or gender-based household maltreatment—should be offered optimal support. This goes well beyond presenting her with a list of contact details for local services.

We have extensive experience managing these challenges, including protocols for responding to threats, access to in-house legal counsel, and strong connections with local police. Interviewers are members of a team that is able to provide a full suite of crisis and counselling services including home visits, medical, surgical and psychiatric referral and negotiation with families, the police and legal representatives.

Psychoscocial interventions are evaluated on the backbone of provision of extensive range of support services. The staff was trained to respond to adverse events. Response protocols were followed by SNEHA community organisers, supervisors and interviewers. Immediate response (active listening, safety assessment, assessment of suicidal ideation, validation and support, psychological first aid, consideration of shelter, admission to hospital if necessary), enlisting of immediate help from line managers, doctors, or the police if required, and then provision of information and referral to an in-house counsellor. Legal support, psychological assessment, mental health counselling and follow up are measures required subsequently.

Box 4: The Importance of Community Level Acceptance in Psychological Interventions

Psychosocial interventions in community settings rely heavily on community-level acceptance. This acceptance is often secured through the buy-in of community gatekeepers such as panchayat leaders, political representatives, community-based organizations, community elders, and religious leaders. However, this acceptance can be fragile and may be withdrawn at any point during implementation.

For example, in one of the clusters involved in our programme, a SNEHA investigator encountered a challenging situation while conducting a survey on the perpetration of violence. The survey included sensitive questions about women's marital and sexual lives. A group of women took offense at these questions, perceiving them as intrusive and intimate, and complained to a political leader in the community. The political leader confronted the investigators, halted the survey, and advised the community women not to participate or entertain the investigators. This incident occurred despite SNEHA having previously obtained consent from community gatekeepers, including political leaders, for the survey.

In response, SNEHA advocated with a higher official in the government machinery, assuring them that the survey was a precursor to a community-level violence prevention intervention and crucial for its successful implementation. This experience highlighted that any psychosocial intervention needs to be long-term, locally grounded, and demonstrably beneficial to community members. Building community and individual-level relationships and trust is essential for the success of such interventions.

Conclusion and Recommendations

What we have tried to do in this chapter is describe our journey from service provision to community mobilisation and evaluation using psychosocial approaches. Programmes to prevent violence against women and to support survivors are necessarily complex. They involve individual actions, group activities, and multiple services and evaluating them is difficult. Two ways of structuring our understanding of how to evaluate them are to categorise activities within a socio-ecologic framework and to develop a theory of change. By doing this, the content of the evaluation is dictated by our understanding of the various levels at which the programme operates and the chain of immediate, intermediate and distal outcomes. The sources of information on whether the programme 'works' emerge from the questions that need to be answered at each level.

These insights support the following directions for future implementation and research:

1. A multifaceted psychosocial approach to preventing violence against women and girls is essential. Such an approach should acknowledge the impact of socio-political and cultural contexts, and encompass primary, secondary, and tertiary prevention interventions across socio-ecologic levels.
2. Visible interventions to support survivors make people aware of the problem and potential solutions. Counselling services and support provided in the beginning of the intervention pave the way for primary prevention in the community.
3. Programmes that focus on the prevention of violence against women and girls need to frame their work in terms of primary, secondary and tertiary interventions along the continuum of psychosocial interventions, with a focus on building competencies of communities to respond and prevent violence. A community-led model for prevention of violence against women and girls can engage in primary prevention activities like surveillance and identification of women and girls survivors of violence, collective actions to stop violence and bystander interventions. Secondary interventions such as psychological first aid, psychoeducation, barefoot counselling, and connecting survivors with police, health care and legal resources can be carried out by community groups and volunteers. Resources such as the GARiMA Package of Care (www.garima.snehamumbai.org) for supporting the mental health of domestic violence and trafficking survivors provide a simple and easy-to-use manual for barefoot counsellors, social workers and mental health professionals working in the community to respond to the needs of violence survivors. When community workers and service providers are trained adequately in addressing and responding to violence, non-profits can focus on providing specialised mental health and legal services to survivors.
4. A community-driven approach empowers communities to address violence against women and girls. It is important to build the capacities of community-based organisations to equip them to work on systematic interventions to effectively address violence against women and girls, mental health challenges, and related issues.
5. Programmes for prevention of violence against women and girls require a multi-disciplinary team to work on a range of psychosocial interventions. This team should include social workers, psychologists, mental health professionals, community workers, anthropologists and sociologists who can understand and assess community dynamics and needs.
6. Solutions and insights shared across civil society organisations will foster collaboration and maximise impact in addressing issues related to gender, mental health, and violence.
7. Finally, SNEHA's experience and monitoring data over the last two decades, as elaborated in Box 5, shows that violence against women cannot be looked at as

a singular issue and any program working on the prevention of violence against women and girls should acknowledge its intersections with violence affecting children.

Box 5: The need to focus on violence affecting children
SNEHA counselling centre data show that 5% of reports are for violence against children compared to 90% for violence against women. Our analysis raised three crucial factors for children not reporting abuse and using these services: (1) the concept of child rights is not understood very well in India and the norms perpetuating violence against children are not often challenged as they fall under the ambit of disciplining the child; (2) children have less agency and access to report violence; and (3) primary prevention activities have focused more on violence against women considering its ubiquity and criticality. Violence against children is usually not reported to our counselling centres until it reaches a point at which the child's security and safety is at stake, often in cases of child sexual abuse. A critical reflection that has emerged from the programme is to focus attention on intersecting norms around violence against women and children.

SNEHA has embarked on a three-year field action research project on ensuring children's safety and well-being by building an ecosystem of non-tolerance of violence against children—a socioecological approach with the involvement of children, parents and community members. The project is nested under a nutrition programme covering 16,500 households. Primary prevention is carried out through awareness campaigns and events in the community, and group education is carried out with children aged 6 to 15 years and their parents on forms of disciplining practices in relation to overt and covert forms of violence, understanding of parenting styles and practices, perceptions of safety and knowledge on child rights and protection and available services. Counselling and mental health services are provided to children identified with abuse to ensure their physical, mental and social well-being.

The project has highlighted the intertwined and complex nature of intersections between violence against children and violence against their mothers. Furthermore, the socio-economic context of residing in these urban informal settlements poses several challenges of inadequate housing, lack of resources and poverty. SNEHA's monitoring data of 275 intensive home visits conducted by field staff to assess family dynamics, the data revealed a distressing environment marked by frequent domestic quarrels, tensions, and conflicts, with the father frequently shouting at and physically abusing the mother. These findings highlight a troubling and abusive atmosphere to which children are exposed causing fear and distress in them. Nearly half of the mothers of these children experienced domestic violence and maltreatment.

Approximately 30% of cases of domestic violence were influenced by the norms that limits reporting of violence, where survivors refrained from disclosing their experiences due to fear of blame, ostracization and lack of external support. In approximately 25% of cases, the acceptance of violence as a form of discipline contributed to the perpetration of domestic violence. These norms were internalised and the act of violence was legitimised by the mother for herself and her children, not only impacting the mother's well-being by contributing to heightened stress, anxiety, and a compromised mental health state, but also influencing her ability to provide nurturing care to her growing children. Around 15% of domestic violence cases were influenced by the norm that limits interventions to stop violence. Witnesses hesitated to intervene as they accepted violence to be a common occurrence and might face sanctions for intervening. Another 30% of cases were affected by norms that increased the use of violence, where individuals justified violence as a way to express love or maintain control.

Box 6: Create community-based models for program sustainability
Our work so far has focussed on providing spaces, methods, and tools to help women access protection and justice against violence, improve their mental health through counselling, and empower both women and men to respond quickly and appropriately to violence within their communities. The program's operating model has gradually shifted from a service-centred approach to community-based solutions on preventing violence against women and girls in clusters where the program has worked for more than 10 years. This is done through education through engagement with women's and men's groups, amplifying and strengthening the volunteer base and capacitating sanginis (volunteers) to deliver secondary interventions for survivors of violence along with development of a cadre of paralegal volunteers. Our aim is to strengthen community stewardship and ownership to address violence against women and girls by integrating and broadening primary and secondary interventions, build sustainability and consolidate the evidence on gender-based violence programs. The program will help people understand the nature of violence, so that survivors make decisions, potential perpetrators think again, and others believe that action is possible. As a result of this, people will stand up against violence, individually and collectively, and community members will act to help survivors, will stop accepting violence, and will strengthen community structures that support a conviction that it is unacceptable.

References

Abramsky, T., Watts, C. H., Garcia-Moreno, C., Devries, K., Kiss, L., Ellsberg, M., Jansen, H. A., & Heise, L. (2011). What factors are associated with recent intimate partner violence? Findings from the WHO multi-country study on women's health and domestic violence. *BMC Public Health, 11*(1), 109. https://doi.org/10.1186/1471-2458-11-109

Alsina, E., Browne, J. L., Gielkens, D., Noorman, M. A. J., & de Wit, J. B. F. (2024). Interventions to prevent intimate partner violence: A systematic review and meta-analysis. *Violence against Women, 30*(3–4), 953–980. https://doi.org/10.1177/10778012231183660

Bacchus, L. J., Ranganathan, M., Watts, C., & Devries, K. (2018). Recent intimate partner violence against women and health: A systematic review and meta-analysis of cohort studies. *British Medical Journal Open, 8*(7), Article e019995. https://doi.org/10.1136/bmjopen-2017-019995

Birckmayer, J., & Weiss, C. (2000). Theory-Based evaluation in practice: What do we learn? *Evaluation Review, 24*, 407–431. https://doi.org/10.1177/0193841X0002400404

Bronfenbrenner, U. (1979). *The ecology of human development: Experiments by nature and design.* Harvard University Press.

Central Bureau of Health Intelligence, M. of H. and F. W. (2015). *National health profile.* https://cbhidghs.mohfw.gov.in/WriteReadData/l892s/NHP-2015.pdf

Chandramouli, C. (2011). *Housing stock, amenities & assets in slums—Census 2011.* https://censusindia.gov.in/nada/index.php/catalog/42602

Chen, H.-T., & Rossi, P. H. (1980). The multi-goal, theory-driven approach to evaluation: A model linking basic and applied social science*. *Social Forces, 59*(1), 106–122. https://doi.org/10.1093/sf/59.1.106

Daruwalla, N., Das, T., Punekar, S., Patil, S., Manjrekar, S., Pantvaidya, S., D'Souza, V., & Osrin, D. (2024). Support needs of survivors of violence against women in urban India: A prospective analysis of client records. *Global Health Research,* 1–14. https://doi.org/10.3310/LKNH2423

Daruwalla, N., Jaswal, S., Fernandes, P., Pinto, P., Hate, K., Ambavkar, G., Kakad, B., Gram, L., & Osrin, D. (2019). A theory of change for community interventions to prevent domestic violence against women and girls in Mumbai, India [version 1; peer review: 2 approved with reservations]. *Wellcome Open Research, 4.* https://doi.org/10.12688/wellcomeopenres.15128.1

Daruwalla, N., Machchhar, U., Pantvaidya, S., D'Souza, V., Gram, L., Copas, A., & Osrin, D. (2019). Community interventions to prevent violence against women and girls in informal settlements in Mumbai: The SNEHA-TARA pragmatic cluster randomised controlled trial. *Trials, 20*(1), 743. https://doi.org/10.1186/s13063-019-3817-2

Davidoff, F., Dixon-Woods, M., Leviton, L., & Michie, S. (2015). Demystifying theory and its use in improvement. *BMJ Quality & Safety, 24*(3), 228–238. https://doi.org/10.1136/bmjqs-2014-003627

Fulu, E., Kerr-Wilson, A., & Lang, J. (2014). *Effectiveness of interventions to prevent violence against women and girls: A summary of the evidence.*

Harbishettar, V., & Math, S. B. (2014). Violence against women in India: Comprehensive care for survivors. *The Indian Journal of Medical Research, 140*(2), 157–159.

Heise, L. (1998). Violence against women: An integrated, ecological framework. *Violence against Women, 4,* 262–290. https://doi.org/10.1177/1077801298004003002

International Institute for Population Sciences (IIPS) and ICF. (2017). *National Family Health Survey (NFHS-4), 2015–16: India.*

Mason, P., & Barnes, M. (2007). Constructing theories of change: Methods and sources. *Evaluation, 13*(2), 151–170. https://doi.org/10.1177/1356389007075221

Michie, S., van Stralen, M., & West, R. (2011). The behaviour change wheel: A new method for characterising and designing behaviour change interventions. *Implementation Science : IS, 6,* 42. https://doi.org/10.1186/1748-5908-6-42

Micklitz, H. M., Glass, C. M., Bengel, J., & Sander, L. B. (2023). Efficacy of psychosocial interventions for survivors of intimate partner violence: Protocol for a systematic review and meta-analysis. *Bjpsych Open, 9*(1), Article e9. https://doi.org/10.1192/bjo.2022.625

Ministry of Home Affairs, G. of I. (2011). *India—Provisional population totals.* https://censusindia.gov.in/nada/index.php/catalog/42611

Ministry of Housing and Urban Poverty Alleviation. (2010). *Report of the committee on slum statistics.* National Buildings Organisation. https://mohua.gov.in/upload/uploadfiles/files/9Slum_Report_NBO(2).pdf

Muluneh, M. D., Francis, L., Agho, K., & Stulz, V. (2021). A systematic review and meta-analysis of associated factors of gender-based violence against women in Sub-Saharan Africa. *International Journal of Environmental Research and Public Health, 18*(9), Article 9. https://doi.org/10.3390/ijerph18094407

Paphitis, S. A., Bentley, A., Asher, L., Osrin, D., & Oram, S. (2022). Improving the mental health of women intimate partner violence survivors: Findings from a realist review of psychosocial interventions. *PLoS ONE, 17*(3), Article e0264845. https://doi.org/10.1371/journal.pone.0264845

Rege, S., & Deosthali, P. (2010). Dealing with spousal violence. *Indian Journal of Medical Ethics, 7*(4), 246–248; discussion 249–250. https://doi.org/10.20529/IJME.2010.091

Rivas, C., Vigurs, C., Cameron, J., & Yeo, L. (2019). A realist review of which advocacy interventions work for which abused women under what circumstances. *Cochrane Database of Systematic Reviews, 6*. https://doi.org/10.1002/14651858.CD013135.pub2

Turner, D. T., Riedel, E., Kobeissi, L. H., Karyotaki, E., Garcia-Moreno, C., Say, L., & Cuijpers, P. (2020). Psychosocial interventions for intimate partner violence in low and middle income countries: A meta-analysis of randomised controlled trials. *Journal of Global Health, 10*(1), Article 010409. https://doi.org/10.7189/jogh.10.010409

UN Habitat. (2003). *The challenge of slums—Global report on human settlements*. https://unhabitat.org/the-challenge-of-slums-global-report-on-human-settlements-2003

Weiss, C. H. (1997). How can theory-based evaluation make greater headway? *Evaluation Review, 21*(4), 501–524. https://doi.org/10.1177/0193841X9702100405

White, S. J., Sin, J., Sweeney, A., Salisbury, T., Wahlich, C., Montesinos Guevara, C. M., Gillard, S., Brett, E., Allwright, L., Iqbal, N., Khan, A., Perot, C., Marks, J., & Mantovani, N. (2024). Global prevalence and mental health outcomes of intimate partner violence among women: A systematic review and meta-analysis. *Trauma, Violence & Abuse, 25*(1), 494–511. https://doi.org/10.1177/15248380231155529

World Health Organisation. (2024). *Violence against women*. https://www.who.int/news-room/fact-sheets/detail/violence-against-women

Dr. Nayreen Daruwalla heads the Research, Partnership and Scaling vertical of SNEHA's Prevention of Violence against Women and Children programme. She holds a doctoral degree in Social Psychology and she has developed models on prevention of violence against women and children in middle-income countries through provision of mental health interventions, community mobilization and influencing public systems response. Her work includes research partnerships with academic and non-government organizations to evaluate, replicate and scale interventions on prevention of violence against women and children. She has developed a research-led curriculum for the police and the innovative GARiMA web-based resource on the mental health of survivors of violence.

Sharanya Gautam is a development practitioner with 12+ years of experience in education, mental health, and preventing gender-based violence. She specializes in program design, qualitative research, curriculum creation, and training material development. Currently, she is a Researcher at SNEHA, leading the SNEHA Knowledge Centre. Previously, she was the Manager for Training and Capacity Building at WorldBeing, India, and Assistant Director of VOICE 4 Girls. A Chevening Scholar, she holds postgraduate degrees from the London School of Economics and the Tata Institute of Social Sciences. Sharanya is also a Prevention Mentor with the Prevention Collaborative.

Gargi Khandekar has been working in the development field for 5 years in Mumbai. In this span she has worked with various students and women's groups—developing and facilitating content on gender-based issues. She currently is working as a Training Coordinator at SNEHA (Society for Health Education and Nutrition for All). As a part of this role, she works with beneficiaries of partner organizations to support them in the identification and addressing of violence. She holds Master's in Women's studies from Tata Institute of Social Sciences.

Vanessa D'Souza has served as CEO of SNEHA since March 2013, following a volunteering stint with the organisation. Prior to that, she worked with Citibank India in various positions, her last role being: Director, Citigroup Private Bank. During her tenure with Citibank she worked across various divisions including Non-Resident Indian Business, Corporate Bank, Project Re-engineering and eventually with the Private Bank. She won the coveted Citicorp Chairman's Service Excellence Award in 1989 for exemplary performance. She has a Bachelors (Honours) degree in Economics and a postgraduate degree in Management with specialization in Marketing. She also holds a postgraduate Diploma in Public Health Nutrition.

Shanti Pantvaidya is the Executive Director of SNEHA. She was the medical teacher for 35 years and Professor/Head of Anesthesiology Services at the Lokmanya Tilak Municipal Medical College & General Hospital. She played a pivotal role in establishing anesthesiology and post-operative intensive care services. She set up the Emergency Medical Services of LTMG Hospital. In SNEHA, Dr. Shanti led the initiative of establishing a maternal and newborn referral systems linking public hospitals of Mumbai and its adjacent six municipal corporations in partnership with the health services of the respective corporations for Child Health and Nutrition, PATH India and DFID.

David Osrin is a Wellcome Trust Senior Research Fellow in Clinical Science, UCL Professor of Global Health, and Honorary Consultant at Great Ormond Street Hospital for Children, with extensive periods in south Asia since 1998. David's current research focuses on urban health and prevention of gender-based violence. His interests include evaluation of complex programmes through a range of methodologies such as programme theory, trials and mixed methods. He has a track record of research into maternal and newborn care and outcomes, nutritional interventions to improve newborn survival, community mobilisation, health service interventions, field surveillance systems for public health indicators, and large-scale evaluation of public health interventions.

Chapter 6
Atmiyata: Community-Led Initiative for Mental Health and Social Care in India

Jasmine Kalha, Nimisha Ajaikumar, Somya Agarwal, Palak Korde, Soumitra Pathare, and Kaustubh Joag

Abstract Data from the National Mental Health Survey (2016) showed that 197 million Indians live with a mental health condition, with 70–92% of them unable to access care in India. This large mental health care gap exists due to both demand (stigma, discrimination), and supply (lack of professionals) factors. Despite the evidence of lay health workers bridging the mental health gap, few interventions provide a scalable and evidence-based model. To reduce the large mental health gap, Atmiyata aimed to create an innovative, community-led intervention enabling communities to address their own mental health and social care. Our randomized implementation trial in one district in the state of Gujarat found that persons who received counselling from Atmiyata volunteers were two times more likely to have recovered from a CMD at 3 months and 3 times more likely at 8 months. Further, the intervention had cost offsets due to substantial use of volunteers. Atmiyata has been recognized by the World Health Organization as one of the 25 good practices for community outreach mental health services that aligns with the rights and recovery-based approach. Since its inception in 2013, the intervention has scaled from 41 to 1890 villages across 7 districts and 5 states covering a total rural adult population of 3.5 million, with immense support from 2500 community volunteers in 2024. The intervention annually reaches out to approximately 25,000 persons with mental health needs within 500 villages in one rural district in India. The chapter will expand on the model of Atmiyata, its use in diverse settings, and future directions.

Keyword Community mental health · Psychosocial interventions · Common mental health conditions

---

J. Kalha (✉) · N. Ajaikumar · S. Agarwal · P. Korde · S. Pathare · K. Joag
Centre for Mental Health Law and Policy, Indian Law Society, Pune, India
e-mail: jasmine@cmhlp.org

U. Vindhya (ed.), *Psychosocial Interventions for Social Issues in Contemporary India*,
https://doi.org/10.1007/978-981-96-6553-2_6

Background

Mental health conditions affect 197.3 million (approximately 14.3%) of the Indian population, with 33.8% and 19% affected by common mental health conditions (CMD) such as depressive and anxiety disorders respectively (Sagar et al., 2020). Despite efforts to improve access to mental health services, limitations in the availability, affordability, accessibility, and quality of services persist. Mental health is determined by the social and cultural factors prevalent in the context. As per the National Mental Health Survey (2016), 85% of the mental health cases were left untreated due to the demand (stigma, discrimination, structural barriers) and supply (lack of mental health professionals) side factors. The scarcity of mental health professionals, combined with societal stigma, discrimination, and limited accessibility to services, further exacerbates the treatment gap [World Health Organization (WHO), 2021].

Furthermore, socio-economic factors affect one's mental health; it has been highlighted in community-based studies that poverty (Lund et al., 2011), gender inequality, and low education (Patel et al., 1999) are interlinked with CMDs. In India, people with mental illness face violations, such as stigma and discrimination in the education and employment sectors, leading to marginalization within the community.

Need for Community-Based Interventions

Reports from around the world have highlighted the existing rights violations and discrimination that exist within mental health care, such as forced admission and treatment (Mental Disability Advocacy Centre, 2014; Ríos-Espinoza, 2018; Turnpenny et al., 2018). Over the past few years, emphasis on a rights-based recovery approach has been fundamental in fighting for human rights within the mental health field as it focuses on the social determinants of mental health (WHO, 2013) and challenges the biomedical approach, i.e., it goes beyond diagnosis and medication (Slade, 2009). The UN Convention on the Rights of Persons with Disabilities (CRPD) further focuses on the importance of protecting and promoting human rights in mental health, with Article 19 of the CRPD emphasizing the necessity of promoting independence and inclusion in the community for people mental health conditions.

Despite the increasing emphasis on self-management and community-based informal networks to support the majority of mental health care for CMDs, mental health systems in countries like India are structured to address treatment largely through specialized in-patient and out-patient settings. These systems are influenced by the biomedical model, which overlooks the social, economic, and cultural factors that shape and affect persons with CMD (Patil et al., 2002).

Additionally, community mental health interventions in India primarily rely on community mental health workers and non-specialized health workers to provide mental health care in rural areas, ranging from active psychosocial support to identification and referrals (Hans & Sharan, 2021). Trained community mental health workers have been recognised in the available literature for delivering effective care to persons with mental health conditions, such as the MANAS intervention for depressive and anxiety disorders in India (Pereira et al., 2011) and Friendship Bench programme for CMD in Zimbabwe (Chibanda et al., 2015). However, few scalable models exist to reduce the ever-growing mental healthcare gap. Despite past programmes by the government such as the District Mental Health Programme (DMHP), scalability remains a challenge, potentially due to concerns about their workload, focus on severe mental disorders, and competing health care tasks (Patel et al., 2009). This is further exacerbated by low mental health budget in the healthcare annual budget (approx. 1% of the budget in 2024) as it has made it difficult to address the gaps for CMDs (Mahashur, 2024).

Task-shifting models have emerged as a potential strategy to address mental health care gaps, leveraging lay health workers to provide counselling and support. However, these models encounter barriers related to acceptability, capacity building, and financial sustainability which hinders their scalability and effectiveness (Kaur et al., 2021). To address these barriers, there is a growing recognition of the need to harness existing informal community resources to enhance access to mental health support and care in rural India.

Research in contexts such as India have demonstrated the effectiveness of community groups in addressing health topics like pregnancy, leading to improved maternal health indicators and reduced depression rates (Nair et al., 2021; Tripathy et al., 2010). Given the social and cultural acceptability of participating in these groups, they offer a unique opportunity for identifying and supporting individuals affected by mental health issues in a supportive community setting. In rural India, community resource groups exist in the form of self-help groups (SHGs) and farmer's clubs (FC), fostering peer support, empowerment, and economic development (Shinogi et al., 2021). These groups, prevalent across many villages, reflect a strong sense of community and a willingness to assist fellow members, especially in the informal economy prevalent in rural areas. Such groups are run democratically, with their leaders belonging to the local communities, hence creating a sense of trust and inclusion (Maheshwari & Goyal, 2014).

These groups, deeply rooted in rural communities, offer a promising avenue for identifying, treating, and caring for individuals experiencing mental health problems. Building the capacity of formal and informal groups to identify, support, and refer individuals in distress or affected by mental health problems holds significant potential for creating sustainable and locally available mental health support options in areas with limited formal treatment options.

Atmiyata, developed by the Centre for Mental Health Law & Policy, Indian Law Society (CMHLP, ILS) aims to leverage existing evidence of using lay health workers to reduce the mental health care gap. Recognising the potential of social capital within rural communities and the existing potential for formal and informal groups, the model aimed to innovate by creating a tiered community volunteer model for addressing mental health and social care needs. Using community volunteers offset challenges of lack of time of the existing community health workers and was economically viable to create a sustainable and scalable model.

It serves as an effective solution for bridging the mental health care gap by empowering communities to address their own mental health needs. The intervention resonates with the vision outlined in the National Mental Health Policy (NMHP, 2014), which emphasizes community involvement and equitable access to mental health services, particularly for underserved populations. Additionally, Atmiyata facilitates the realization of the right to access mental health care and services, as stipulated in Sect. 18 of the provisions of the Mental Healthcare Act (MHCA). Furthermore, it contributes to achieving Sustainable Development Goal 3 (SDG 3): Good Health and Well-being by improving mental health outcomes and overall quality of life. Through these contributions, Atmiyata emerges as a vital component in advancing mental health equity and well-being on both national and global scales. Recognized by the WHO (2021) for its rights and recovery-based approach, Atmiyata aimed to develop, implement and scale an evidence-based, low-cost, and scalable approach to mental health and social care delivery.

The Atmiyata Model

There are a multitude of community-based intervention models established for mental health and well-being that have undergone rigorous experimental evaluation (Killaspy et al., 2022; Moroz et al., 2020; Porteny et al., 2020). However, documentation regarding the practical implementation of these evidence-based interventions in real-world settings is scarce (Shidaye et al., 2016). Atmiyata, meaning empathy and shared compassion, was developed by the CMHLPS in 2013.

The initial Atmiyata pilot programme (Joag et al., 2020) was implemented in 41 villages in the Peth block of Nashik district, Maharashtra, targeting approximately 14,000 adults. In total, 59 Champions and 264 Mitras received training, along with follow-up mentoring and support from the project team. The intervention was scaled to cover an entire district of approximately 500 villages covering 0.8 million adults in Mehsana, Gujarat, to evaluate the effectiveness of lay health workers at scale to improve mental health and social care in rural communities from 2017–19.

To improve mental health and social outcomes, Atmiyata taps into the existing social capital, to identify and train community volunteers (Champions) through four main activities:

(i) provide counselling to persons with common mental health conditions (CMD) like depression and anxiety, using evidence-based techniques,
(ii) link persons with severe mental health conditions (SMD) to the public mental health system,
(iii) facilitate access to national and state-based social benefits (SB) such as pension, employment under the Mahatma Gandhi National Rural Employment Guarantee Scheme, and disability support, and

(iv) create awareness by narrowcasting short films that speak to social factors influencing mental health and wellbeing.

Structure of the Intervention

The Atmiyata intervention follows a structure of intermediaries who are given specialised structured training to prepare them for their responsibilities. The training is typically conducted face to face and in an interactive format. All training manuals are developed internally with inputs from experts in animation training (Fig 6.1).

I. The first tier are the **Champions**, who form the core of the intervention. They are community leaders, approachable within their villages, often serving as leaders of self-help groups or community figures. Each Champion trains 4–5 Mitras and is responsible for approximately 1000 to 1200 community members. They receive 35 h of training over 3 weeks, covering the mental health spectrum which includes stress/distress, CMD, SMD, counselling skills and understanding social determinants of mental health, with refresher trainings provided

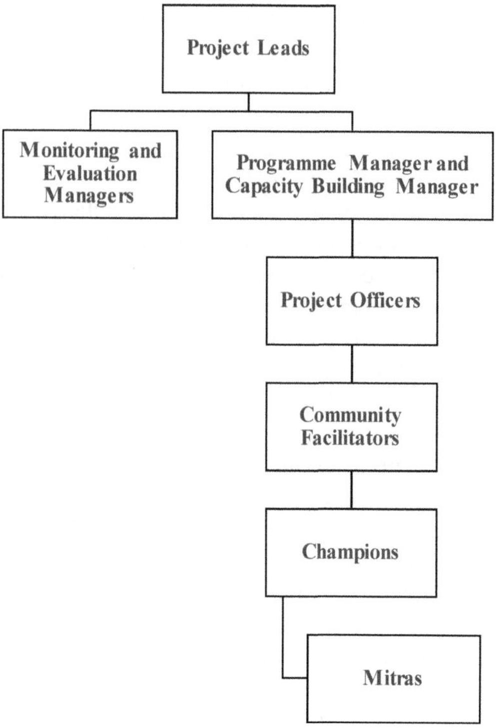

Fig. 6.1 Structure of team at a district level

every 4 months. It builds on the questions like *"what can you do as a counselor?" and "what are some of the skills that we can use while we are having the sessions with the end user?"*

The selection criteria for Champions prioritise qualities such as leadership, commitment to voluntary work, communication skills, and an understanding of community needs. These Community volunteers play a vital role in delivering structured counselling to persons they have identified with CMD. They are also responsible for building referral pathways for persons with SMD, facilitating access to SB, and promoting community awareness through discussions and films. While monetary compensation is not provided, Champions are given smartphones to narrowcast the Atmiyata mental health awareness films in the community and collect end-user data in the Atmiyata app.

II. The second tier are **Mitras**, meaning "friends," who are community volunteers from diverse caste and religious backgrounds. Mitras accentuate the programme's reach and coverage across the entire village, to ensure that the intervention is accessible to individuals from various castes, genders and religions. They receive 4 h of training to equip them with skills for identifying persons with CMD and SMD.

III. The **Community Facilitators (CFs)**, who are paid employees with bachelor's or master's degrees in humanities or social work. They reside locally within the district which enhances their understanding of socio-cultural realities. CFs receive comprehensive training over 2 weeks, focusing on effective supervision, mentorship, and various aspects of programme management. CFs are tasked with mentoring, supervising, and training 40–50 Champions within their allotted villages. They play a crucial role in identifying eligible Champions, providing training, and maintaining their motivation to volunteer. Additionally, CFs map villages with a comparable population of potential end-users and build relationships with community stakeholders. During monitoring visits, CFs inquire about counselling sessions and, with consent, sometimes meet end-users to understand the counselling process and ensure fidelity to intervention delivery.

IV. Next, **Project Officers (POs)** oversee the operations. They are typically residents of the selected district and hold a master's degree in social work or humanities with 3–4 years of relevant work experience. They are responsible for identifying, training, and mentoring 16–17 CFs each. POs ensure the quality and fidelity of the programme by leveraging their understanding of the local community, language, and culture. The POs report to the Programme Manager (PrM) and Capacity Building manager (CB).

V. Ultimately, the Atmiyata Core team ensures adherence to strict protocols of quality assurance, logistics, timelines, and feedback sessions to check whether there are any gaps in communication and issues during the training and implementation. The core team is headed by the Project Leads, to whom the PrM, CB and Monitoring and Evaluation managers' report.

The methodology of the training is reflective, participatory, and interactive based on adult learning principles. Atmiyata's Capacity Building Manager provides an insight into how the training influences intermediaries' understanding of mental health:

> What the training does mainly is we talk about everyone in the room, what their experiences are with stress, distress and we try to bring it together to say that you know, mental health conditions are not like some alien concept like they exist within us, within our communities.

Voices from the Field: Atmiyata's Stakeholders

This section includes narratives of Atmiyata stakeholders including the lay health workers/Champions and their supervisors/Community Facilitator based at Mehsana, Gujarat. They describe the intervention from their perspectives.

Champion 1: Meer Joharaben Manubhai

Atmiyata Champion, Joharaben, who has been actively engaged with the programme for the past 1.5 years. Joharaben is a homemaker aged 47 years and a member of the Other Backward Classes (OBC) community from the village of Sartanpur. Her involvement began when the community health worker introduced her to the Atmiyata programme. Intrigued by the opportunity to contribute to her community's mental well-being, she eagerly joined as a champion.

Joharaben shares, "As a Champion, my work focuses on addressing mental health concerns in the community. I provide counseling sessions to the end-users I identify in my village, and I've seen positive changes in their quality of life. I approach end-users with the help of the observant Mitras (second tier of Atmiyata community volunteers). My training has significantly refined my ability to identify changes in the mental state of the people around me. Additionally, I attribute much of my success to the support I receive from my family, which has been a crucial facilitator in my role."

Joharaben shares that the Atmiyata training equipped her with the skills to improve not only the lives of others but also of her family. She used to quarrel with her husband and two daughters and was in a distressed state at the time of joining Atmiyata, but the training helped her navigate her approach towards family life. She reflects over gaining the self-awareness to learn from her own mistakes and the ability to empathise with her family's concerns.

The Champion mentioned one of many cases of positive changes among end-users, wherein a woman, stressed by her child's ill-health and other familial issues, was referred to her by one of her friends. She conducted sessions with her, resulting in significant improvements. The end-user was able to restart her discarded hobbies, and now works in a beauty parlour.

Joharaben mitigates end-users concerns around their confidentiality through consistent reassurance, which gives them the safe space to open up to her.

Champion 2: Rameshji Thakor

Rameshji Thakor is a 28-year-old farmer from the OBC community in the village of Gothva, who joined the Atmiyata programme as a Champion 5 years ago. The Panchayat committee of his village had nominated his name for the project. He was introduced to the CF, and after learning about the intervention, he expressed his interest in joining as a Champion.

Rameshji adds, "The Atmiyata training helped me empathize with my fellow villagers undergoing psychological distress and changed my perspective on mental illness. I also learned how to identify signs of distress so that I could provide timely intervention. As a Champion, I even shared my reflections on the training with my family members to improve their understanding of mental health. The training educated me on ways to appropriately respond to those in need, including my family members."

Rameshji takes great pride in his role as a Champion, citing a grateful end-user who considers him like a 'God-like' figure for the help he had provided to them during tough times. He believes that a Champion performs a more important service than a doctor. He recalls an end-user diagnosed with kidney failure, whom, with Rameshji's help, was able to regain his sense of control in life by restarting past pleasurable activities. Rameshji is committed to his role as an Atmiyata Champion to make a positive impact in his community.

Community Facilitator 1: Malek Mohammedmoinuddin Sikandarbhai

Moin has been working in Atmiyata as a CF for the past 4 years, currently managing 81 Champions from 26 villages in 6 primary health centres (PHCs). He is 31 years old, from a Muslim, OBC community. According to him, a CF bridges the gap between the Champion and the Atmiyata team. He mentioned that a CF's role includes village mapping and training, recruitment and management of Champions. He spends his days meeting 6–8 Champions per day and resolving any issues that they may face regarding their work in the project.

According to Moin, "Atmiyata aims to bring mental healthcare to rural areas. During my visits, I've encountered community members who have a basic understanding of mental health, often seeing mental ill health as something that can be treated. Building trust and rapport with these communities has been crucial to gaining acceptance for our interventions." In fact, Moin pinpoints community support and the positive attitude towards community service as the facilitators for the project.

During his years working as a CF, Moin had faced certain challenges, but he eventually learned to prevent and mitigate them with experience. It is difficult to gain support from new villages to establish an intervention like Atmiyata, especially when there is a stigmatised perspective towards mental health. Nevertheless, he shares that

Panchayat members and community health workers aid this process because of their prioritisation of the welfare of their villages. Champion dropouts are also a pressing issue for which Moin recommends ensuring proper communication. Thus, from his long-term work experience, Moin has noted the positive influence of Atmiyata in the community.

Community Facilitator 2: Sohina Solanki

Sohina Solanki joined Atmiyata as a CF almost 3 years ago. She is in charge of 36 Champions across 26 villages in 3 PHCs. She is a 32-year-old woman from the Scheduled Castes community. As a CF, her days are spent communicating with stakeholders and mapping villages where Atmiyata is yet to be implemented. As per her training, she employs simple and destigmatising language when introducing the project to a new community. Instead of using mental health jargon, she refers to mental illness in terms of stress and distress. Discussing examples of psychological distress helps the community members relate to the need for this intervention, making it more welcome in their village. After receiving some nominations from the community, for the role of the Champion, she reaches out to them and describes the Atmiyata intervention. Those interested and available for training, which is scheduled on weekends as per the nominee's convenience, are encouraged to attend.

After training the Champions, she acts as a supervisor to them, helping them navigate the sessions that they conduct with end-users. She also guides them on the strategies employed when working with end-users with social benefits and referrals. Sohina attributes the success of the Atmiyata intervention to enablers like community interest in public health services and the present reputation of Atmiyata. Some of the challenges in implementing the intervention have been around the end-users' fear of the breach of confidentiality and their reluctance to accept referrals for alcohol addiction.

Sohina reflects, "I joined Atmiyata as a Community Facilitator because of my deep interest and education in psychology and mental health. During my intensive CF training, I learned Problem Solving skills that I immediately began applying to my own life. The training not only enhanced my ability to navigate emotional challenges but also taught me effective ways to manage familial conflicts with greater ease."

Sohina has also noticed positive changes among her champions and the end-users they work with, even preventing multiple cases of suicide attempts. She provided two examples of people dealing with alcohol addiction following the death of their fathers, who recovered after undergoing the CMD sessions. Sohina has observed an immense positive impact not only in her personal life but also among the end-users, Champions and communities with whom she has worked.

Components of the Atmiyata Intervention

The Atmiyata intervention adopts a stepped care and support approach, utilizing trained community-based volunteers to conduct four primary activities:

I. ***Identification and counselling***

Trained Champions have a pivotal role in identifying community members experiencing CMD and providing them with 4–6 counselling sessions spread over 6 to 12 weeks. The philosophy behind the *Atmiyata* approach lies in its emphasis on tapping into social capital (leaders of formal and informal groups) and encouraging community members to assist their fellow community members by enhancing their own social networks and status within their communities as a result of contributing to the greater wellbeing of the community. More details on the intervention have been mentioned in the programme paper (Shields-Zeeman, 2017).

During their training, Champions are taught how to identify the signs and symptoms of the spectrum of mental health, from wellbeing to common to severe mental health conditions, and potential socio-cultural situations that can be distressing for the community members (death of a loved one, a woman moving into a new home post marriage, loss of employment).

These sessions offer flexible scheduling and durations ranging from 20 to 40 min. In the initial session (Session 0), Champions builds trust and rapport to gauge whether the individual falls under the criteria for CMD and is willing to engage in counselling. Sessions are tailored to individual needs, incorporating evidence-based techniques such as active listening, behavioural activation, and problem-solving. Behaviour activation involves scheduling pleasurable and meaningful activities towards building a routine, whereas problem-solving assists in setting goals and identifying solutions to resolve life challenges.

The final session focuses on reviewing progress and discussing future coping strategies. Should the end-user require more than six sessions, they are referred to a mental health professional for additional support. Champions conduct sessions in the local language, typically Gujarati, and deliver interventions either at the end-user's residence or a preferred location, such as a community hall or temple. The real-life implementation of the intervention allows for variations in the frequency and duration of sessions. Champions are provided broad guidelines during their training to ensure consistency and enable exploration of dose–response effects.

II. ***Referral to specialized services***

Champions refer individuals with SMD, addiction issues, suicidal ideation, or history of attempted suicide to district mental health services, specifically psychiatrists at district hospitals or community health centers. The Champions provide information about available services, but the decision to seek specialized assistance rests with the individual and their family. CFs receive de-identified information about referrals to facilitate follow-up support if needed.

III. ***Enabling access to social benefits***

Champions assist individuals and families in accessing government-provided social benefits, including pensions, rural employment opportunities, disability schemes, and financial assistance. They assess the eligibility of end-users, facilitate the acquisition of their documents, assist them in application processes, and monitor their progress until the benefits are received. Additionally, Champions may connect individuals with paid work opportunities through government schemes.

IV. ***Narrow-casting films on social determinants***

Champions disseminate four 10-min films on smartphones within the community. These films address four prevalent social issues that impact mental health, namely unemployment, family conflicts, domestic violence, and alcoholism. These films are shown in community gathering places and aim to raise awareness about the social determinants of mental health. Viewers may self-refer or refer others experiencing distress to the programme after viewing the films.

Atmiyata App

In August 2022, the Atmiyata App was created to simplify data collection for monitoring and evaluation purposes. the app streamlines data collection through built-in questionnaires which enables the project team to monitor engagement and evaluate the impact of the intervention. Before the introduction of the app, data collection relied on manual methods employed by Champions, CFs and POs. However, starting from 2022, the Atmiyata app has been gradually rolled out across Mehsana, Sabarkantha, and Patan districts in Gujarat.

By December 2023, all stakeholders transitioned to utilizing the app for real-time data storage and monitoring.

Key Elements of Atmiyata

The Atmiyata intervention holds significant value from a health system perspective for several reasons.

- It uses a distress paradigm and not an illness model of care that increases the acceptability and feasibility of the model
- It is complementary to health systems and therefore created a referral pathway that channels those who need specialised services to reach the available district-based specialists
- It enhances the community's ability to address their own mental health needs by applying evidence-based techniques
- It uses a quality assurance and fidelity check to ensure that the community is receiving good quality, evidence-based service at their doorstep, free of cost

- It enables ownership of the communities by the volunteers and stakeholders investing their time and effort towards the intervention
- It enhances acceptability and reduces associated stigma by engaging community volunteers and embracing a social model of mental distress;
- It creates a sustainable pathway for the community to channel its own resources without relying on outside experts.

Evaluation of Atmiyata Using a Stepped-Wedge Cluster Randomized Controlled Trial

The Atmiyata team had conducted a Stepped Wedge Cluster Randomized Controlled Trial (SW-CRCT) (Pathare et al., 2023) between April 2017 and August 2019. The following significant findings were discovered, alluding to the effectiveness of this intervention in alleviating symptoms of depression and anxiety among individuals in Gujarat, India:

- Persons with CMD who received the Atmiyata intervention were three times more likely to experience a reduction in symptoms related to depression and anxiety. This positive impact was not only significant but also sustained over time.
- Persons with CMD who received the Atmiyata intervention were two times more likely to show improvement at three months and three times more likely to improve at eight months.
- The Atmiyata intervention demonstrated effectiveness not only in reducing symptoms of depression and anxiety but also in enhancing the overall quality of life and social participation of the end-users.
- Champions exhibited a 58% accuracy rate in identifying individuals with common mental health conditions. This accuracy improved as Champions gained more experience and expertise.
- The Atmiyata intervention has a good return on investment (ROI), as per our ongoing evaluations (unpublished). This ROI reflects the improved health and productivity of individuals who received the intervention, underlining its economic value. With every US$1 investment for the intervention, there is a US$9.35 return in terms of improved health and productivity of the individuals (work prepared for publication but not submitted).

The encouraging positive results have motivated the team to think of further scaling with the necessary adaptations to the contextual realities as described below. The team is now working on unpacking the implementation research questions that can assist in understanding the intervention package.

Pathways to Scale

Direct Implementation

Post the evaluation at scale at Mehsana, Gujarat, the team intended to increase the reach and impact to other rural and urban-poor geographies. Right after the evaluation results, we witnessed the pandemic due to which implementation was in itself a challenge. We began with expanding the intervention in the neighbouring districts of Mehsana, Gujarat where the team had already worked on strong collaboration across the State and district level.

As of March 2024, 537 villages in Mehsana with the help of 16 CFs, 658 Champions, and 500 Mitras have been covered. Services to 64,374 end-users with CMD, 5119 end-users with SMD, and 16,291 end-users with SB were provided. 1,44,506 community members viewed the narrowcasting films on social determinants. Atmiyata was scaled up in the Patan district of Gujarat in 2023. As of March 2024, 255 villages in Patan have been covered with the help of 11 CFs, 194 Champions and 371 Mitras. Services to 109 end-users with CMD, 35 end-users with SMD and 75 end-users with SB were provided. 453 community members viewed the narrowcasting films on social determinants. In the same year, Atmiyata was also scaled up in Sabarkantha district, India. As of March 2024, 537 villages in Sabarkantha have been covered with the help of 8 CFs, 197 Champions and 245 Mitras. Services to 403 end-users with CMD, 174 end-users with SMD and 211 end-users with SB were provided. 1,791 community members viewed the narrowcasting films on social determinants. On an average, with full district coverage, the Champions reach out to 25,000 adult population approximately.

Scaling Atmiyata Through Partnerships

One of the intended pathways to scale the intervention is to leverage the networks and strengths of the existing community-based organisations. The Atmiyata model provides a framework and structure to implement community mental health, while allowing for the necessary tweaks and adaptations to the unique needs of the community.

In line with the collaborative and participatory approach of Atmiyata, the model can be integrated into existing community programmes by recruiting and training either existing or new community-based volunteers or community health workers to deliver mental health interventions. The team has been working with a range of community-based partners to take this work forward. We enlist a few examples to demonstrate the range of interventions that have integrated Amiyata into three ongoing community programmes by involving their existing community workers.

I. ***Pilot of Atmiyata's counselling model at Ambuja Cement Foundation.*** The partnership between CMHLP and the Ambuja Foundation (AF) signified a collaborative effort to enhance mental health interventions within AF's operational areas. It mobilised on the synergy between CMHLP's expertise in community mental health intervention and AF's established community infrastructure. AF's cadre of frontline workers, known as *Sakhis*, deliver a interventions for hypertension and diabetes where Atmiyata's package of intervention was integrated successfully.

   Through this collaboration, CMHLP undertook scoping exercise to evaluate the process to ensure the intervention's effectiveness and feasibility within ACF's operational framework. The implementation strategy unfolded over three years, targeting four sites across India, namely Chhattisgarh, Maharashtra, Himachal Pradesh, and Uttarakhand. Activities included scoping, community mapping, adaptation of training materials, selection and training of trainers and frontline workers, field implementation, supervision, monitoring, and process evaluation. The phased approach allowed for gradual scale-up, ensuring adequate coverage, quality assurance, and sustainability of the intervention. The collaboration is being sustained and scaled to other geographies.

II. ***Pilot of Atmiyata's counselling model in urban poor communities, Hasiru Dala, Bangalore.*** The Atmiyata intervention was integrated into the Hasiru Dala (HD) programme to address the mental health needs of waste picker communities in urban poor communities in Bangalore, Karnataka. The collaboration between Atmiyata and HD sought to achieve several specific objectives, including assessing the feasibility of integrating Atmiyata into HD's existing work, improving access to mental health services, enhancing the mental health of individuals with CMD and potentially expanding Atmiyata across HD's work sites.

   The evaluation conducted in December 2023 highlighted the need for further adaptation and contextualisation of the intervention model to better address the mental health needs of waste pickers in urban poor communities facing several other structural determinants to mental health.

III. ***Pilot of Atmiyata's counselling model at Mahila Panchayats, Delhi Commission for Women, New Delhi.*** The partnership ofCMHLP and Mariwala Health Initiative (MHI), Mumbai,aimed to integrate Atmiyata's counselling model within the Delhi Commission for Women (DCW) programme of Mahila Panchayat (MP) programme. The MP programme focuses on empowering women and providing crisis intervention and legal assistance. Over the course of one year, the project unfolded across 12 urban poor communities, involving activities such as scoping, training, field implementation, and ongoing support.

   The integration of Atmiyata's intervention components into the MP programme included providing evidence-based counselling for persons with CMD and referral pathways for persons with SMD. The pilot phase assessed the feasibility, acceptability, and impact of the intervention. The evaluation underscored the ease of layering a mental health intervention on those working on gender based violence in communities. The training was further scaled-up to cover the entire 62 MPs in New Delhi, India.

Further Innovation

One of the key challenging issues highlighted by the Champions while working on Atmiyata was of improving the mental health response to domestic violence (DV). in India, with approximately 41% of women reporting lifetime experiences of DV, and nearly 30% reporting recent incidents (Kalokhe et al., 2017), the Champions often felt like they were not 'doing enough' for domestic violence and reported the need to improve our respond towards the same.

The COVID-19 pandemic has exacerbated this crisis, leading to an increase in DV cases due to factors such as prolonged physical confinement, reduced access to social support, economic insecurity, and stress (Ghoshal, 2020). The consequences of DV extend beyond immediate physical harm, encompassing long-term mental health effects, reproductive health complications, economic productivity loss, and adverse child outcomes (Malathesh & Das, 2020). Rural Gujarat, including Mehsana, faces specific challenges due to poverty, limited access to legal recourse, and cultural acceptance of violence (Kamimura et al., 2017).

The team wanted to leverage on the rich history of work done by gender-focused organisations at the community, institutional, and legal frameworks and work towards reducing the inter-sectoral gap between mental health and domestic violence work. Amongst the various needs of the communities, the team prioritised attempts to address gender related familial conflicts that impact mental health, layering on the foundational work of Atmiyata in Mehsana, Gujarat. The team intends to work with exploring arts-based methods to address group settings, in addition to enhancing the skills of the Champions to respond to DV during their one-on-one sessions.

This initiative aims to enable a conversation on familial conflict, including domestic violence and its impact on mental health and check for the feasibility and acceptability of integrating DV intervention within AtmiyataThe initiative holds promise for addressing DV and mental health at scale within community-based interventions in rural India.

The Atmiyata Course

In continuing the spirit of reducing the large mental health care gap in India, the team has worked towards creating a brief online course using Atmiyata's learning. The course began in the pandemic where there was an urgent need for people to effectively respond to the mental health needs of themselves and of people around them. The team worked on a simplified version based on evidence-based skills, knowledge and practice from Atmiyata and opened it to the public across urban communities.

Launched in October 2020, the Atmiyata Course equips participants with skills in evidence-based counselling techniques to identify, reach out to, and support individuals experiencing distress. As of 2024, the course has completed seven batches, having trained a total of 83 individuals to date. The course spans across 20 h over seven days, is currently open only to Indian citizens and aims to enhance participants' capacity for self-care, informal mental health care including support to family, friends, and colleagues. It aimed to reach out to individuals with lived experiences, caregivers, educators, managers, human resource management professionals, medical practitioners, mental health professionals, and nonprofit organizations.

Sessions are conducted online on weekends and ensure interactive and practice-based sessions, with small groups to provide individualized attention. The methodology includes open discussions, engagement through case studies, role plays, reading materials, and the participants are provided with a workbook to summarise key messages. The modules cover topics such as mental health spectrum, common and severe mental health conditions, suicide awareness, social determinants of mental health, qualities of a good mental health supporter, evidence-based techniques, relaxation techniques, and self-care tips. Additionally, a check-in session two weeks post-completion allows participants to share their real-life application of course learnings.

Looking Ahead

Shifting the Mental Health Narrative

In the attempt to bring a paradigm shift in mental health services to a rights-based and recovery-oriented care, enabling communities to address their own mental health and social care is the low-cost, high-impact, scalable and sustainable pathway.

The COVID-19 pandemic had brought to light the profound impact of social isolation, economic instability, and uncertainty on mental health (Radfar et al., 2021). Where structural barriers, stigma, discrimination remain significant barriers in accessing care and support for millions worldwide, psychosocial interventions such as Atmiyata play a crucial role in offering support, and resilience-building strategies to mitigate the adverse effects of such unprecedented circumstances (Barbui et al., 2020).

In fact, they can further be customised and tailored for unique needs of marginalised and vulnerable populations. While such psychosocial interventions may not solve the structural barriers and all social determinants of mental health disparities, the model provides pathways in which we can acknowledge and recognise the structural factors of mental health while promoting mental well-being within a rights-based framework.

The strength of the intervention is in building collaboration and alliances with a diverse range of stakeholders. For instance, at the village level: the emphasis on community involvement and capacity building fosters a sense of ownership and empowerment within the community. The training of village-based or community-based Champions and Mitras reduces the dependence on external resources and instead builds local expertise. The involvement of gram panchayats, community health workers are essential in the success of the acceptance from the community.

At the District and State level: Building collaborations with the district and State collaborations enhance the referral pathways for people to access the services they need is crucial and critical to its success. The model is complementary to health systems.

At the implementation team level: The training and regular supervision from CFs ensures that Champions receive the necessary support to maintain fidelity to the intervention model.

At the partner level: The adaptation to the intervention to suit the local context cannot be done without tapping into the expertise of the community-based organisations.

Overall, the Atmiyata Toolkit describes the essential ingredients of the 'how-to-implement the Atmiyata model'. This can be integrated into existing community programs, like those by partner organisations. This demonstrates a sustainable approach to scaling up interventions by leveraging existing infrastructure and resources. Besides, utilising technology with the Atmiyata app and films continues to expand our knowledge and assessment based on the data collection and reach of the intervention respectively.

Preliminary research points to Atmiyata being an economically sound investment in communities, creating even more evidence-based and low-cost interventions to scale. The continuous monitoring and evaluation allow for refinement of the intervention to better meet the evolving needs of the communities.

Implications for Future Directions

Atmiyata's positive trial results leave scope for further implementation research questions in the field of community-based mental health care. The team is working on exploring the reasons and motivation for the Champions, understand the specific interventions from the entire package of interventions that is supporting the community members. There are open questions on whether the intervention can be applied to similar low-resources contexts across a diverse country such as India, in addition to exploring the possible adaptation and implementation of the intervention to high-low-middle-income country contexts.

The team also intends to explore diverse research questions on exploring diverse settings of urban communities in addition to rural settings, exploring the different kinds of volunteers, with different kinds of incentives that can be engaged within this model. We are also exploring how we can review and redesign the tasks of the volunteers, such as using community volunteers who are working on gender-based violence, livelihood, can integrate the work of mental health onto their existing tasks. We are also exploring if changing the elements of the intervention package has an impact on mental health outcomes. We also aim to explore whether the model can be enhanced further to provide a response to structural factors such as gender and caste-based discrimination and unemployment.

With the growing scale of the intervention, the focus is on ensuring quality assurance and fidelity checks on the existing intervention across all the sites. The team is working towards integrating the EQUIP, Ensuring Quality in Psychological Support, a joint WHO/UNICEF project to improve the competence of mental health providers and to ensure the consistency and quality of training and service delivery. We see Atmiyata as a living and ever-evolving intervention that needs consistent improvements, evaluation, and ensuring no harm is done to the communities.

The team is also working towards exploring further innovative research trials to assess pathways for integration of Atmiyata within the health systems. For instance, would it be possible to engage the existing community health workers to adapt and use the elements of Atmiyata package. Would it be possible for this integration to have the same impact on the end-users once the intervention is placed within the health systems, are some of the questions that the team continues to explore.

We aim to expand our reach to all community settings that might benefit from Atmiyata's evidence-based approach. We plan to explore several pathways to achieve the scale, either through partnerships with existing organisations, implementation research grants, or integration within health systems. We will continue to enhance the model further to support more unique needs of the communities. The team aims to explore more research questions on whether we can expand our scope and approach with volunteers.

Acknowledgements We express our gratitude to the communities who have collaborated and partnered with us to improve the mental health and social care. We extend our appreciation to the Department of Health and Family Welfare, Government of Gujarat, and the Civil Hospital, Mehsana, Gujarat, and all health care services for consistent and supportive collaboration to make Atmiyata possible. We thank our funding partners who have supported this work and continue to support the work of the Champions.

References

Barbui, C., Purgato, M., Abdulmalik, J., Acarturk, C., Eaton, J., Gastaldon, C., Gureje, O., Hanlon, C., Jordans, M., Lund, C., Nosè, M., Ostuzzi, G., Papola, D., Tedeschi, F., Tol, W., Turrini, G., Patel, V., & Thornicroft, G. (2020). Efficacy of psychosocial interventions for mental health outcomes in low-income and middle-income countries: An umbrella review. *The Lancet Psychiatry, 7*(2), 162–172. https://doi.org/10.1016/S2215-0366(19)30511-5

Chibanda, D., Bowers, T., Verhey, R., Rusakanika, S., Abas, M., Weisee, H.A., & Araya, R. (2015). The Friendship Bench programme: acluster randomized controlled trial of a brief psychological intervention for common mental disorders delivered by lay health workers in Zimbabwe. *International Journal of Mental Health Systems, 9*, 21, 2–7.

Ghoshal, R. (2020). Twin public health emergencies: Covid-19 and domestic violence. *Indian Journal of Medical Ethics, 5*, 1–5.
Gururaj, G., Varghese, M., Benegal, V., Rao, G. N., Pathak, K., Singh, L.K., ... & Misra, R. (2016). National mental health survey of India, 2015–16: mental health systems. Bengaluru: National Institute of Mental Health and Neurosciences.
Hans, G., & Sharan, P. (2021). Community-based mental health services in India: Current status and roadmap for the future. *Consortium Psychiatricum, 2*(3), 60–68.
Joag, K., Shields-Zeeman, L., Kapadia-Kundu, N., Kawade, R., Balaji, M., & Pathare, S. (2020). Feasibility and acceptability of a novel community-based mental health intervention delivered by community volunteers in Maharashtra, India: The Atmiyata programme. *BMC Psychiatry, 20*(1), 48. https://doi.org/10.1186/s12888-020-2466-z
Kalokhe, A., Del Rio, C., Dunkle, K., Stephenson, R., Metheny, N., Paranjape, A., & Sahay, S. (2017). Domestic violence against women in India: A systematic review of a decade of quantitative studies. *Global Public Health, 12*(4), 498–513.
Kamimura, A., Ganta, V., Myers, K., & Thomas, T. (2017). Intimate partner violence, childhood abuse, and in-law abuse among women utilizing community health services in Gujarat India. *Journal of Interpersonal Violence, 32*(24), 3778–3796.
Kaur, A., Kallakuri, S., Kohrt, B. A., Heim, E., Gronholm, P. C., Thornicroft, G., & Maulik, P. K. (2021). Systematic review of interventions to reduce mental health stigma in India. *Asian Journal of Psychiatry, 55*, Article 102466.
Killaspy, H., Harvey, C., Brasier, C., Brophy, L., Ennals, P., Fletcher, J., & Hamilton, B. (2022). Community-based social interventions for people with severe mental illness: A systematic review and narrative synthesis of recent evidence. *World Psychiatry, 21*(1), 96–123.
Lund, C., De Silva, M., Plagerson, S., Cooper, S., Chisholm, D., Das, J., Knap, M., & Patel, V. (2011). Poverty and mental disorders: Breaking the cycle in low-income and middle-income countries. *The Lancet, 378*(9801), 1502–1514.
Mahashur. (2024, March 7). *The interim Union Budget FY 2024–25: Where does mental health stand?* Centre for Mental Health Law & Policy.
Maheshwari, M., & Goyal, S. (2014). Role of self help groups in socio-economic empowerment of women: A review of studies. *Pacific Business Review International, 2*(7), 85–93.
Malathesh, B. C., Das, S., & Chatterjee, S. S. (2020). COVID-19 and domestic violence against women. *Asian Journal of Psychiatry, 53*(1), Article 102227.
Mental Disability Advocacy Centre (2014). https://www.mdac.org
Moroz, N., Moroz, I., & D'Angelo, M. S. (2020). Mental health services in Canada: Barriers and cost-effective solutions to increase access. In *Healthcare management forum* (Vol. 33, No. 6, pp. 282–287). SAGE Publications.
Nair, N., Tripathy, P. K., Gope, R., Rath, S., Pradhan, H., Rath, S., Kumar, A., Nath, V., Basu, P., Ojha, A., Copas, A., Houweling, T. A., Haghparast-Bidgoli, H., Minz, A., Baskey, P., Ahmed, M., Chakravarthy, V., Mahanta, R., & Prost, A. (2021). Effectiveness of participatory women's groups scaled up by the public health system to improve birth outcomes in Jharkhand, eastern India: a pragmatic cluster non-randomised controlled trial. *BMJ Global Health, 6*(11), e005066.
National Mental Health Policy (NMHP) (2014). Ministry of health and family welfare, Government of India.
Patel, V., Araya, R., de Lima, M., Ludermir, A., & Todd, C. (1999). Women, poverty and common mental disorders in four restructuring societies. *Social science & medicine (1982), 49*(11), 1461–1471. https://doi.org/10.1016/s0277-9536(99)00208-7

Patel, V., Goel, D. S., Desai, R., & Singh, D. (2009). Scaling up services for mental and neurological disorders in low-resource settings. *International Health, 1*, 37–44. https://doi.org/10.1016/j.inhe.2009.02.002

Patil, A. V., Somasundaram, K. V., & Goyal, R. C. (2002). Current health scenario in rural India. *Australian Journal of Rural Health, 10*(2), 129–135.

Pathare, S., Joag, K., Kalha, J., Pandit, D., Krishnamoorthy, S., Chauhan, A., & Shields-Zeeman, L. (2023). Atmiyata, a community champions led psychosocial intervention for common mental disorders: A stepped wedge cluster randomized controlled trial in rural Gujarat India. *Plos ONE, 18*(6), Article e0285385.

Pereira, B., Andrew, G., Pednekar, S., Kirkwood, B.R., & Patel, V. (2011). The integration of the treatment for common mental disorders in primary care: experience of health care providers in the MANAS trial in Goa, India. *International Journal of Mental Health Systems, 5*, 26, 2–9.

Porteny, T., Alegría, M., Del Cueto, P., Fuentes, L., Markle, S. L., NeMoyer, A., & Perez, G. K. (2020). Barriers and strategies for implementing community-based interventions with minority elders: Positive minds-strong bodies. *Implementation Science Communications, 1*, 1–13.

Radfar, A., Ferreira, M. M., Sosa, J. P., & Filip, I. (2021). Emergent crisis of COVID-19 pandemic: Mental health challenges and opportunities. *Frontiers in Psychiatry, 12*, Article 631008.

Ríos-Espinoza, C. (2018). They stay until they die. A lifetime of isolation and neglect in institutions for people with disabilities in Brazil. *Human Rights Watch.* https://www.hrw.org/report/2018/05/23/theystay-until-they-die/lifetime-isolation-and-neglect-institutions-people

Sagar, R., Dandona, R., Gururaj, G., Dhaliwal, R. S., Singh, A., Ferrari, A., … & Dandona, L. (2020). The burden of mental disorders across the states of India: The Global Burden of Disease Study 1990–2017. *The Lancet Psychiatry, 7*(2), 148–161.

Shidhaye, R., Shrivastava, S., Murhar, V., Samudre, S., Ahuja, S., Ramaswamy, R., et al. (2016). Development and piloting of a plan for integrating mental health in primary care in Sehore district, Madhya Pradesh, India. *British Journal of Psychiatry, 208*, s13–s20.

Shields-Zeeman, L., Pathare, S., Walters, B. H., Kapadia-Kundu, N., & Joag, K. (2017). Promoting wellbeing and improving access to mental health care through community champions in rural India: The *Atmiyata* intervention approach. *International Journal of Mental Health Systems, 11*, 6. https://doi.org/10.1186/s13033-016-0113-3

Shinogi, K. C., Jayashree, K. M., Varghese, E., Srivastava, S., Rashmi, I., Balakrishnan, R., & Gills, R. (2021). Empowerment of smallholder women farmers through self-help groups in south-west India. *Indian Journal of Extension Education, 57*(2), 31–37.

Slade, M. (2009). *Personal recovery and mental illness: A guide for mental health professionals.* Cambridge University Press.

Solotaroff, J. L., & Pande, R. P. (2014). *Violence against women and girls: Lessons from South Asia.* World Bank Group.

Tripathy, P., Nair, N., Barnett, S., Mahapatra, R., Borghi, J., Rath, S., Gope, R., Mahto, D., Sinha, R., Lakshminarayana, R., Patel, V., Pagel, C., Prost, A., & Costello, A. (2010). Effect of a participatory intervention with women's groups on birth outcomes and maternal depression in Jharkhand and Orissa, India: A cluster-randomised controlled trial. *The Lancet, 375*(9721), 1182–1192.

Turnpenny, A., Petri, G., Finn, A., Beadle-Brown, J., & Nyman, M. (2018). Mapping and understanding exclusion: Institutional, coercive and community-based services and practices across Europe.

United Nations. (2006). *Convention on the rights of persons with disabilities.* Retrieved from https://www.un.org/development/desa/disabilities/convention-on-the-rights-of-persons-with-disabilities.html

United Nations General Assembly. (1948). *Universal Declaration of Human Rights.* Retrieved from https://www.un.org/en/universal-declaration-human-rights/

United Nations. (2015). *Transforming our world: The 2030 agenda for sustainable development.* Retrieved from https://sdgs.un.org/goals

World Health Organization. (2013). *Comprehensive mental health action plan 2013–2020*. World Health Organization.
World Health Organization. (2021). *Community outreach mental health services: Promoting person-centred and rights-based approaches*. Retrieved from https://iris.who.int/handle/10665/341644. License: CC BY-NC-SA 3.0 IGO

Jasmine Kalha Jasmine Kalha is a Program Director and Research Fellow at the Centre for Mental Health Law & Policy, Indian Law Society, Pune. With a background in Social Work and Sociology, she works on innovative, evidence-based implementation research interventions at-scale for rights-based approaches to mental health in low resource settings. She co-leads the scale-up and evaluation of Atmiyata, a community-led intervention for mental health and social care. She has worked on peer support and implemented the WHO's QualityRights scale-up in India for mental health systems reform. She continues to provide capacity building support to countries implementing the QualityRights framework globally.

Nimisha Ajaikumar is a Project Officer and Research Associate at the Centre for Mental Health Law & Policy, Indian Law Society, Pune. She is a counselling psychologist with an M.Sc. Clinical Psychology from Amity University and a B.Sc. Honours Psychology with Counselling Skills from Middlesex University. Nimisha oversees the monitoring and evaluation of Atmiyata, and educational programmes at CMHLP-Learn, including the International Diploma in Mental Health, Human Rights & Law. She has worked on Project SIREN for suicide prevention at the Keshav Desiraju India Mental Health Observatory. Nimisha has multiple academic publications in psychology, going on to win SHAPES India's PSYNTHESIS COPIOUS 2021.

Somya Agarwal as an Assistant Project Manager and Research Associate at the Centre for Mental Health Law & Policy, Indian Law Society, Pune. At the Centre, she has worked as a Youth Advisor for the Being Initiative project and is currently working on the gender-based violence intervention within the Atmiyata project. Prior to joining CMHLP, she led a psychoeducational project for a mental health app. She has also developed a curriculum on dating violence for high school students in California and has facilitated mental health training workshops in Ladakh. Somya holds a Master's in Applied Psychology from the University of Delhi.

Palak Korde is a Project Manager and Research Coordinator at the Centre for Mental Health Law & Policy, Indian Law Society, Pune. Her educational background is in social and cultural anthropology. In her role at Atmiyata, a community-led intervention for mental health and social care, Palak is responsible for designing, implementing, and supervising the capacity-building aspect at intervention sites and with partners. She has also been involved in implementing UPSIDES, a peer support intervention for people with severe mental illness, across high-, middle-, and low-resource settings in India.

Soumitra Pathare is a consultant psychiatrist and the Director of the Centre for Mental Health Law and Policy at Indian Law Society Pune. He played a key role in drafting India's Mental Health Care Act, 2017 and the National Mental Health Policy, 2014. which takes a rights-based approach to mental healthcare. He has served as a WHO consultant in many low and middle-income countries (Botswana, Seychelles, Lesotho, Samoa, Vanuatu, Eritrea) assisting them in drafting and implementing mental health legislation and national mental health policy. He is Co-Director of SPIRIT (an implementation research project on suicide prevention in Gujarat funded by NIMH, USA) and PI of CASP (a suicide prevention project in collaboration with Government of Chhattisgarh funded by Mariwala Health Initiative), co-Lead on Outlive (a youth suicide prevention project funded by Comic Relief, UK) and co-Lead on ENGAGE (a suicide prevention gatekeeper training for school teachers implementation research project in Chhattisgarh funded by Grand Challenges Canada) He enjoys travelling, meeting new people and dreams of being a cheese maker one day.

Kaustubh Joag is a trained psychiatrist and serves as the Program Director and Senior Research Fellow at the Centre for Mental Health Law & Policy, Indian Law Society, Pune. He co-leads Atmiyata and has been involved in the project since its inception: initially as the Co-Principal Investigator during its proof-of-concept stage, and later as Principal Investigator for the transition-to-scale stage. Currently, he co-leads the partnership model with Ambuja Cement Foundation. Kaustubh also coordinates the Centre's International Diploma in Mental Health, Human Rights & Law.

Chapter 7
Common Mental Disorders in Primary Health Care Settings: Implementation of Brief Counselling as a Psychosocial Intervention

Nalini Bikkina, Sumati Guntaka, and U. Vindhya

Abstract Over the past three decades or so, there has been increasing evidence of common mental disorders (CMD) constituting a significant public health problem in India. Presenting themselves as somatic symptoms and associated with considerable morbidity including psychosocial disability, diminished productivity, economic and psychological costs for the affected, care givers and for society at large, the distress of CMD is however, often disguised and unrecognized. Studies have also reported that a significant proportion of patients in primary health care settings (PHCs) have CMD although they are not identified as such, since the PHCs are not designed or equipped with psychological service providers to deal with mental health concerns. This study reports on the prevalence of CMD, its association with socio-demographic factors, and the implementation of a psychosocial intervention called Brief Counselling in two PHCs in the city of Visakhapatnam in the southern state of Andhra Pradesh. Findings indicated a significantly high prevalence of CMD; fairly equal distribution of all three categories of physical health, psychological problems, and social and interpersonal concerns (such as domestic violence) across the sample, underscoring the fact that it is not physical health alone, but rather a range of underlying issues

This paper is based on a major research project, sponsored by the University Grants Commission, done by U.Vindhya, with research assistance provided by Nalini Bikkina and Sumati Guntaka.

N. Bikkina
School of Humanities and Social Sciences, GITAM, Visakhapatnam, India
e-mail: nbikkina@gitam.edu

S. Guntaka
KL University, Guntur, India
e-mail: sumati.guntaka@kluniversity.in

U. Vindhya (✉)
Independent Researcher, and Former Professor, Tata Institute of Social Sciences, Hyderabad, Telangana, India
e-mail: u.vindhya@gmail.com

U. Vindhya (ed.), *Psychosocial Interventions for Social Issues in Contemporary India*,
https://doi.org/10.1007/978-981-96-6553-2_7

of distress that manifest as physical health complaints for which people consult PHC facilities; and the most frequently used counselling interventions, reflecting the needs of the sample, were *ventilation*, followed by *problem-solving*. The findings are discussed in the context of the intertwining and bidirectional linkages of multiple social and economic inequalities with the burden of psychological distress as seen at this level.

Keywords Common mental disorders · Primary health care settings · Brief counselling

Introduction

Common mental disorders (CMD), defined as a range of anxiety and depressive disorders (Goldberg & Huxley, 1992), and classified in the International Classification of Diseases (ICD) as "neurotic, stress-related and somatoform disorders" (World Health Organization, 2018a), are commonly seen disorders in primary health care settings, and contributing significantly to the burden of disease (Nirisha et al., 2023; Patel & Kleinman, 2003; Patel et al., 2008; Pothen et al., 2003). Recent estimates of the global prevalence of CMD show depressive and anxiety disorders to be contributing to 7.5% and 3.4% of years lived with disability respectively (World Health Organization, 2017). In India, data from the first multisite nationwide household survey (National Mental Health Survey of India, 2015–16) (NIMHANS, 2016) show the weighted prevalence of current CMD to be 5.1%, with around 60% of them reporting disabilities of varying severity (Jayasankar et al., 2022). While the contribution of mental disorders in general to the total disability adjusted life years (DALYs) has been found to have increased from 1990 to 2017 in India, depressive disorders was found to be contributing the most to the total mental disorders DALYs, followed by anxiety disorders, indicating CMD to be a significant public health problem (India State-Level Disease Burden Initiative Mental Disorders Collaborators, 2020).

The central aim of this research was to study CMD in the primary health care (PHC) setting and the application of a psychosocial intervention termed 'Brief Counselling' in this setting. Primary care has been defined as the point of first-time care provided to patients who access the health care system and is said to have four key components: first time care, continuity of care, direct care for common health concerns, and coordination and collaboration with specialists where necessary (WHO, 2018b; WHO & UNICEF, 2018). Studies have reported that around 20–50% of all patients in PHC settings have CMD and are associated with considerable morbidity such as psychosocial disability in family and social life, reduced productivity, economic and psychological costs both for the affected and their caregivers (Miranda & Patel, 2005; Patel, 2005; Patel & Kleinman, 2003; Shankar et al., 2006). Further, it is important to note that although CMD may not be characterized by extensive cognitive breakdown and personality fragmentation as in the case of severe mental disorders (SMD), they are nevertheless characterized by a high degree of personal distress and impairment of social functioning. Calling a set of behaviors as 'common' does not necessarily entail that they are mild or that they cause very little personal suffering. Indeed, as Goldberg and Huxley (1992) note in the case of CMD, "there is no hard and fast line between where normality ends and mental disorders begin" (p. 58); and they can profoundly affect one's sense of personal and social well-being, and may be associated with severe disability (Goldberg & Huxley, 1992). Another key distinction between SMD and CMD is that the former are determined more by bio-genetic causes, deserving the designator, 'illness' while CMD are psychosocial in origin and could be determined to a great extent and influenced by social circumstances (e.g., Patel & Kleinman, 2003; Stansfeld et al., 2016; World Health Organization, 2017). While the clinical picture of SMD is thus explicitly visible and therefore better referred to as 'illness', that of CMD on the other hand, is such that mental distress is often 'masked' (Davar, 1999). Despite its reportedly high prevalence, the accumulated evidence so far shows that CMD are often unrecognized, disguised, and generally go untreated since the PHCs in India are not designed or equipped with psychological service providers to deal with mental health problems (Jayasankar et al., 2022); these conditions also often go undetected and untreated since those consulting the health care facility at this level do so primarily for somatic symptoms.

Furthermore, the burden of psychological distress as seen at the level of PHCs has also been found to be linked closely with the social and economic inequalities and multiple deprivations in development contexts that create mental health problems (Lund, 2020; Lund et al., 2018; Jorm et al., 2017; Patel et al., 2020). It is perhaps useful in this context to remind ourselves of the historical evolution of the primary health care approach as conceptualized by the Alma Ata Declaration (1978) that had emphasized on the following:

- *A comprehensive* approach to health by emphasizing interventions that promote and protect health, such as food security, women's literacy, access to clean water, etc.,
- *Integration* of different programmes and services at all levels of the health care system.
- *Equity* and recommended addressing of imbalances at different levels.
- *Use of'appropriate'* health technology, and health care that is socially and culturally acceptable.
- *Appropriate and effective community involvement* in the health care system.
- *A strong human* rights perspective on health by affirming that health is a fundamental human right and by placing the responsibility on governments to act on this.
- *Peace, reduced military expenditure and a 'New International Economic Order'* to reduce the health status gap between developing and developed countries.

The philosophy and vision of the Declaration with emphasis on—equity, community participation in decision making, health promotion, and need for multi sectoral approach to health—resonates with the social model of health subsequently espoused by international agencies such as the World Health Organization, and reiterated by the United Nations Convention on Rights of People with Disabilities of 2006 (and ratified by India in 2007). Further, the emphasis on integration of mental health services within the existing health system using the primary care approach, based on principles of universal access, equity and rights-based care, and intersectoral coordination, amongst others, is encapsulated in recent mental health policy and legislations in India too such as the Mental Health Policy of 2014, the Rights of Persons with Disabilities Act of 2016, and the Mental Healthcare Act of 2017 (Hans & Sharan, 2021; Ranade & Bertotti, 2021).

The primary health centres in India have the following functions: Mother and child health care; Family Welfare Activities; Medical Termination of Pregnancy (M.T.P.); Nutrition; Communicable diseases—Prevention, control and treatment; Immunization; Antenatal (ANC) and postnatal (PNC) care; Emergency treatment; Birth and death registration; and Maintenance of reports and records. Although the operationalization of mental health care integration into primary care was sought to be implemented by the National Mental Health Programme (NMHP) (Directorate of Health Services, 1982), the challenges however, to the integration of mental health care in primary care settings and its delivery have been documented as several including dearth of resources, infrastructure, trained personnel and so on (Goel, 2011; Shastri, 2021).

Psychosocial Intervention

This study is located in the conceptual framework of the 'psychosocial model' and illustrates the current shift in research interest from mortality and illness to examining morbidity, quality of life, and well-being and their correlates. The term 'psychosocial' has been in use for some time now and refers to the interaction of psychological factors and social circumstances impacting on mental health; and the term 'psychosocial intervention' has come to refer to any programme that aims to improve the psychosocial well-being of people. In recent decades, it has come to be increasingly used by international organizations such as WHO to indicate the appropriateness and relevance of its usage and its commitment to non-medical approaches. The term is also said to be more appropriate for developing countries because of the overwhelming context of social determinants such as poverty and social disadvantage influencing mental health of their populations (Ommeren et al., 2005). Further, in recent decades, developments such as the new economic policies being followed since the neo-liberal economic reforms were launched since the 1990s, and the resultant widening of socio-economic disparities (Dev, 2007), the gradual erosion of traditional and community norms in interpersonal relationships have been found to have had varying impacts on the psychosocial health of people (Barua, 2009; Fu et al., 2013; Patel & Kleinman, 2003; Patel et al., 1998, 2006; Skapinakis et al., 2013).The psychosocial emphasis on social as well as psychological aspects of well-being also ensures that state policies, distribution and allocation of resources in the community, and individuals' access and control over these resources are fully brought into the picture.

Brief Counselling is a key form of psychosocial intervention and differs from more traditional forms of therapy/counseling in that it emphasizes (1) a focus on a specific problem and (2) direct intervention. Rather than the formal analysis of historical causes of distress, the primary objective of brief counselling is to help the client to view the present from a wider context and to utilize more functional understandings. By becoming aware of these new understandings, it is expected that successful clients will de facto undergo spontaneous and generative change (Osborn & Johanson, 2001).

The essential underlying principles of brief counseling are as follows.

- Change can take place quickly if interventions are specific and targeted to particular goals
- Emphasis is on the present rather than on the past
- The approach is flexible and pragmatic in its means for solving problems
- The counselor adopts an active, directive approach in attempting to break dysfunctional patterns and to establish new ones
- Attention is directed toward not only what is wrong but also to what is working well (Kottler, 2008).

Brief counselling is often highly strategic, exploratory, and solution-based rather than problem-oriented. It is less concerned with how a problem arose than with the current factors sustaining it (Babor & Higgins-Biddle, 2000). Coping questions are designed to elicit information about client resources that will have gone unnoticed by them. Even the most hopeless story has within it examples of coping that can be drawn out: "*I can see that things have been really difficult for you, yet I am struck by the fact that, even so, you manage to get up each morning and do everything necessary to get the kids off to school. How do you do that?*" Validation of clients' experience can help to highlight strengths without appearing to contradict the client's view of reality, such as an initial summary statement such as "*I can see that things have been really difficult for you*". The second part "*you manage to get up each morning* etc." is also a truism, but one that counters the problem focused narrative. Undeniably, they cope and coping questions start to gently and supportively challenge the problem-focused narrative (Mac Donald et al., 2007).

A key task in brief counselling is to help clients identify and attend to their skills, abilities, and external resources (e.g., social networks). This process not only helps to construct a narrative of the client as a competent individual, but also aims to help the client identify new ways of bringing these resources to bear upon the problem. Resources can be identified by the client and the worker will achieve this by empowering the client to identify their own resources. Resources can be *internal*: the client's skills, strengths, qualities, beliefs that are useful to them and their capacities or they may be *external*: supportive relationships such as, partners, family, friends, faith or religious groups and also support groups (Eatock & Gus, 2007; Macdonald, 2007).

Thus, the following sequential steps are adopted in brief intervention techniques (Kottler, 2008):

1. Identifying what the problem is and focusing primarily on the presenting complaint.
2. Identifying the positive aspects of the individual's life situation, current circumstances of his or her personality and way of functioning and more importantly, communicating this to the individual.
3. Enforcing boundaries to stay within the presenting problem because of the time constraints.
4. Identifying what strategies have worked and what have not in order to save time by not repeating what have already been tested.
5. Developing interventions that are aimed to get the person moving and not be stuck in the same groove.
6. Finally, to make the individual be stimulated to seek out new options.

Method

The central aims of this study were to examine the prevalence of common mental disorders in the primary health care setting, their association with socio-demographic factors, and to implement a psychosocial intervention for the distress experienced by those who consulted the health care facility primarily for physical health problems. The primary advantage of conducting a study of this kind at the primary health care level is that it helps us to identify individuals who present themselves at PHCs with predominantly physical health problems with underlying psychological distress that is largely unrecognized, unidentified and thereby untreated.

Sample

This study was based in the coastal port city of Visakhapatnam in the southern state of Andhra Pradesh and conducted in two PHCs in the urban and peri-urban areas of the city. The sample comprised 300 patients visiting the two PHCs for consultation as consecutive attendees over a period of one year. The inclusion criteria were a) patients above 18 years of age; and b) those with presenting complaints of predominantly physical ailments. The exclusion criteria were consultation for vaccinations and injuries and emergencies; and pregnant women consulting for routine check-ups.

Tools Employed

a) A socio-demographic data sheet, designed for the purpose of the study was used to gather information on age, sex, religion, caste, education, occupation, financial status, marital status, residential status, type of family. Additionally, there were two items on experience of domestic violence and on consumption of alcohol keeping in view the variables that had to be taken into consideration in this particular context.

b) Self-Reporting Questionnaire-20 (SRQ-20) for detection of psychological morbidity: The SRQ-20 is derived from four psychiatric morbidity instruments from a wide variety of cultural backgrounds. Developed by Harding et al., (1980) for a WHO collaborative study to screen for CMD in primary health care, it can be self-administered but in low-income population-based studies, it is the interviewer who usually administers it. It indicates probable cases of mental disorder. The SRQ-20 can only indicate probable cases of mental health concerns, and reflects the multidimensional nature of 'mental illness' with factor analysis showing that one group of the questions taps into a ***somatic factor*** (headaches, appetite, digestion, sleep); another into ***depressive/anxiety*** symptoms (frightened, unhappiness, crying, feelings of worthlessness); while a third captures a more ***cognitive/decreased*** energy factor (cannot think or make decisions, work being affected adversely, cannot enjoy daily activities) (Lacoponi & Mari, 1989; Sen et al., 1987; Tafari et al., 1991). The SRQ-20 is composed of 20 "yes–no" questions, 4 on physical symptoms and 16 on psycho-emotional disturbance. The SRQ-20 has been used as both a mental health screening instrument at an individual level, and as a way in which to establish the mental ill-health prevalence in a community (Harpham et al., 2003). In the present study the questionnaire was translated into the local language, Telugu. As majority of the sample were not formally educated, the questionnaire was not administered to the patients; instead, responses to each item were elicited individually from the respondents by asking them.

c) Selected (15) items of WHO's Psychiatric Disability Assessment Schedule (WHO/DAS) were adapted and modified to assess social functioning of individuals affected by psychological morbidity. Applicable in a variety of cultural settings (WHO, 1988), it has been used for mental health evaluation assessment in India too (e.g., Srinivasan et al., 2001).

d) The CAGE Questionnaire, developed by Ewing (1984) is a simple 4-question test, and an internationally used and validated assessment instrument for detecting the use or abuse of alcohol is (e.g., Girela et al., 1994; Kitchens, 1994).

e) Short-form Social Support Questionnaire (SSQ), developed by Sarason et al (1987) was used to categorize people into those with high and low social support. Respondents list the people they can rely on for support in a given set of circumstances, and indicate overall level of satisfaction with the support provided.

f) A semi-structured interview protocol used for initiating the brief counseling intervention and consisted of the following questions: What do you think is the central concern/problem in your life at present? What do you think can be done to overcome this situation? What are the factors that facilitate you? What are the obstacles? What do you think are the most positive aspects in your life and in your personality?

Procedure

The study utilized a cross-sectional survey design. Patients consulting the two PHCs were recruited upon fulfilling the inclusion criteria. Their socio-demographic information data were gathered by interviewing the patients. The SRQ-20, 15 items adapted and modified from the WHO-DAS, CAGE and SSQ, translated into Telugu were then administered to each respondent individually. The semi-structured interview was then conducted to explore the central and current concerns in the individual's life in order to initiate the counseling intervention. Finally, brief supportive counseling was provided based on the identified needs of the individual respondents.

Informed consent was obtained from the patients recruited for the study including providing information about the nature and purpose of the study, and assuring them that their responses would be kept strictly confidential and would be used only for research purposes. The instructions for the SRQ-20 were read out orally and explained to the respondents individually, to reinforce and facilitate better understanding and to clarify doubts if any.

Responses to the questions in the semi-structured interview schedule were noted and at the end of each interview, the researcher recorded (a) the kind of complaint—whether it was physical health, psychological, or social and interpersonal and (b) the predominant intervention employed subsequently—Providing space for *ventilation*; *Problem-solving* through identifying central problem of client's life, obstacles and options in the domains of work, economic situation, relationships, health, and social context; Providing *psycho-education* for antenatal care, nutrition related issues and for alcohol dependence for those who reported such dependence. The technique of psycho-education for antenatal care and nutrition related issues was considered useful and appropriate keeping in view the primary needs of women who consulted the facility.

The notings of the researcher were subsequently grouped into the categories with the above-mentioned descriptive labels. For instance, if in an interview session emotional relief and the space and time given to the individual was the predominant intervention provided by the researcher, it was noted down as emotional relief. Subsequently all such responses were labeled as 'ventilation'. Similarly, if some information concerning legal assistance or accessing government schemes was given for problems such as domestic violence it was noted as 'addressing informational needs' and later on classified as 'problem-solving'.

Analyses of Data

The socio-demographic variables were analyzed in terms of significant representation across the various categories using frequencies and chi-square test.

With the SRQ-20 method of scoring the cutting score that gives optimum discrimination between those identified as 'cases' and those who are not is that between 7 and 8, so that respondents with 8 or more symptoms are considered as 'cases'.

Fifteen items were adapted and modified from the WHO/DAS based on their relevance to the objectives of the present study. The presence or absence of each of these items as reported by the respondents was considered as presence or absence of the disability or dysfunction in that particular area.

CAGE is scored by allocating '1' point to each 'yes' answer. Total scores of 2 or above are thought to be clinically significant and may indicate alcohol dependence. Prevalence of alcoholism was calculated and scores on CAGE were correlated with scores on SRQ-20, WHO/DAS and responses to SSQ.

The responses to the SSQ were scored for the presence or absence of social support, and the perceived adequacy or inadequacy of support.

The responses to the semi-structured interview were qualitatively analyzed. Content analysis was used for the qualitative data. For quantitative analysis, the Statistical Package for Social Sciences (version 16) was used.

Findings of the Study

Prevalence of Common Mental Disorders

Of the total sample 207 (69%) manifested CMD as measured by SRQ-20, while 93 (31%) did not report symptoms of significant psychological distress. The mean score of the sample of 300 respondents on SRQ-20 was 9.95 while the mean SRQ-20 score of the ***cases*** was 12.45.

The high prevalence of CMD as identified by the SRQ-20 in our sample is in accordance with our hypothesis that individuals consulting the PHC would be reporting significantly high symptoms of psychological distress, that are however not detected or identified as such by the health care providers in this setting. This finding of high prevalence is not only similar to earlier investigations reported, but is also a pointer to the importance of economic inequalities and low social capital in impacting health outcomes. Considering that an overwhelming majority of the present sample is from low-income groups with different levels of disadvantage such as lack of formal education, opportunities for skill development and economic participation, this finding represents the complex bidirectional relationship between multiple deprivations and mental health problems. The high levels of morbidity identified in this sample indicate that poverty and the multiple deprivations and disempowering factors that it is associated with constitutes a significant high risk for people.

This finding therefore underscores the fact that CMD are a significant public health problem and the importance of recognizing sites of health care such as the PHCs as locations wherein psychological distress is manifested but regrettably goes undetected and hence untreated. This is because the service providers at the PHC level, usually the first point of health service contact for economically disadvantaged populations in particular, are not equipped to screen, identify and treat psychological distress. The present findings therefore have implications for our mental health care policy and delivery of services.

Distribution of the Socio-Demographic Variables Across the Sample

Frequency distributions along with chi-squares were used to arrive at the distribution of the socio-demographic variables including personal characteristics, socio-economic status variables, and family variables cross the sample. The proportional distribution of the sample of 300 across cases and non-cases based on SRQ-20 scores across personal characteristics of age, gender, religion, caste and residence is presented in Table 7.1.

Taking personal characteristics into consideration, it was found that age and gender were significantly associated with psychological symptoms as measured by the SRQ-20 with the two largest groups represented in those who were identified as cases were the 31–50 years age group and female respondents. The finding of female gender being a risk factor for CMD is in line with several earlier investigations in the area and is a pointer to the disempowering conditions in many women's lives in our country, leading to considerable psychological distress that goes unrecognized and unidentified.

Table 7.2 presents the frequency distribution of the sample across the socio-economic status variables of education, occupation, income, marital status and age at marriage. It was found that among these variables, the ones that were significantly associated were education, income, marital status, and age at marriage. Those who were significantly affected by psychological distress, as identified by the SRQ-20 were those with no formal education, those with an income range of Rs. 1001 to Rs. 3000, those who were married and those who were married below the legal age of marriage.

These findings are a pointer to the association between psychological distress and the combination of disempowering factors of lack of education and economic opportunities. In addition, the findings also demonstrate that being married and married below the legal age of marriage in particular also have a significant impact on psychological distress.

There is by now a wealth of relationship between social class or socio-economic status and mental health (e.g., Kuruvilla & Jacob, 2007; Chadda & Gupta, 2012; Gupta & Coffey, 2020; Kallivayalil & Enara, 2022). The epidemiological research

Table 7.1 Frequency distribution of personal characteristics across the sample

Variable	**Non-cases**		**Cases**		**Chi-square**
	N	%	**n**	%	
Age					df = 3 10.756*
Below 18	6	6.5	11	5.3	
19–30	51	54.8	74	35.7	
31–50	24	25.8	80	38.6	
51 & above	12	12.9	42	20.3	
Gender					df = 1 18.459**
Female	43	46.2	149	72	
Male	50	53.8	58	28	
Religion					df = 2 0.179
Hindu	85	91.4	190	91.8	
Muslim	3	3.2	5	2.4	
Christian	5	5.4	12	5.8	
Caste					df = 3 1.062
Upper caste	25	26.9	46	22.2	
BC	55	59.1	135	65.2	
SC	12	12.9	24	11.6	
ST	1	1.1	2	1.0	
Residence					df = 2 0.196
Rural	34	36.6	81	39.1	
Urban	45	48.4	95	45.9	
Semi-urban	14	15.1	31	15.0	

* significant at 0.05 level; ** significant at 0.01 level

is largely based on correlational investigations—the question of the direction of causality remains contested about some aspects of the overall picture. The most contentious in this relationship between social class and mental health is that while the class gradient in mental health statistics is unequivocal (as is the unequal pattern of mental health service delivery) the direction of causality is open to debate. Those retaining a strong biodeterminist approach to mental illness argue that patients become poor because of their social incompetence (the *downward drift hypothesis*). The opposing view is that of *social causation*: poverty makes people mentally ill. A third position is that genetically vulnerable individuals are differentially exposed to social stressors. The controversy essentially applies to the causality of psychosis. It does not apply to stress reactions or to psychosomatic reactions. Here the evidence is unambiguous. For example, low paid and unemployed people are disproportionately likely to suffer from a range of anxiety and depressive symptoms and are more likely to commit suicide and abuse drugs and alcohol. When psychosomatic symptoms are taken as a proxy for mental health (e.g., cardiovascular disease) then lower pay and

Table 7.2 Distribution of non-cases and cases across socio-economic status variables

Variable	Non-cases		Cases		Chi-square
	N	%	n	%	
Education					df = 4 17.523**
No formal education	18	19.4	79	38.2	
Primary education	13	14.0	40	19.3	
Secondary education	39	41.9	61	29.5	
Inter & graduation	18	19.4	24	11.6	
Above graduation	5	5.4	3	1.4	
Occupation					df = 7 10.652
Student	9	9.7	17	8.2	
Home maker/daughter	22	23.7	71	34.3	
Unemployed	3	3.2	4	1.9	
Agriculture/Daily labour	17	18.3	48	23.2	
Skilled worker	7	7.5	12	5.8	
Petty business	8	8.6	13	6.3	
Clerical	3	3.2	13	6.3	
Services	24	25.8	29	14.0	
Income					df = 4 13.764**
Up to Rs. 1000	12	12.9	44	21.3	
Rs. 1001–3000	43	46.2	111	53.6	
Rs. 3001–5000	20	21.5	21	10.1	
Rs. 5001 & above	12	12.9	12	5.8	
Don't know	6	6.5	19	9.2	
Marital Status					df = 3 18.047**
Unmarried	22	23.7	20	9.7	
Married	68	73.1	153	73.9	
Widowed	2	2.2	23	11.1	
Separated/divorced	1	1.1	11	5.3	
Legal Age at marriage					df = 3 15.705**
Yes	44	47.3	85	41.1	
No	24	25.8	92	44.4	
Not applicable	22	23.7	20	9.7	
Don't know	3	3.2	10	4.8	

* * significant at 0.01 level

lower task control in work are factors in the development of hypertension, strokes and heart attacks. This picture of unemployment and low pay adversely affecting mental health also parallels the picture of physical health (Pilgrim, 2006).

The significant relationship between low educational attainments and the manifestation of CMD is in line with several earlier findings that demonstrate the risk factor of less schooling (Barros, 2005; Marin-Leon et al., 2007; Rojas et al., 2005). Individuals with less schooling are perhaps usually less able to cope with adversities. Low literacy can also be a recognized barrier to efficient and effective health care, and in mental health care, it may have additional detrimental effects. Furthermore, a higher level of education favours health as it provides better job opportunities and living conditions, while illiteracy and low level of education are associated with poor living conditions that make access to treatment difficult. In this connection, it needs to be pointed out that literacy programs have been found to positively influence mental health by reducing hopelessness and insecurity (Patel & Kleinman, 2003).

The multiple deprivations that dearth of education and economic opportunities entail and the associations they have with the likelihood of being affected by CMD underscore the necessity of making policy changes and investments in these sectors for enhancement of both physical and mental health.

The next set of findings of marital status and age at marriage being related to manifestation of CMD implicate the institution of marriage and its role in creating or exacerbating conditions of psychological distress. The stresses and strains associated with being married, combined with having been married at a young age (below the legal age of 18 years for girls and 21 years for boys) demonstrate the necessity of examining the structure and conditions of married life and the socially accepted practice of marrying off girls (and boys too) below the legally sanctioned age at marriage. Though it would be too sweeping a generalization to indict marriage per se for its role as a risk factor for CMD, it does appear that early marriage sets off a chain of disempowering factors, curtailing opportunities and imposing disproportionate burden of responsibilities when the individual is not yet in a state of preparedness and readiness to assume them.

The distribution of cases and non-cases across the type of family—nuclear, extended, or single—did not show any significant difference between cases and non-cases.

Areas and Extent of Disability/Dysfunction Based on Responses to WHO-DAS

The following table presents the extent and nature of disability/dysfunction reported by the sample of patients who were consulting the PHCs, based on their responses to the WHO/DAS. As can be seen from the table, there were several areas of dysfunction, contributing to the experience of psychological distress, and to diminished productivity.

Table 7.3 Areas and extent of disability/dysfunction based on responses to WHO/DAS

	N		%	
Areas of Dysfunction	Present	Absent	Present	Absent
Interpersonal interaction	121	179	40.3	59.7
Participation in regular household activities	54	239	18.0	79.7
Participation in decision making	84	208	28.0	69.3
Interaction with spouse	135	154	45.0	51.3
Attending to child care	47	212	15.7	70.7
Conflicts outside the home	113	187	37.7	62.3
Attending to work duties in time	77	223	25.7	74.3
Interested in working	143	157	47.7	52.3
Efforts made to obtain a job	192	108	64.0	36.0
Interest in current affairs	138	162	46.0	54.0
Entertainment/recreation	54	246	18.0	82.0
Responsiveness to health issues of family members	45	254	15.0	84.7
Participation in supportive groups	231	69	77.0	23.0
Sharing personal problems	176	124	58.7	41.3
Anger/Aggression	160	140	53.3	46.7

All the items tapped by the WHO-DAS pertained to the level of social functioning of the individuals. Although this schedule is purportedly for assessing the psychiatric disability of patients in hospital settings, disability in the sense adopted in the DAS means dysfunctional social behavior and disturbance in the performance of social roles, resulting or impacted by some form of mental disorder. One of the objectives of the study was also to examine the nature and to what extent mental health disturbances affect social roles and responsibilities, and interpersonal functioning of individuals. The scores indicate that lack of responsiveness to the health concerns of members of their family, inability to participate in recreational activities, as well as in regular activities, attending to child care responsibilities, and participating in decision making involving key areas in social and interpersonal life were some of the important areas in which the respondents showed some deficit (Table 7.3).

The five areas that indicated presence of highest dysfunction were the following: Responsiveness to health issues of family members; Entertainment/recreation activities; Participation in regular household activities; Attending to child care responsibilities; and Participation in decision making.

Distribution of the CAGE Scores Across the Sample

This section deals with the distribution of the sample who reported substance abuse, based on the CAGE scores, across personal characteristics, socio-economic variables,

Table 7.4 Distribution of cases and non-cases based on CAGE scores

	N	%
Non-case	10	20.4
Case	39	79.6
Total	49	100

family variables, and variables of spousal substance abuse and domestic violence. Of the total sample of 300, 49 respondents reported substance abuse and answered the CAGE questionnaire. Of the 49 respondents who reported substance abuse and answered the CAGE questionnaire, 39 were found to be substance abusers based on the CAGE cut-off score of 2, as shown in Table 7.4.

Although, none of the personal characteristics, socio-economic status and type of family variables were found to be significantly associated with substance abuse as measured by the CAGE questionnaire, the single largest groups represented among those identified as cases were found in the 19–30 age group, male, Hindus, belonging to the backward castes, from urban locations, those with secondary education, working as daily wage laborers, those who were married, and those from nuclear family.

Social Support and Manifestation of CMD

The availability of social support systems that can serve as potential protective buffers for the affected individuals is well-recognized in the literature. As defined by Caplan (1974) social support systems consist of enduring interpersonal ties to a group of people who can be relied upon to provide emotional sustenance, assistance and resources in times of need. It has also been observed that deficiencies in support systems will not in themselves contribute to susceptibility to illness in the absence of social stressors. The converse is also probable. Social stressors in the presence of strong social support systems are considered to have only minor effects on health (Rabkin & Struening, 2004). The findings of the present study however, were in an unexpected direction. The perceived presence and adequacy of social support did not seem to have any relationship with manifestation of CMD.

Nature of Complaints

The classification and frequency distribution of complaints reported by individuals who consulted the PHCs were done on the basis of the semi-structured interviews with them. The responses to the question "What do you think is the central concern/problem in your life at present?" were classified as either belonging to the categories of (a) physical health, (b) psychological well-being, and (c) social and interpersonal issues. Frequency of these complaints was noted in order to examine the significant representation of these concerns across the sample.

Although the individuals consulting the health facility were purportedly for physical health complaints, the interviews with them elicited a range and variety of concerns extending from those related to physical health to those concerning psychological and social and interpersonal issues.

The *physical health* issues which were causes of concern for the individual respondents ranged from aches and pains, allergies, asthma, blood pressure, fatigue and weakness, fever, cold and cough, gynecological problems, injuries, insomnia, kidney problems, loss of appetite, to tuberculosis. As can be seen from Table 7.5, aches and pains, fatigue and weakness, and sleep and eating problems (insomnia and loss of appetite) were the most frequently reported complaints, indicating the somatization of psychological distress. These responses indicate the somatization of psychological distress, a trend that has been reported and noted in several earlier investigations, in the context of developing countries in particular. Medically unexplained symptoms, preoccupation with physical illness, and not having the required vocabulary and psychological-mindedness to express psychological distress may constitute culturally shaped idioms of distress, and may be employed to express concerns about a broad range of personal and social problems that are psychological in origin (Venkoba Rao, 1978).

The *psychological* issues that emerged from the interview narratives included depression, anxiety, anger, frustration and guilt. The *social and interpersonal* concerns that emerged from the interview narratives included domestic violence by spouse, burden of domestic responsibilities and work, relationship problems, and substance abuse in the home. As expected, depression emerged as the single largest concern with anxiety closely following, and both of them together are a pointer to the presence of significant levels of psychological distress in the sample. The high reporting of symptoms associated with depression and anxiety underscore the point that people who consult physical health facilities come with underlying psychological distress as well, which need to be addressed. Once again, the presence of this kind of a psychological distress implicates the lack of appropriate health care services to address such distress at the primary health care level. These findings emphasize the need to provide mental health care at the level of PHCs in order to alleviate feelings of psychological ill-being and also to prevent likely scaling of full-blown disorders.

The social and interpersonal concerns emerging out of the narratives included domestic violence, economic problems, substance abuse at home, relationship issues, and the burden of domestic responsibilities (Table 7.5). These findings reiterate the widespread prevalence of domestic violence as a significant risk factor for women's mental health, and with CMD in particular, as attested by several studies from both the global north and south (e.g., Astbury, 2001; Fischbach & Herbert, 1997; Heise et al., 2002; Patel et al., 2006).

Table 7.5 Distribution of complaints—physical, psychological, and social and interpersonal

Physical Complaints	n	%
Aches & Pains	145	48.3
Allergies	14	4.7
Asthma	9	3.0
Blood Pressure	17	5.7
Fatigue & Weakness	130	43.3
Fever, cold & cough	53	17.7
Gynaecological problems	12	4.0
Injuries	6	2.0
Kidney Problems	2	0.7
Tuberculosis	7	2.3
Insomnia	84	28
Loss of appetite	93	31
Psychological Complaints	**n**	**%**
Anger	33	11.0
Anxiety	164	54.7
Depression	171	57.0
Frustration	31	10.3
Social and Interpersonal Concerns		
Domestic violence	139	46.3
Economic problems	104	34.7
Substance abuse at home	129	43.0
Relationship Issues	109	36.3
Burden of domestic responsibilities	74	24.7

Brief Counseling Intervention

The types of individuals who commonly consult primary health care facilities are those who can be described as suffering from distress ranging from 'mild' to 'moderate' mental health problems. The present study is a modest attempt to build a case for introducing providing of psychological services—of a brief intervention kind—in order to provide some relief from the distress of those who consult these health facilities. The brief counselling intervention developed in the present study was based on the assumptions and principles detailed above. On the basis of the pilot study, the following techniques were found appropriate for individuals consulting primary health care facilities. These techniques were (a) providing space and some time for ventilation of their problems; (b) focusing on a problem-solving mode for identifying the central problem/concern in their current life circumstances, identifying the obstacle(s) to resolving the problem, and then looking at the other options or alternatives available to them; and (c) providing psychoeducation for concerns related to antenatal care, nutrition, and for alcohol dependence for those who reported such dependence.

The ventilation technique did not only aim to provide emotional space and relief. It also included pointing out and highlighting the positive aspects of the individual's life situation and/or his or her personality. Positive aspects included resources that could be used to his or her advantage such as education or specific wage-earning skills or supportive ties with individuals who could be relied upon or aspects of personality such as evidence of resilience in earlier adversities, or assertiveness or patience and so on. By pointing out to such resources and strengths, the person's attention could be more effectively directed to such sources from which they could look for solutions to their current life problems.

The technique of problem-solving consisted of identifying the central concern in his or her current life situation, knowing in brief what strategies have worked and what have not in the past, and stimulating the person to look for newer options if the earlier alternatives have not worked.

Antenatal care included attention to compliance with diet, medication, and hygiene, some information about physiological changes during pregnancy, and the need to follow nutritious diet for good health of the others. Information on diet and other methods such as adequate exercise for a healthy life style was provided to the individuals who consulted the facility. For those with alcohol dependence, the adverse health and social consequences including the care giving burden for the spouse were pointed out, without any underlying value judgments.

Table 7.6 presents the distribution of counselling techniques used in the present sample depending on the needs of the individuals who were consulting the health facilities. As the table shows, it was *ventilation* that was used the most, followed by techniques of *problem solving and psychoeducation.*

In this connection, it must be mentioned here that the proportion of women in the total sample was very large at 72%. Given this kind of a composition of the sample, it is perhaps not too surprising that the predominant needs of the women were for space to ventilate their concerns for emotional relief. This finding reiterates once again the importance of ventilation in individuals' perceptions of emotional relief

Table 7.6 Techniques of brief counselling

Intervention	N	Chi-square
Ventilation	253	141.453**
Problem solving	169	4.813*
Psycho education	131	4.813*
Ventilation & Problem solving	86	54.613**
Ventilation & Psycho education	66	94.080**
Problem solving and Psycho education	5	280.333**
Ventilation, Problem Solving and Psycho education	51	130.680**

when they unburden their distress onto an objective third party who is free from the 'baggage' of family associations.

Problem-solving technique was the second most frequently preferred one, indicating the appropriateness of the intervention for locating the central problem in the life of the individual, searching for a solution from a range of possible alternatives, and encouraging the individual to reach for this solution instead of being stuck in the same position. Problem-solving also included providing information on issues such as government schemes on a range of items such as housing and shelter, pension benefits, scholarships for economically disadvantaged sections, and availability of vocational courses. The information provided to the individuals also included resources for legal assistance for domestic violence, and deaddiction centres for alcohol and other forms of substance abuse. It was felt that by addressing the informational needs of the individuals and providing them specific information on a range of their needs, it would be easier for them to get into the problem-solving mode instead of lamenting their fate, or by being passive and not take recourse to any concrete steps for redressal of their problems. Studies to this extent have reported positive outcomes with brief counseling interventions (Babor et al., 1994). Additionally, brief supportive interventions that can be integrated into daily routines reportedly brought about clinically significant modifications amongst the populations seeking primary care for a large number of risk factors (Whitlock et al., 2022). This is particularly so in the non-Western contexts which accentuate didactic guidance (Hurley et al., 2017).

Summing up and Conclusion

To reiterate the rationale and context of the study once again, they are as follows: (a) CMD are most commonly encountered in PHC settings; however, because primary health care service providers are not equipped or mandated to handle problems of this kind, such mental health problems often go undetected and unrecognized, and therefore untreated; (b) The prevalence and presence of CMD point to unmet needs of vulnerable groups such as those from socially and economically disadvantaged populations since these are the people likely to consult PHC facilities; (c) CMD present themselves as somatic symptoms and are associated with considerable morbidity including disability, diminished productivity, economic and psychological costs for the affected, care givers and for society at large.

The prevalence of CMD as identified by the SRQ-20 in patients visiting the PHCs showed that 69% were identified as affected by CMD. Second, the association between socio-demographic variables and CMD indicated that age, gender, education, income, and marital status were significantly related to CMD. Third, the nature and extent of disability/dysfunction in the sample indicated the following concerns in their social and interpersonal life: lack of responsiveness to the health concerns by members of their family, inability to participate in regular and recreational activities, and participating in decision making involving key areas in social and interpersonal life. Fourth, the single largest groups represented among those identified as cases of alcohol dependence and abuse were the 19–30 age group and male. Fifth, the nature of complaints reported by the sample underscoring the fact that it is not physical health alone that is foregrounded, but rather a range of underlying issues of distress experienced by those who consult the health facilities. While aches and pains, and fatigue and weakness were the most commonly reported concerns among *physical health* complaints, depression and anxiety were the most commonly voiced concerns in the *psychological* category; and domestic violence and substance abuse the most frequently reported complaints in the category of *social and interpersonal* concerns—issues that are of close concern to a vast majority of women in Indian society. Finally, the finding related to the counseling intervention indicated that *ventilation* was the most frequently used technique, reflecting the needs of the respondents, followed by *problem-solving.* Although no outcome evaluation or assessment of users' satisfaction with the counselling intervention could be done, the findings attest to the importance of providing non-threatening space for people to express and emotionally unburden themselves even in the context of physical health care settings.

The findings point to the compelling need for integration of mental health care in primary health care settings so that mental health problems such as CMD can be detected, recognized and addressed. The significance of the present study is therefore located in the context of the necessity of signaling the importance of catering to the unmet health needs of vulnerable groups in particular who consult these facilities. The application of a psychosocial intervention, termed Brief Counselling was an attempt, however, modest and limited, to address the psychosocial needs of individuals consulting the PHC facilities. The study findings would hopefully be useful for designing and initiating similar interventions in primary care elsewhere.

References

Astbury, J. (2001). Gender disparities in mental health. In *Mental Health. Ministerial Round Tables 2001*, 54th World Health Assemble. World Health Organization.

Babor, T. F., et al. (1994). A randomized clinical trial of brief interventions in primary health care: Summary of a WHO project. *Addiction, 89*, 657–660.

Babor, T. F., & Higgins-Biddle, J. C. (2000). Brief intervention for hazardous and harmful drinking: A manual for use in primary care. *Addiction, 95*(5), 677–686.

Barros, M. B. (2005). Transtorno Mental Comum. In C. L. Cesar (Ed.), *Saude e condicao de vida em Sao Paulo: inquerito multicentrico de saude no Estado de Sao Paulo:* Faculdade de Sauda Publica (pp. 163–171). University of Sao Paulo.

Barua, A. (2009, January–June). Need for a realistic mental health programme in India. *Indian Journal of Psychological Medicine, 31* (1), 48–49.

Caplan, G. (1974). *Support systems and community mental health: Lectures on concept development.* Behavioral Publications.

Davar, B. V. (1999). *Mental health of Indian women. A feminist agenda.* Sage Publications.

Dev, S. M. (2007). *Inclusive growth in India: Essays on agriculture, poverty, and human development*. Oxford University Press.

Directorate General of Health Services. (1982). *National mental health programme for India*. Government of India.
Eatock, J., & Gus, A. (2007). Managing patient adherence and quality of life in epilepsy. *Neuropsychiatric Disease and Treatment, 3*(1), 117–131.
Ewing, J. A. (1984). Detecting alcoholism: The CAGE Questionnaire. *Journal of American Medical Association, 252*(14), 1905–1907.
Fischbach, R. L., & Herbert, B. (1997). Domestic violence and mental health: Correlates and conundrums within and across cultures. *Social Science and Medicine, 45*(8), 1161–1176.
Fu, T. S., Lee, C. S., Gunnell, D., Lee, W. C., & Cheng, A. T. (2013). Changing trends in the prevalence of common mental disorders in Taiwan: A 20-year repeated cross-sectional survey. *Lancet, 381*, 235–241.
Girela, E., Villanueva, E., Hernandez-Cueto, & Luna, J. D. (1994). Comparison of the CAGE questionnaire versus some biochemical markers in the diagnosis of alcoholism. *Alcohol and Alcoholism, 29*(3), 337–343.
Goel, D. S. (2011). Why mental health services in low- and middle-income countries are underresourced, under-performing: An Indian perspective. *National Medical Journal of India, 24*(2), 94–97.
Goldberg, D., & Huxley, P. (1992). *Common mental disorders: A biosocial model*. Routledge.
Groh, C. J. (2007). Poverty, mental health and women: Implications for psychiatric nurses in primary care settings. *Journal of the American Psychiatric Nurses Association, 13*(5), 267–274.
Gupta, A., & Coffey, D. (2020). Caste, Religion and Mental Health in India. *Population Research and Policy Review, 39*(6), 1119–1141.
Hans, G., & Sharan, P. (2021). Community-based mental health services in India: Current status and roadmap for the future. *Consortium Psychiatricum, 2*(3), 60–68.
Harding, T. W., Arango, M. V., Baltazar, J., et al. (1980). Mental disorders in primary health care: A study of the frequency and diagnosis in four developing countries. *Psychological Medicine, 10*, 231–242.
Harpham, T., et al. (2003). Measuring mental health in a cost-effective manner. *Health Policy and Planning, 18*(3), 344–349.
Heise, L., Ellsberg, M., & Gottmoeller, M. (2002). A global overview of gender-based violence. *International Journal of Gynecology & Obstetrics, 78*, S5–S14.
Hurley, E. A., et al. (2017). MHSU-provider communication styles in HIV treatment programs in Bamako, Mali: A mixed-methods study to define dimensions and measure MHSU preferences. *SSM-Population Health, 3*, 539–548.
India State-Level Disease Burden Initiative Mental Disorders Collaborators. (2020). The burden of mental disorders across the states of India: The Global Burden of Disease study 1990–2017. *Lancet Psychiatry, 7*(2), 148–161.
Jorm, A. F., Patten, S. B., Brugha, T. S., & Mojtabai, R. (2017). Has increased provision of treatment reduced the prevalence of common mental disorders? Review of the evidence from four countries. *World Psychiatry, 16*, 90–99.
Kitchens, J. M. (1994). Does this patient have an alcohol problem? *Journal of American Medical Association, 272*(22), 1782–1787.
Kottler, J. A. (2008). *A brief primer of helping skills*. Sage Publication.
Kuruvilla, A., & Jacob, K. S. (2007). Poverty, social stress and mental health. *Indian Journal of Medical Research, 126*(4), 273–278.
Jayasankar, P., Manjunatha, N., Rao, G., Gururaj, G., Varghese, M., Benegal, V. (2022). Epidemiology of common mental disorders: Results from "National Mental Health Survey" of India, 2016. *Indian Journal of Psychiatry, 64*(1), 13–19.
Kallivayalil, R. A., & Enara, A. (2022). Mental health in an unequal world—The role of social determinants. *Indian Journal of Social Psychiatry, 38*(1), 3–6.
Lacoponi, E., & Mari, J. J. (1989). Reliability and factor structure of the Portuguese version of Self-Reporting Questionnaire. *The International Journal of Social Psychiatry, 35*(3), 213–222.

Lund, C. (2020). Mental health and the sustainable development goals. https://globaldev.blog/mental-health-and-sustainable-development-goals/
Lund, C., Brooke-Sumner, C., Baingana, F., Baron, E. C., Breuer, E., Chandra, P., Haushofer, J., Herrman, H., Jordans, M., Kieling, C., Medina-Mora, M. E., Morgan, E., Omigbodun, O., Tol, W., Patel, V., & Saxena, S. (2018). Social determinants of mental disorders and the Sustainable Development Goals: A systematic review of reviews. *The Lancet Psychiatry, 5*(4), 357–369. https://doi.org/10.1016/S2215-0366(18)30060-9
Mac Donald, E., Fitzsimons, E., & Walsh, P. N. (2007). Use of respite care and coping strategies among Irish families of children with intellectual disabilities. *British Journal of Learning Disabilities, 35*(1), 62–68.
Marin-Leon, L., Oliveira, H. B. D., Barros, M. B. D. A., Dalgalarrondo, P., & Botega, N. J. (2007). Social inquality and common mental disorders. *Brazilian Journal of Psychiatry, 29*, 250–253.
Miranda, J. J., & Patel, V. (2005). Achieving the Millennium Development Goals: Does mental health play a role? *PLoSMedicine, 2*, 291.
NIMHANS. (2016). National mental health survey of India, 2015–2016 (2016). Author.
Nirisha, L. P., Malathesh, B. C., Jayasankar, P., Aswatha, P., Parthasarathy, R., Manjunatha, N., Kumar, N. C., Thirthalli, J., & Math, S. B. (2023). Analyzing psychiatric disorders from rural primary health centers: A clinical epidemiological study from a district of south India. *Journal of Psychiatry Spectrum, 2*(1), 35–40.
Ommeren, M. V., Saxena, S., & Saraceno, B. (2005). Mental and social health during and after acute emergencies: Emerging consensus? *Bulletin of the World Health Organization, 83*(1), 71–77.
Osborn, C., & Johanson, G. A. (2001). Development and validation of the theoretical orientation scale for clinicians: Reflecting solution-focused principles. *Assessment, 8*(3), 301–313.
Patel, V. (2005). Social origins, biological treatments: The public health implications of common mental disorders in India. *Indian Journal of Psychiatry, 47*, 15–20.
Patel, V., Flisher, A., Nikapota, A., & Malhotra, S. (2008). Promoting child and adolescent mental health in low and middle income countries. *The Journal of Child Psychology and Psychiatry, 49*(3), 313–334.
Patel, V., & Kleinman, A. (2003). Poverty and common mental disorders in developingcountries. *Bulletin of the World Health Organization, 81*, 609–615.
Patel, V., Kirkwood, B. R., Pednekar, S., Weiss, H., & Mabey, D. (2006). Risk factors for common mental disorders in women: Population-based longitudinal study. *The British Journal of Psychiatry, 189*, 547–555.
Patel, V., Pereira, J., Coutinho, L., Fernandes, R., Fernandes, J., & Mann, A. (1998). Poverty, psychological disorder and disability in primary care attenders in Goa, India. *British Journal of Psychiatry, 172*, 533–536.
Patel, V., et al. (2020). The Lancet Commission on global mental health and sustainable development. *The Lancet, 392*(10157), 1553–1598.
Pilgrim, D. (2006). Social class. In C. Feltham & I. Horton (Eds.), *The Sage handbook of counseling and psychotherapy* (pp. 36–40). Sage.
Pothen, M., Kuruvilla, A., Philip, K., Joseph, A., & Jacob, K. S. (2003). Common mental disorders among primary care attenders in Vellore, South India: Nature, prevalence and risk factors. *International Journal of Social Psychiatry, 49*(2), 119–125.
Ranade, A., & Bertotti, B. M. (2021). Implementation of the right to health in Brazil and India: A comparative study. *Revista Eurolatinoamerican De Derecho Administrativo, 8*(2), 27–46.
Rojas, G., Araya, R., & Lewis, G. (2005). Comparing sex inequalities in common affective disorders across countries: Great Britain and Chile. *Social Science and Medicine, 60*(8), 1693–1703.
Sarason, I. G., Sarason, B. R., Shearin, E. N., & Pierce, G. R. (1987). A brief measure of social support: Practical and theoretical implications. *Journal of Social and Personal Relationships, 4*, 497–510.
Sen, B., Wilkinson, G., & Mari, J. J. (1987). Psychiatric morbidity in primary health care. A two-stage screening procedure in developing countries: Choice of instruments and cost-effectiveness. *British Journal of Psychiatry, 151*, 33–38.

Shankar, B., Saravanan, B., & Jacob, K. S. (2006). Explanatory models of common mental disorders among traditional healers and their patients in rural south India. *International Journal of Social Psychiatry, 52*(3), 221–233.

Shastri, M. (2021). *Deconstructing the DMHP: Part I. Introduction to India's district mental health programme*. India Mental Health Observatory.

Skapinakis, P., Bellos, S., Koupidis, S., Grammatikopoulos, I., Theodorakis, P. N., & Mavreas, V. (2013). Prevalence and sociodemographic associations of common mental disorders in a nationally representative sample of the general population of Greece. *BMC Psychiatry, 13*, 163.

Stansfeld, S., Clark, C., Bebbington, P., King, M., Jenkins, R. & Hinchliffe, S. (2016). Common Mental Disorders. In S. McManus., P. Bebbington., R. Jenkins., T. Brugha (Eds.), *Mental health and wellbeing in England: Adult psychiatric morbidity survey 2014* (pp. 37–68). NHS Digital.

Srinivasan, T. N., Rajkumar, S., & Padmavathi, R. (2001). Initiating care for untreated schizophrenia patients and results of one year follow-up. *International Journal of Social Psychiatry, 47*(2), 73–80.

Tafari, S., Aboud, F. E., & Larson, C. P. (1991). Determinants of mental illness in a rural Ethiopian adult population. *Social Science & Medicine, 32*(2), 197–201.

Venkoba Rao, A. (1978). Epidemiology of depression. *Indian Journal of Psychological Medicine, 1*, 37–52.

Whitlock, E. P., Orleans, T., Pender, N., & Allan, J. (2022). Evaluating primary care behavioral counseling interventions: An evidence based approach. *American Journal of Preventive Medicine, 22*(4), 267–284.

World Health Organization. (1988). *WHO Psychiatric Disability Assessment Schedule (WHO/DAS)*. Author.

World Health Organization. (2017). *Depression and other Common Mental Disorders: Global Health Estimates*. Author.

World Health Organization. (2018a). ICD-11 for mortality and morbidity statistics (ICD-11 MMS) 2018 version. WHO. https://icd.who.int/browse11/

World Health Organization. (2018b). *Continuity and coordination of care: A practice brief to support implementation of the WHO Framework on integrated people-centred health services*. Author

World Health Organization (WHO) and the United Nations Children's Fund (UNICEF). (2018). *A vision for primary health care in the 21st century: Towards universal health coverage and the Sustainable Development Goals*. World Health Organization. https://iris.who.int/handle/10665/328065

Nalini Bikkina is Professor at GITAM School of Humanities and Social Sciences, Visakhapatnam. An ICSSR Doctoral Fellow, her research interests are in the interdisciplinary social sciences with an emphasis on public policy. She worked on projects funded by the UGC and the ICPR in her capacity as a Project Fellow. She was also the Principal Investigator in projects funded by the Indian Institute of Management, Ahmedabad and the SPARC Scheme of the Ministry of Education. She is a Fulbright Academic and Professional Excellence Fellow and a Fellow of the Royal Society of Arts, London. She won the Fulbright Alumni Award.

Sumati Guntaka has a Ph.D. in Psychology from Andhra University, Visakhapatnam, and was a research assistant in a UGC-funded project on prevalence of common mental disorders in primary healthcare settings.

U. Vindhya Independent Researcher, and Former Professor, Tata Institute of Social Sciences, Hyderabad, Telangana, India.

Chapter 8
Young Adult Resilience for Recovery to Substance Addiction in Assam, India: Practitioner Reflections on Pathways to Recovery Model

Sangeeta Goswami and Anna Madill

Abstract India has more than 50% of its population below the age of 25 years. This is a huge potential human resource. However, the mental health report, National Mental Health Survey (NMHS) for the state of Assam, on which this chapter is based, highlights that in 2015–2016, nearly 5.85% of people aged 18 years and above required active interventions for one or more mental health issues including substance use disorder (SUD). This data reflects that mental wellbeing can be a hindering factor for sustainable socio-economic development and should be considered a public health priority. This chapter focuses on 'The Big Picture' project that was aimed at understanding the lived experience of young Assamese people around risk, recovery and resilience in relation to substance misuse. The bedrock of the project was the use of psychosocial visual participatory methods involving photo-led interviews which centralizes the lived experience of our participants. In total 15 young Assamese people (11 men; 4 women) aged 19–24 years provided detailed information about their journey to recover from SUD. This allowed the development of a multi-route, multidirectional pathways to recovery model comprising three phases: Recreational Use, Addiction (Relaxed, Chaotic, Strategic) and Supported Recovery. This chapter provides a summary and practitioner reflection in the context of Assam on the pathways to SUD recovery model developed in 'The Big Picture.'

Keywords Substance use disorder · Youth · Positive behaviour formation · Resilience · Recovery · Sustainable development

---

S. Goswami (✉)
Institute of Positive Mental Health & Research, MIND India, Guwahati, Assam, India
e-mail: sangeetamind@gmail.com

A. Madill
University of Leeds, Leeds, UK

U. Vindhya (ed.), *Psychosocial Interventions for Social Issues in Contemporary India*,
https://doi.org/10.1007/978-981-96-6553-2_8

Introduction

India has more than 50% of its population below the age of 25 years. This is a huge potential human resource. However, the National Mental Health Survey (NMHS), the first and largest population-based representative sample survey in India (Gautham et al., 2020), with reference to the state of Assam, the focus of this chapter, indicates that nearly 5.85% of people aged 18 years and above require active interventions for one or more mental health issues including substance use disorder (SUD). This data (for 2015–2016) reflects that mental wellbeing concerns can be a hindering factor for sustainable socio-economic development and should be considered a public health priority.

Substance abuse especially amongst youth has been a concern throughout the world. Rapid industrialization, urbanization and changing life styles have left the youth struggling for their survival, forcing many to seek refuge in the dark world of substance abuse. India, too, is facing a similar situation that has attracted attention of policy makers and researchers (Juyal et al., 2006). Before the turn of the century, the World Health Organisation estimated that globally 25–90% of children and adolescents indulge in substance abuse (WHO, 2012). This has, at last, become of matter of priority to the government, parents, teachers, non-governmental organization and other relevant agencies (Chesang, 2013). Alcohol, cannabis (bhang) and tobacco are increasingly being abused by school going children showing a steady upward trend. Those between 16–30 years of age, a critical period in one's development, are most affected. This assumes greater relevance in developing countries like India which is already burdened with inadequate health-care facilities (Goswami, 2015). However, SUD is not confined to young people from a certain geographical area or socio-economic background. It affects both urban and rural areas and across classes, more so in the urban areas. Recent studies have shown that children of affluence, who are generally presumed to be at low risk, have problems in several domains—notably, substance use, anxiety, and depression, and the potential causes are pressures to achieve and isolation from parents. (Luthar, 2003).

Thus, as substance abuse is increasingly becoming a public health problem, we face an almost overwhelming need to understand prevention, risk reduction and treatment of SUD.

Assam, Meghalaya, Sikkim, Tripura, Arunachal Pradesh, Manipur, Mizoram, Nagaland comprise all the eight northeastern states. The last four states share a common international border with Myanmar, the world's second largest illicit opium producing country. From the early 1970's drug use among local youth of North East India, particularly in the states closer to Myanmar, took a new turn. Alcohol is the most commonly used substance in all states except Mizoram, where Cannabis has the highest use. Children and adolescent population often experiment with drugs for fun and amusement in the company of friends, particularly in the urban areas (Goswami, 2015). As a practitioner, similar instances have been observed where youth between the age group pf 18–30 years use substances for recreational purposes and there is strong peer pressure to do so. A high stake is placed on scholastic achievement and material affluence, while structural inequalities and lack of opportunity to develop life skills contribute to college dropout, suicide and SUD. In fact, the Assam State Report of the National Mental Health Survey of India identifies adolescent SUD as an urgent public health problem (Pathak et al., 2017).

According to a prevalence study, 13.1% of the people involved in substance abuse in India are below 20 years of age. (*Child Protection and Child Rights. Vulnerable Children Affected by Substance Abuse. Childline 1098,* 2008). As a practitioner's observation as well as a clinic-based survey revealed that 63.6% of the substance users seeking treatment were introduced to drugs at a young age when they were 15 years or younger. (Stockings et al., 2016). Early initiation of drug use is often associated with poor prognosis and lifelong pattern of disturbed behaviour. The fall out of SUD is associated with a variety of psychosocial problems such as poor educational achievement, loss of employment or unemployment, depression, and disharmony in family relationships it can have long-lasting effects on the developing brain and may interfere with positive family and peer relationships and school performance. (Tripathi & Lal, 1999). Thus, the problem of substance abuse is multi-dimensional and solutions entail more than the legal and health arenas. It is difficult to find statistics on adolescent SUD in Assam, particularly by gender. However, a review of the limited literature available suggests that youth 10–19 years living in a border area, use alcohol and 3.2% (only males), use drugs such as heroin and solvents while it is reported that 80% of street children in Guwahati aged 5–18 years abuse substances, 87.4% of whom abuse solvents (Madill et al., 2023).

Community based responses to SUD in the northeastern states ranged from coercive measures against drug users by local pressure groups to various drug reduction approaches, including central and state government initiatives. Some of them being Launching of Drugs Free Assam Mobile App developed by NIC, (Kavita Barkakoty, Assam, December 27, 2021, https://informatics.nic.in/news/1389#:~:text=10%20Dec%202021%20Guwahati%20%3A%20Drugs,Director%20General%20%2D%20Narcotics%20Control%20Bureau), Scheme of Assistance for the Prevention of Alcoholism and Substance (Drugs) Abuse for the State of Assam (https://socialwelfare.assam.gov.in/frontimpotentdata/scheme-of-assistance-for-the-prevention-of-alcoholism-and-substance-drugs-abuse).

The element common to all these responses has been the active participation of local non-governmental organisations and community-based organisations, the formation of which are often catalysed by addicts in recovery. One such organisation is Nirmaan Rehabilitation Facility which was central to the recruitment of participants in 'The Big Picture' project. Prevention is better than cure when it comes to SUD and the family and community plays an important role in both preventing SUD in young people and helping them to sustain recovery from addiction. This chapter provides a summary and practitioner reflection in the context of Assam on the pathways to SUD recovery model developed in 'The Big Picture.'

India has a comprehensive SUD treatment programme which includes 'detoxification, pharmacotherapy, individual therapy, family therapy, group therapy, multifamily therapy, 12-Step programmes. (Perumbilly & Anderson, 2017). Some programmes also integrate Indian cultural practices such as yoga, spirituality and an emphasis on social interdependence including support groups for families. (Greene, 2021). However, more research is required to understand these programmes in the Indian context in the rehabilitation facilities, especially in the context of women addicts, who are usually underserved and disproportionately stigmatized (Kermode et al., 2012).

The Big Picture Project

The aim of 'The Big Picture' project was to understand the lived experience of young Assamese people around risk, recovery and resilience with regard to substance misuse and develop a model of pathways to recovery. Its goal is to check for possible transferability of the model to a wider range of contexts, increase knowledge, enhance the voice of young people, and inform practice through impacting policy and promoting public awareness. The developed model enhances psycho-socio-cultural insights into the experience of risk and recovery, and informs prevention and treatment for youth substance misuse in Assam. This is the first model of its kind and an important public health resource (Madill et al., 2023).

The project took place between September 2018 and February 2022, with researchers from the University of Leeds and University of Brighton UK, supporting the main activities in Assam through the project partner organisations MIND India, Nirmaan Rehabilitation Centre, and Hope Foundation Rehabilitation Center. Both the centres are residential rehabilitation facilities that has been started with the aim of treating individuals suffering from chemical dependence such as drug addiction and alcoholism. They are run by experienced professionals in the field of substance abuse prevention and they are supported by volunteers who are recovering from addictions and gave been maintaining sobriety. They focus not only on the patient but also supports the families too.

The bedrock of The Big Picture was the use of psychosocial visual participatory methods involving photo-led interviews which centralizes the lived experience of our participants. We generated rich information through interviewing total of 30 young people. Fifteen high school students aged 15–18 years (7 males; 8 females) took part and explored with us during interview how they had successfully resisted substance use despite experiencing a high-risk environment such as friends and/or family using addictive substances (excluding tobacco) (Hugh-Jones et al., in press). A further 15 young Assamese people (11 males; 4 females) aged 19–24 years provided detailed information about their journey to recover from SUD. It is this latter group on which we focus in this chapter because their interviews allowed the development of a multiroute, multidirectional pathways to recovery model of three phases: Recreational Use, Addiction (Relaxed, Chaotic, Strategic) and Supported Recovery (Madill et al., 2023). Our participants also collaborated with us to create posters and films to convey their experiences, Most of the recruitment of participants for the project was referral from the two rehabilitation centres who were part of the project, some were referred by MIND India and through word of mouth.

Pathways to Recovery Model: Summary and Practitioner Reflections

We describe the rigorous and systematic way in which we generated our pathways to recovery model in a previous publication (Madill et al., 2023). In short, this entailed a thematic analysis (Braun & Clarke, 2006) in which each transcript was analysed independently by two researchers who discussed and came to an agreement about their findings. These agreed upon analyses were then integrated into a model through discussion with the wider research team. The posited model was then reviewed by a mental health professional and senior rehabilitation practitioner and his team in Assam. This led to some refinements to the model including, for example, an additional pathway from 'strategic self-management' to 'abstinence'. Finally, four original participants—two men and two women—were invited to test the model to see if they could trace their own journey through its pathways. This test was successful and led to a further refinement through the suggestion by one that the path between 'in recovery' and 'abstinence' should be two-way.

We now provide a summary of our pathways to recovery model and offer reflections on it from the perspective of an experienced mental health practitioner working in the context of northeast India (i.e., the first author Dr Sangeeta Goswami). While exposition requires us to work through the phases sequentially, we try not to lose the multiroute and multidirectional nature of the model as is illustrated in Fig. 8.1.

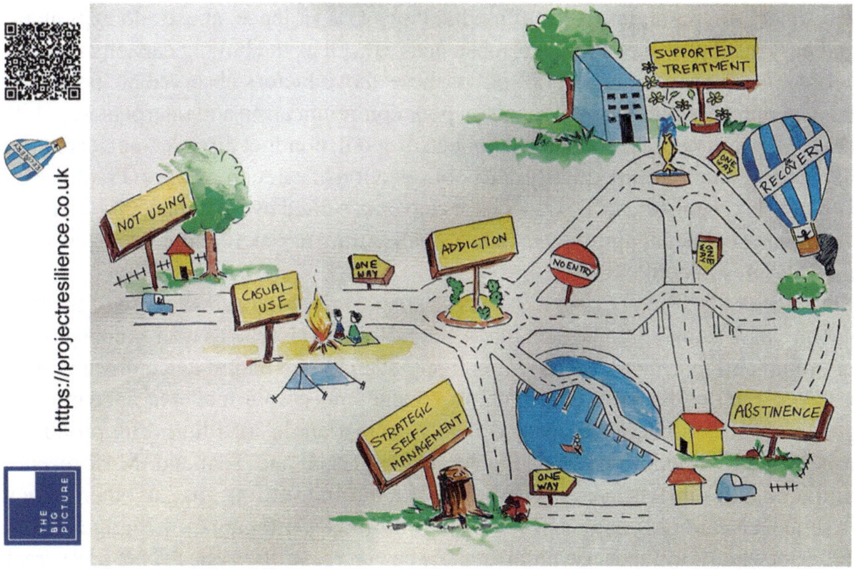

Fig. 8.1 Pathways to Recovery. Non-commercial license https://licensing.leeds.ac.uk/product/pathways-to-recovery-model-of-substance-use-disorder-youthassam-comics-type-images-and-animations

Phase 1: Recreational Use

In the phase of Recreational Use, participants had the opportunity to cycle between two stages: that of 'not using' and of 'casual use' (Fig. 8.1). Importantly, it was not apparent often that a transition had occurred into the phase of Addiction until an individual experienced difficulty getting hold of their needed substance(s).

Substance use is one of the leading causes of death and disability adjusted life years and affects the lives of individuals, families, and society at the large. There are multifarious factors associated with initiation of substance misuse including biological, psychological, behavioural and sociocultural milieu in which the individual lives. Gururaj et al. (2016) report that SUD is prevalent in 22.4% of the Indian adult population and is 2.5 times more common in men than women. Thirteen percent of those abusing substances are children and adolescents, (Katoki et al., 2016), with only 5% of those under 20 years old seeking treatment (National Survey on Extent, Pattern and Trends of Drug Abuse in India. United Nations Office on Drugs and Crime, 2004). The most common substances abused by young people apart from tobacco, are alcohol, cannabis and opioids, with initiation typically between 13 and 15 years (Dhawan et al., 2016). This shows the trend towards decrease in the entry age of young people into substance misuse.

Guwahati, Assam was initially an agrarian society but with rapid change brought about by urbanization, there is a rapid change in the geo-socio-scenario. Some of the critical concerns which acts as vulnerability factors as far as youth is concerned are increasing economic disparity, regional economic unbalance, lack of equal opportunity, unemployment, influence of media, impact of violence, abuse and exploitation and easy availability of addictive substances as well as the buying capacity of young people. As a practitioner, the fall-out of these above factors observed are poor anger management, poor coping mechanism, poor communication and interpersonal skills, negative peer pressure, school and college dropout, conduct disorder, anxiety, stress, depression, suicide vulnerability and poor selection of career pathways (Practitioner's clinical observation). Similar risk factors have been cited by Mackinzie M Bachand in "Familial, social, and individual factors contributing to risk for adolescent substance use" (Whitesell et al., 2013).

Traditionally, locally prepared liquors are prevalent in the social life of the tribal peoples of Assam (e.g., rice beer like Apong, Ruhi and Haria) as well as consumption of opium and marijuana because it is freely available in nature and cultivated in the villages. Gradually, substance such as cocaine and heroin made an appearance as geographical boundaries expanded the 'golden triangle' of illicit drug production was formed, including parts of Burma, China, Laos, and Thailand. Most recently, initiation into substance use is commonly via 'huffing sniffing glue' or other solvents in school children as young as 9 years old followed by smoking from the age of about 14 years when substance use unfortunately can increase often due to peer pressure. In fact, in Guwahati, the largest urban area in Assam, peer influence, 'fun,' and curiosity are key reasons reported for substance use, with highest rates among middle-school children (Goswami, 2015).

The overall economic growth in Assam and other northeast states like Mizoram, Nagaland, Arunachal Pradesh, Meghalaya, Manipur have changed the social scenario too. The influence and impact of urbanisation and easy flow of money have led to a change in the lifestyle of people. The peer pressure of upkeeping a certain lifestyle is not only seen with the children but also with the parents as parenting style has shifted from authoritative or democratic towards permissive and laissez-faire. This led to more spending power and buying capacity in the hands of young people. One the other hand, late adolescence and early adulthood can bring academic pressure, competition in employment, and increased family responsibilities and associated family disharmony, feelings of financial, emotional, and life opportunity deprivation which, alongside negative peer pressure can lead some young people to substance misuse. And those most vulnerable to addiction include children with a family history of substance use and/or those with emotional and behavioural problems (Mahanta et al., 2016). Some, however, demonstrate resilience even when at high risk of SUD, and conversation with some young people in the clinic setting, revealed that they did not want to experiment with substances because they had seen their siblings, other family members, and peers suffering from withdrawal symptoms and struggling to recover. Some were even reticent to try cigarettes due to childhood memories of being hugged by their father smelling of cigarette smoke and making them feel suffocated.

Phase 2: Addiction (Relaxed, Chaotic, Strategic)

The second phase, Addiction, can be conceptualised as a kind of negative event horizon from which there is no return to the phase of Recreational Use per se. Addiction consists of three possible sub-phases: Relaxed Addiction, Chaotic Addiction, and Strategic Addiction.

Relaxed Addiction. At first, there may be no motivation to quit because the substance(s) of addiction are available and the positives of using substances are perceived generally to outweigh the negatives. Here the young person is reasonably happy to live in the stage 'in addiction' because it does not cause them a problem and may indeed bring perceived benefits such as peer acceptance.

Various forms of addictive substances such as cannabis, opium, opiates and cough syrups are abused in northeast India, with tobacco and alcohol abuse very high in some states (Mahanta et al., 2016). Most often, it has been observed that there is no motivation to quit because the substance(s) of addiction are available and the positives of using substances are perceived generally to outweigh the negatives. This is seen particularly during the formative period of life, when boys and girls start to use substances to fit in with peers, by dint of general inquisitiveness, and growing-up with the norm of substance use in their family and wider community. With regard to the latter, for example, in rural areas, homemade alcoholic drinks are used by parents and elders in social functions without inhibition and in which contexts many young people to try alcoholic drinks. They continue in tolerable doses, some graduating to commercially available alcoholic drinks, and gradually becoming habitual drinkers.

Children of parents with SUD are at increased risk for abuse or neglect, physical problems, poor behavioural or impulse control, poor emotional regulation, conduct or oppositional disorders, poorer academic performance, psychiatric problems such as depression or anxiety, and substance abuse (Daley, 2013). The risk of substance abuse is relatively higher among those who had never been to school and more common in those from a joint family when compared to others. Though not found to be statistically significant, substance use is more common in case of deaths of both parents. This may be again due to lack of family support and to be 'forced' into adulthood before they are ready (Duara et al., 2021). Most importantly, easy access to substances and available pocket money apart from other factors make youth and adolescent boys and girls vulnerable to slip into relaxed addiction.

Chaotic Addiction. There is the possibility that an individual shows Chaotic Addiction, cycling between the stages of 'in addiction' and 'abstinence' because the needed substances or not available and/or because there is an attempt to quit on one's own (Fig. 8.1).

As part of the Indian socio-economic and cultural context, parents are entrusted with supporting their children at least until they are financially independent (Sinha, 1995). In turn, children have responsibility to respect their parents' position and expectations (Hofstede, 2011; Sinha, 1995). This can be a double-edged sword. Young people feel responsible for meeting social expectations to look after elderly parents and helping them financially, since they raised them and paid for their education and this may come be in conflict with the young person pursing their own personal goals.

For example, a young Nepalese man of 32 years from Mizoram was brought to the clinic by a relative because he had started abusing marijuana and alcohol. From a humble background, his father had died while he was in the final year of college, and he had to take up a job immediately and support his mother. The pressure of work and lack of contact with friends led him to feel exhausted and frustrated and he had turned to substances. At the same time, he did not neglect work but was aware that his efficiency was declining and that, to meet his responsibilities, he needed to improve. However, he found it impossible to quit on his own and got stuck in Chaotic Addiction cycling between the stages of being 'in addiction' and mere 'abstinence' that never reached true recovery. Hence, he sought help from his family who then reached out to mental health professionals.

In Chaotic Addiction, the tendency is to think that they do not need external help. This may be due to lack of knowledge about the effects of withdrawal and feeling that seeking help is a sign of weakness and poor will power. Attempts at recovery, but which results in episodes of mere 'abstinence' include removing substances from their home and vicinity, looking for a steady job, avoiding drug taking peers, and avoiding personal triggers.

Strategic Addiction. These is also a possibility that an individual shows Strategic Addiction and this can be very hard to spot and it takes its toll on well-meaning family and friends. In Strategic Addiction, there is another kind cycling: that is, between the stages of 'in addiction' and 'strategic self-management' (Fig. 8.1). What can be so difficult about this sub-phase is that, although it looks like a real effort to quit, the person addicted has no intension of doing so and, instead, engages with interventions—particularly medical substitution therapy—in order to sustain their habits and to mollify other people.

There is a thin line between Chaotic Addiction and Strategic Addiction and both sub-phases bear heavily on family and friends. Many studies and reports document adverse effects of SUD on individual family members and on the family system (Daley, 2013). This includes high relationship distress, tension and conflict related to the SUD. While in the stage 'in addiction', the young person may express many negative emotions such as anger, frustration, anxiety, fear, worry, depression and may act out through violence towards family members. Other destructive behaviours include selling household items and stealing, or borrowing money with no real intension of return, to buy the required substances. This can create fear, despair and shame throughout the family.

SUD impacts the social functioning of the individual and becomes a burden for society as well. Social problems associated with SUD include unemployment, inability to maintain a job, criminal behaviours, vulnerability to exploitation and crime, incarceration, HIV transmission due to drug injecting and high-risk sexual behaviours—all of which create dependency on the family. The focus of rehabilitation is usually for men suffering from SUD and there is little residential support for women in addiction. This may be due to the greater social taboo and social expectation attached to how women should act. For example, a few young women aged between 20–30 years who came to the clinic, mentioned that, although like their brothers, they smoked weed and consumed alcohol they kept this knowledge from their parents because, as women, they would receive a more negative response. This anticipation of strong judgement stops women from seeking help and getting the support they need from family and society as a whole.

It has been observed that families of drug users are often characterized by parental substance abuse, parental disharmony, parental aggression, and poor attachment between parent and child leading to poor interpersonal relationships and less emotional support available for many young people with SUD. Thus, the family system itself can become a hindrance against recovery. Further complicating the issue of substance abuse, psychiatric disorders are prevalent in people with SUD. For example, it has been found that antisocial personality disorder and borderline personality disorder are especially comorbid with SUD (Mirin et al., 1991). Though this holds true, it is to be noted that young people with SUD and with no personality disorder, can demonstrate destructive manipulation to secure family resources to support their addiction while in the sub-phase Strategic Addiction. Specifically, mostly unknown to their family, they cycle between the stages of 'in addiction' and 'strategic self-management' to support their habit. Strategic self-management imitates real intention to quit but is used by the young person to sustain themselves when, for example, they do not have the money to purchase substances or when their substance of choice is unavailable. A major strategy widely available in northeast India is to leverage family hope that they will recover by engaging with the medical intervention of Oral Substitution Therapy (OST). The young person with SUD may undergo OST scores of times unsuccessfully before their family is able to understand that they are being manipulated into supporting the addition and misdirecting their resources.

In summary, there are three possible sub-phases of Addiction: Relaxed Addiction, Chaotic Addiction, and Strategic Addiction. It is essential to understanding the sub-phase in which a young person is at any moment because that provides insight into the young person's motivation with regard to substances and viable, and non-viable, approaches to intervention. Families can benefit from mutual support organisations such as Al-Anon or Nar-Anon which provide opportunities to learn from others affected by SUD. These services have started in Guwahati a decade ago, who also extends their services to the families too. However, these services are few and far between in Assam and needs to be expanded. These support groups are helpful to reduce the emotional burden on the family, allowing members to focus on their own lives and the wellbeing of each other while their family member with SUD is undergoing treatment.

Phase 3: Supported Recovery

Real change can occur when an individual moves in the phase of Supported Recovery. This involves engaging meaningfully with the stage 'supported treatment' and subsequently, if fortunate, progressing to the stage 'in recovery' (Fig. 8.1). A central feature of this transition is acceptance of the support needed to quit. However, despite engaging with meaningful treatment, there is the possibility of relapsing to 'in addiction' before being 'in recovery' or after a period of being 'in recovery', directly or via 'abstinence' defined merely as an interlude of not using the substance of addiction (Fig. 8.1).

Even though phase 3 involves the idea of *supported* recovery, most substance users do not engage with this willingly, at least at first. Many will have tried to quit on their own unsuccessfully through, what we have identified above as Chaotic Addiction, and been disheartened. Many will also have utilised the pretence of engaging in recovery through Strategic Addiction and be cynical and nihilistic towards recovery opportunities. However, for the fortunate, the time will come when the young person is ready to grapple sincerely with what is required to begin the true journey to recovery, understanding that they cannot do this alone.

Entering Supported Recovery usually requires persistence from family and in the direction of professional services that are realistic in not promising a quick fix. This most likely means a quality residential facility with staff who understand the life-long effort required. As well as dealing with physical withdrawal, Support Recovery helps the young person with SUD create a new approach to life that mitigates the need for substances and distance from drug using context. Hence, rehabilitation facilities in Assam involve medical and psychiatric interventions but, importantly, alongside a structured routine of activities including yoga, meditation, and group discussion. There is a need to develop effective group psychological interventions for young people with SUD in the context of northeast India. One such intervention in recent times (2023) is MiCBT: an evidence-based therapy approach using core principles of Cognitive Behavioural Therapy through mindfulness-based exposure practices that directly challenge schematic beliefs. This has been piloted at MIND India, Guwahati by Ms Sandamita Choudhury, Consultant of MIND India and Founder of Spreeha Wellness Centre) with promising results. Further exploration will provide evidence based data, which will help to establish MiCBT as an alternative group therapy in the rehabilitation centres.

Supported Recovery is difficult to sustain and there is always a risk of relapsing back into the stage 'in addiction' before reaching the stage 'in recovery' and, sadly, even after some of years after. For example, in the clinic, some addicts in recovery mention that they find it difficult to keep on track when they return home from residential rehabilitation because they re-enter a social context which includes still using peers. This highlights the importance of integrating fully with a recovery community focused on the goal of staying clean and providing alternative, meaningful activities. Quality rehabilitation facilities enable integration with appropriate community support, but there is a need for better medical and professional psychosocial follow up after a residential rehabilitation period.

The importance of community approaches to rehabilitation of young people with SUD has been recognised for some time given their resource efficiencies and the inclusion in the healing process of family and neighbourhood, often severely impacted by the drug misuse of members (Tripathi & Lal, 1999). However, although understandably, many people are suspicious of people known to be in recovery from substance addiction and, for example, are unwilling to offer them employment. Hence, as part of their recovery journey, some addicts in recovery support themselves to reintegrate into society by demonstrating their sincerity and reliability through volunteering and, for some, eventually gaining employment in the rehabilitation sector. Understanding this need, similar programmes and initiatives have been taken in other states to mitigate substance use which is a serious issue. For example, in 2022, one of the efforts taken by Government of Punjab was to train counsellors working under Directorate of Health & Family Welfare, National Health Mission on counselling skills and mental health with special reference to alcohol and substance use disorders and on how to support addicts, recovering addicts and their family members. The technical support for this project was provided by MIND India, Guwahati, Assam and ECHO India, New Delhi.

For many, this is a path that provides them new meaning and purpose in life and a way of giving value to the community as they stabilise a lifestyle of sobriety. Although rehabilitation work is extremely valuable, wider training is required in employability skills, vocational skills, and general life skills to enable addicts in recovering to reintegrate into society. Such training increases 'psychological capital' comprising the positive psychological resources of hope, self-efficacy, resilience, and optimism. "Research shows that psychological capital can be a predictor of substance abuse with a significant negative relationship between psychological capital and relapse tendency (e.g., Krasikova et al., 2015; Zeng & Wei, 2023).

What Next?

The Ministry of Social Justice and Empowerment, Government of India, introduced the Minimum Standards of Care in the field of Addiction Treatment / Prevention since 1987. This includes prevention efforts, creating awareness, early identification, treatment and rehabilitation, sustained follow-up care, and also involving and mobilising the community. The scheme provides financial assistance to support NGOs to offer treatment of addiction and provide composite or integrated services for the rehabilitation of substance dependent people. It aims for 'whole person recovery' and has guidelines for the structure and functioning of these centres.

Regular assessment of these centres is important to check that guidelines are being implemented effectively and that the objectives of the centre are being met (Tripathi & Ambekar, 2009). Based on these prescribed standards, in September 2022 the Ministry of Social Justice and Empowerment, Government of Assam, compiled guidelines to regulate rehabilitation and de-addiction centres and, subsequently, to monitor their functioning (Government of Assam, 2022). Following this action, an appropriate Standard Operating Procedure has been developed for the rehabilitation centres which is however, yet to be finalised.

The Big Picture project, some of the outcomes of which have been described above, has therefore been timely in providing evidence-based information to support state policy in the region. We outline the following major policy-related implications of our work on psychosocial interventions for substance abuse.

First, *investment in family and community education and peer-to-peer support* is likely an economical and effective strategy for preventing youth SUD and enabling rehabilitation. Positive support systems are one of the foremost requirements for recovery from addiction and there is a significant positive association between perceived friendship quality and resilience. Specific actions include government investment in: (i) community education on substance abuse prevention and rehabilitation pathways; (ii) family support programmes to address the impact of SUD on the family system; and, (iii) peer advisors within school and colleges who can educate and support other young people to avoid, or to see help in relation to, addictive substances.

Second, *financial support is needed from the government for setting-up high-quality rehabilitation centres.* Interventions are best geared towards encouraging a young person to accept support to quit. Effective interventions, including medical treatment, require also long-term psychosocial support to have the best chance of sustaining sobriety. Although providing a valuable service, many personnel in private rehabilitation facilities and providing long term support are volunteer addicts in recovery without adequate training. Specific actions include: (i) working with medical professionals to integrate long-term psychosocial support in a package of care and to avoid reliance on short-term, medical-only treatment; (ii) building on current policy for alcohol and substance use rehabilitation centres so that there is a high standard of service delivery and accountability; and, (iii) ensuring the monitoring of compliance with standards of care, including the training of rehabilitation personnel and their continuing professional development.

Third, *investment in women's rehabilitation* is needed due to the immense stigma women experience, even when in recovery, and will have the additional potential benefit of contributing to the well-being of their current and future children. Specific actions include: (i) acknowledging the need for women-only rehabilitation facilities and encouraging these through preferential start-up grants; and, (ii) implementing recommendations of the Assam State Report of the National Mental Health Survey (Pathak et al., 2017) to work closely with addiction rehabilitation services to decreasing stigma and encourage help-seeking through better public awareness.

Conclusion

In Assam, people with SUD and associated mental health challenges are often stigmatized and lack adequate support from families, government aid and society at large. As an educational tool, the pathways to recovery model, described and reflected on here, has the potential to challenge myths about SUD, enhance the effectiveness of SUD management, and act as a prevention measure by increasing awareness of the pitfalls amongst youth. With government investment, sustained recovery from SUD can be envisioned for young people with appropriate support from their family, rehabilitation facilities, medical professionals, voluntary sector, and community. We suggest that key policy developments to enhance recovery from SUD to the benefit of all should include: (i) investment in family and community education and peer-to-peer support; (ii) financial support for setting-up high-quality rehabilitation centres; and, (iii) investment in women's rehabilitation. Future research may include a trial of the effectiveness of our pathways to recovery education package and extending our understanding of the pathways to long term recovery from SUD in Assam.

Acknowledgements This work was funded by the UK Economic and Social Research Council and the Arts and Humanities Research Council award number ES/S00047X/1. Approval was obtained from the Ethics Committee of the LGB Regional Institute of Mental Health, Assam and from the Ethics Committee of the School of Psychology, University of Leeds, UK. We thank, in particular, Dr Raginie Duara who was the Research Fellow on the project and Mr Ratul Dey of Nirmaan Rehabilitation Facility for facilitating so expertly participant recruitment to the project. Further information can be found at https://projectresilience.co.uk/ and intervention materials downloaded for free from https://licensing.leeds.ac.uk/product/pathways-to-recovery-model-of-substance-use-disorder-youthassam-comics-type-images-and-animations. The data that support the findings of this study are openly available in ReShare at https://reshare.ukdataservice.ac.uk/855418/.

References

Braun, V., & Clarke, V. (2006). Using thematic analysis in psychology. *Qualitative Research in Psychology, 3*(2), 77–101. https://doi.org/10.1191/1478088706qp063oa

Chermack, S. T., Stoltenberg, S. F., Fuller, B. E., & Blow, F. C. (2000). Gender differences in the development of substance-related problems: The impact history of alcoholism, family history of violence and childhood conduct problems. *Journal of Studies of Alcohol, 61*, 845–852.

Chesang, R. K. (2013). Drug abuse among the youth in Kenya. *International Journal of Scientific and Technology Research, 2*(6), 126–213.

Child Protection and Child Rights. (2008). Vulnerable Children Affected by Substance Abuse. Childline 1098, http://www.childlineindia.org.in/children-affected-by-substance-abuse.htm

Cooke, P., Duara, R., & Madill, A. (2022). 'The Big Picture': Participatory video as a tool for developing community-led approaches to substance use disorder in Assam. *Journal of Applied Arts & Health, 13*(2), 179–193. https://doi.org/10.1386/jaah_00099_1

Daley, D. C. (2013). Family and social aspects of substance use disorders and treatment. *Journal of Food and Drug Analysis, 21*(4), S73–S76.

Dhawan, A., Pattanayak, R., Chopra, A., Tikoo, V., & Kumar, R. (2016). Injection drug use among children and adolescents in India: Ringing the alarm bells. *Indian Journal of Psychiatry, 58*(4), 387–393. https://doi.org/10.4103/0019-5545.196701

Duara, R., Hugh-Jones, S., & Madill, A. (2021). Forced adulthood': An aspect of 'quarterlife crisis' suffered by young English and Assamese adults. *Qualitative Studies, 6*(1), 11–37.

Duara, R., Chowdhury, D., Dey, R., Goswami, S., & Madill, A. (2022). Using co-created visually-informed community mental health education in low-and-middle-income-countries: Case study of youth substance misuse in Assam India. *Health Expectations, 25*(4), 1930–1944. https://onlinelibrary.wiley.com/doi/10.1111/hex.13550

Goswami, H. (2015). Substance abuse among youths at Guwahati City, Assam (India): Major instigator and socio-demographic factors. *International Education & Research Journal, 1(4). Retrieved from* https://ierj.in/journal/index.php/ierj/article/view/35

Government of Assam. (2022, September 29). Regarding implementation of decisions of the meeting held on 3/09/2022; Chaired by the Hon'ble Minister, Department of Social Justice & Empowerment, Assam Beltola, Guwahatl-28; No. DSJE(G) 65/2022/3.

Graber, R., Duara, R., Hugh-Jones, S., Goswami, S., Chowdhury, D., & Madill, A. (in press). Resilience for recovery to substance addiction in Assam, India: Lived experience insights from a photo-led interview study. *Journal of Community and Applied Social Psychology.*

Gautham, M. S., Gururaj, G., Varghese, M., Benegal, V., Rao, G. N., Kokane, A., Chavan, B. S., Dalal, P. K., Ram, D., Pathak, K., Singh, R. K. L., Singh, L. K., Sharma, P., Saha, P. K., Ramasubramanian, C., Mehta, R. Y., & Shibukumar, T. M. (2020). The national mental health survey of India (2016): Prevalence, socio-demographic correlates and treatment gap of mental morbidity. *International Journal of Social Psychiatry, 66* (4), 361–372. https://doi.org/10.1177%2F0020764020907941

Greene, D. (2021). Revisiting 12-step approaches: An evidence-based perspective. In W. M., Meil & J. A., Mills (Eds.), *Addictions: Diagnosis and Treatment. IntechOpen,* https://doi.org/10.5772/intechopen.95985

Gururaj, G., Varghese, M., Benegal, V., Rao, G. N., Pathak, K., Singh, L. K., Mehta, R. Y., Ram, D., Shibukumar, T. M., Kokane, A., Lenin Singh, R. K., Chavan, B. S., Sharma, P., Ramasubramanian, C., Dalal, P. K., Saha, P. K., Deuri, S. P., Giri, A. K., Kavishvar, A. B., Sinha, V. K., Thavody, J., Chatterji, R., Akoijam, B. S., Das, S., Kashyap, A., Ragavan, V. S., Singh, S. K., Misra, R., & NMHS collaborators group. (2016). National MentalHealth Survey of India, 2015–2016: Prevalence, patterns and outcomes. Bengaluru, NationalInstitute of Mental Health and Neuro Sciences, NIMHANS Publication No. 129, 2016.

Hofstede, G. (2011). Dimensionalizing cultures: The Hofstede model in context. *Online Readings in Psychology and Culture, 2* (1), 2307–0919. https://indianmhs.nimhans.ac.in/phase1/Docs/statereports/Assam-NMHS-Report.pdf

Hugh-Jones, S., Graber, R., Goswami, S., & Madill, A. (online). What protects at-risk young people in India from using and abusing substances? A photo-led study of lived experience. *Journal of Adolescent Research*. https://doi.org/10.1177/07435584241231376

Juyal, R., Bansal, R., Kishore, S., Negi, K. S., Chandra, R., & Semwal, J. (2006). Substance use among inter college students in district Dehradun. *Indian Journal of Community Medicine, 31*(4), 252–254.

Katoki, K., Bhagabaty, S. M., & Kalita, M. (2016). Silhouette of substance abuse amongst an adolescent sample group from urban slums of Guwahati metro, North East India. *International Journal of Medical Research and Health Sciences, 5*(3), 1–8.

Kavita Barkakoty, Assam, (2021, December 27). *Scheme of Assistance for the Prevention of Alcoholism and Substance (Drugs) Abuse for the State of Assam.* https://informatics.nic.in/news/1389#:~:text=10%20Dec%202021%20Guwahati%20%3A%20Drugs,Director%20General%20%2D%20Narcotics%20Control%20Bureau), (https://socialwelfare.assam.gov.in/frontimpotentdata/scheme-of-assistance-for-the-prevention-of-alcoholism-and-substance-drugs-abuse)

Kermode, M., Songput, C. H., Sono, C. Z., Jamir, T. N., & Devine, A. (2012). Meeting the needs of women who use drugs and alcohol in North-east India: A challenge for HIV prevention services. *BMC Public Health, 12*, 825. https://doi.org/10.1186/1471-2458-12-825

Krasikova, D. V., Lester, P. B., & Harms, P. D. (2015). Effects of psychological capital on mental health and substance abuse. *Journal of Leadership and Organizational Studies, 22*(3), 280–291. https://doi.org/10.1177/1548051815585853

Luthar, S. S. (2003). *The culture of affluence: Psychological costs of material wealth, society for research in child development 2003*, https://doi.org/10.1046/j.1467-8624.2003.00625.x

Luthans, F., & Larson, M. (2006). Potential added value of psychological capital in predicting work attitudes. *Journal of Leadership & Organizational Studies, 13*(1), 1–27.

Madill, A., Duara, R., Goswami, S., Graber, R., & Hugh-Jones, S. (2023). Pathways to recovery model of youth substance misuse in Assam India. *Health Expectations, 26*(1), 318–328. https://doi.org/10.1111/hex.13658

Mahanta, B., Mohapatra, P. K., Phukan, N., & Mahanta, J. (2016). Alcohol use among school-going adolescent boys and girls in an industrial town of Assam India. *Journal of Psychiatry, 58*, 157–163.

Merwin, D. S. (2003). *Emotional empathy and reasons for living in substance-using college students.* A thesis presented to the faculty of the Department of Psychology East Tennessee State University; In partial fulfilment of the requirements for the degree Masters of Arts in Psychology.

Mirin, S. M., Weiss, R. D., Griffin, M. L., & Michael, J. L. (1991). Psychopathology in drug abusers and their families. *Comprehensive Psychiatry, 32*, 36–51.

National Survey on the Extent, Pattern and Trends of Drug Abuse in India (Book on 08.05.2019.cdr, 2004).

Pathak, K., Deuri, S. P., Gogoi, V., et al. (2017). Assam State Report, National Mental Health Survey, (2015–16). LGBRIMH, http://indianmhs.nimhans.ac.in/Docs/statereports/Assam-NMHS-Report.pdf

Perumbilly, S. A., & Anderson, S. A. (2017). Indian perspectives on treating substance use disorders. *Alcoholism Treatment Quarterly, 35*(3), 298–314. https://doi.org/10.1080/07347324.2017.1322433

Stockings, E., Hall, W. D., Lynskey, M., Morley, K. I., Reavley, N., Strang, J., et al. (2016). Prevention, early intervention, harm reduction, and treatment of substance use in young people. *Lancet Psychiatry, 3*, 280–296.

Sinha, S. R. (1995). Childrearing practices relevant for the growth of dependency and competence in children. *Child Development within Culturally Structured Environments*, 105–135.

Tripathi, B. M., & Lal, R. (1999). Substance abuse in children and adolescents. *Indian Journal of Pediatrics, 66*, 569–575.

Tripathi, B. M. & Ambekar, A. (2009). Minimum standards of care for the Government deaddiction centres. National Drug Dependence Treatment Centre, All India Institute of Medical Sciences.
Tripathi, R., Singh, S., Sarkar, S., Lal, R., & Balhara, Y. P. S. (2021). Pathway to care in co-occurring disorder and substance use disorder: An exploratory, cross-sectional study from India. *Advances in Dual Diagnosis, 14*(1), 20–32. https://doi.org/10.1108/ADD-10-2020-0023
United Nations Office on Drugs and Crime. (2004). *National Survey on Extent, Pattern and Trends of Drug Abuse in India.* https://www.unodc.org/pdf/india/presentations/india_national_survey_2004.pdf
Whitesell, M., Bachand, A., Peel, J., & Brown, M. (2013). Familial, social, and individual factors contributing to risk for adolescent substance use. *Journal of Addiction, 2013*, 579310. https://doi.org/10.1155/2013/579310. Epub 2013 Mar 20. PMID: 24826363; PMCID: PMC4008086.
Word Health Organisation. (2012, June). *Working with street children: A training package on substance use and sexual and reproductive health including HIV-AIDS (Technical Document).* At https://www.who.int/publications/i/item/working-with-street-children-a-training-package-on-substance-use-sexual-and-reproductive-health-including-hiv-aids
Zeng, X., & Wei, B. (2023). The relationship between the psychological capital of male individuals with drug abuse and relapse tendency: A moderated mediation model. *Current Psychology, 42*, 10334–10343. https://doi.org/10.1007/s12144-021-02325-y

Sangeeta Goswami is a trailblazer in the field of Counselling Psychology in North East India, particularly in Assam, founding the region's first independent counselling clinic, MIND India, Institute of Positive Mental Health & Research in 2006. Her 28 years of experience focus on mental health awareness and research, with two specialized counselling skills courses developed to address regional needs. Her efforts significantly enhance mental health education, earning her the Distinguished Service Award as Psychologist 2021 from AHPI. This accolade underscores her profound impact on enhancing mental health services and resources in Assam and beyond.

Anna Madill is Chair in Qualitative Inquiry in the School of Psychology at the University of Leeds UK. She is the School Internationalisation Lead and former acting Head of the School. She specialises in qualitative research methods with a particular interest in visual methods and her research is broadly in the area of well-being. She is a Fellow of the British Psychological Society and Fellow of the Academy of Social Sciences. She Co-Founded and Chaired (2008–11) the British Psychological Society Qualitative Methods in Psychology Section. Extended information about her research projects can be found at University of Leeds Project Resilience—People, Systems, Places.

Chapter 9
Embedding Psychosocial Support in Youth Suicide Prevention: Suicide Prevention Implementation Research IniTiative (SPIRIT) Program, Gujarat, India

Nikhil Jain, Isha Lohumi, and Soumitra Pathare

The SPIRIT program is a multilevel community-based integrated model that addresses psychological and social aspects of suicide risk. It focuses on identifying and supporting individuals displaying suicidal behaviour, enhancing resilience, and providing support through its varied interventions. The Youth Aware of Mental Health (YAM) is part of the SPIRIT program, which was implemented in 47 public schools in rural Gujarat, reaching 2,474 students aged 14–16 by certified instructors from the local community. Its success lies in its culturally sensitive, community-driven approach, leveraging local psychosocial networks. The findings highlight the effectiveness of the YAM program in addressing mental health challenges, supporting at-risk adolescents, and promoting well-being through psychosocial approaches. By addressing psychological and social determinants of suicide risk, SPIRIT offers a scalable model for youth suicide prevention, particularly in low-resource settings.

N. Jain (✉)
Indian Law Society, Pune, India
e-mail: nikhil@cmhlp.org

I. Lohumi
Indian Law Society, Pune, India

S. Pathare
Indian Law Society, Pune, India

U. Vindhya (ed.), *Psychosocial Interventions for Social Issues in Contemporary India*,
https://doi.org/10.1007/978-981-96-6553-2_9

Youth Suicide from an Indian Perspective

Adolescence is a period of rapid changes encompassing physical, social, emotional, cognitive, and intellectual development (Balaji et al., 2023; Senapati et al., 2024). These changes are often intensified by societal norms and inequalities, leading to stressful situations manifesting as mental health issues, including self-harm and suicidal behaviour (Aggarwal et al., 2020; Balaji et al., 2023). Suicidal behaviour in youth is rooted in a complex interaction between personal characteristics, formative experiences due to various life events, and a wider sociocultural context (Mueller et al., 2021). These multifaceted factors interact across various levels of a person's ecosystem spanning across individual, proximal, and distal ecological dimensions and evolve throughout their lifespan, predisposing them to suicide risk (Senapati et al., 2024). In the Indian context, these issues are pertinent, considering that suicide rates among Indian youth (15–29 years) are among the highest in the world (Balaji et al., 2023) and are the leading cause of death in this age group (WHO, 2021). According to the World Health Organization, the suicide rate among young Indian males is twice the global rate while among young Indian females, it is about six times the global rate (WHO, 2021). Given the high prevalence of suicide, addressing youth suicide in India becomes a priority focus area for intervention.

India's societal structure, diverse cultural norms, complexities such as relationship issues, caste affiliations, gender-based discrimination and societal expectations, coupled with fear of social exclusion and shame, underscores the intricate societal pressures faced by youth (Arun & Chavan, 2009; Bhosle et al., 2015; Sidhartha & Jena, 2006; Verma et al., 2021). The pressures to succeed, crucial for identity development and socioeconomic progress, can cause feelings of alienation and increase the risk of suicidal behaviour. This pressure is evident in the career pursuit of Indian youth, where conventional career paths like engineering, medicine or administrative services are highly sought after and often are seen as the only pathways to "successful life" as per existing social norms. However, this pursuit comes with immense pressure, leading many students to spiral into persistent anxiety and depression and, in tragic cases, self-harm or take their own lives. The gravity of the issue among Indian students is highlighted by the fact that suicides among students rose by 68.78% between 2011 and 2022 according to the report on suicide deaths published by the National Crime Report Bureau (NCRB, 2012, 2023).

Harrowing cases of student suicide reported across different levels ranging from medical, engineering and administrative services aspirants appearing in competitive examinations, to students enrolled in various premier academic institutions, universities or schools are anyway rife (Chowdhury, 2024; Jaiswal, 2024). These cases are often worse off among the youth from marginalized groups as seen vividly in the past few years (Moizee, 2023). The inherent stereotyping, discrimination, and harassment, reveal the deep-rooted social inequalities in such academic settings exacerbated by various individual-level vulnerabilities among students from poor economic backgrounds, sexual minorities, inadequate linguistic skills or being first-generation learners influencing their identities and self-worth and amplifying the risk of suicide (Moizee, 2023; Mungekar, 2023).

Another contemporary challenge contributing to suicidal behaviour is the increased affordability and accessibility of internet services (Sedgwick et al., 2019). Though technical advancements have been fruitful in increasing access and connectivity, rampant use of social networking sites, social media platforms, online gaming, gambling and digital technology have emerged as new risk factors for suicidal behaviour (Sedgwick et al., 2019). Mediating mechanisms include gaming addiction, online risky behaviour, body dysmorphia, cyber victimization, and cyberbullying intensified by the preexisting vulnerabilities among youth (John et al., 2018; Sinha et al., 2021; Tsui & Cheng, 2021). Social contagion effects can be detrimental when self-harming behaviour is modelled, normalized, and reinforced in media depictions that perceive maladaptive self-injurious behaviour as an effective coping strategy (Khasawneh et al., 2020).

The conventional biomedical model primarily relies on medication-based interventions for the treatment of psychiatric disorders, but it may not be sufficient on its own (Engel, 2012). In contrast, the psychosocial approach acknowledges the limitations and emphasizes the significance of addressing the psychological and social factors associated with suicide risk. It posits various risk factors such as deficit in emotional regulation, maladaptive personal coping strategies, inadequate problem-solving skills, and the adverse dynamics of the social environment, including family, peers, culture, and socioeconomic challenges (Gray & Otto, 2001). By addressing these immediate aspects of individual-level risk conditions within their social context, psychosocial interventions offer a comprehensive approach to suicide prevention by recognizing the intricate interplay between individual psychological factors and social determinants. Strategies aimed at promoting social connections, reducing the stigma surrounding mental health, and encouraging help-seeking behaviours have demonstrated promising results in reducing suicidal tendencies (Balaji et al., 2023; Naslund & Deng, 2021; Ratnayake & Hyde, 2019). By enhancing a supportive social environment and empowering individuals to seek help, the psychosocial approach addresses both the immediate and underlying factors contributing to suicide risk.

To enhance the effectiveness of suicide prevention efforts, it is essential, therefore, to adopt an integrated approach that combines pharmacological treatments with psychosocial interventions. This comprehensive approach acknowledges the importance of both biological and psychosocial factors in understanding and preventing suicide and provides an integrated framework for addressing both the psychological and social aspects of mental health.

Theoretical Underpinnings of Psychosocial Approach for Youth Suicide Prevention

Various theories and models have endeavoured to explain the complexity of suicidal behaviour that are equally applicable to youth. Durkheim's sociological theory of suicide first articulated in 1897, continues to be a foundational concept in the study of suicide. This theory emphasizes the crucial role of social integration and regulation in shaping suicide research, highlighting the relevance and importance of Durkheim's insights more than a century after their introduction (Durkheim, 2005; Kushner & Sterk, 2005). Building on this, further developments such as Shneidman's concept of psychological pain (Tossani, 2013) and Joiner's interpersonal theory of suicide (IPTS) (Stewart et al., 2017), have underscored the importance of addressing subjective experiences and the necessity for psychosocial interventions to alleviate feelings of burdensomeness, thwarted belongingness, and the capability for attempting suicide (O'Connor & Kirtley, 2018). IPTs have explained the protective role of perceived social network support against psychological distress and suicidal behaviours, distinguishing between emotional, instrumental, informational, and social support.

Ecological models, including Bronfenbrenner's Ecological Systems Theory (Eriksson et al., 2018), Zayas' Eco-developmental Model (Gulbas et al., 2015), and Cramer and Kapusta's Social-Ecological Suicide Prevention Model (SESPM) (Cramer & Kapusta, 2017) also postulate the integrated approach considering both general and population-specific risk and protective factors. Emphasizing the importance of contextual factors in shaping individual susceptibilities to suicidal risk, these models accentuate the critical role of the system of relationships forming one's environment, from immediate settings like family, peers and school (microsystem) to broader societal and cultural influences (macrosystem), necessitating a multi-level approach to interventions (Cramer & Kapusta, 2017). Various theoretical approaches are constantly evolving and being refined over time to understand different complexities linked with suicidal behaviour. The recent developments in this regard point towards multifactorial causation and thus underscore the need for interventions following a broader framework of psychosocial approach.

Various theories of suicidal behaviour with an "ideation-to-action" framework, call for a differential, though synergistic intervention approach to address the diverse pathways and risk factors associated with suicidal behaviour (Klonsky et al., 2021). Drawing from this theoretical perspective, the proposed national suicide prevention strategy (Ministry of Health and Family Welfare, 2022) incorporates a combination of universal, selective, and targeted interventions, with a specific approach tailored to the context, scope, and current state of suicide risk. The universal interventions have the widest scope, aiming to address the broader social, cultural, and systemic factors that influence suicide risk within the general population. These programs focus on removing barriers to care, enhancing mental health literacy, increasing access to support services, and strengthening protective processes like social connectedness and adaptive coping skills.

Complementing the universal approach, the selective interventions are tailored to address the specific needs of various high-risk groups, such as youth, elderly, or agrarian communities. These targeted programs account for the unique vulnerabilities and predispositions of these populations, involving collaborative efforts across sectors like education, healthcare, and local governance structures (Bunney et al., 2002). Finally, the targeted interventions focus on providing individualized, evidence-based care and support for those already experiencing suicidal ideation or behaviours. These programs leverage clinical expertise and community-based resources to deliver timely, tailored interventions that address the complex interplay of factors contributing to suicidal crises (Bunney et al., 2002).

Effective implementation of this multi-tiered approach requires extensive adaptations and sustained collaborations across various systems and stakeholders, ensuring cultural congruence and leveraging existing community resources and infrastructure for long-term sustainability and impact.

Suicide Prevention Implementation Research Initiative (SPIRIT) Program—A Case Study for an Embedded Psychosocial Approach to Youth Suicide Prevention

The Suicide Prevention and Implementation Research Initiative (SPIRIT), consisted of targeted interventions based on an approach that integrates psychosocial support into various tenets of suicide prevention interventions (Pathare et al., 2020). The program was conceptualised and implemented by a consortium of researchers across academic institutions from India (Centre for Mental Health Law and Policy, Pune and SNEHA, Chennai), Bangladesh (Bangladesh Centre for Communication Programs) and the Netherlands (Trimbos Instituut). Designed as a cluster-randomized trial, the SPIRIT trial has used mixed methods to evaluate the implementation, effectiveness, and costs of an integrated suicide prevention programme. Through its multi-faceted approach, the integrated interventions aim to address the complex nature of suicide across the lifespan including adolescence and early to late adulthood period (Pathare et al., 2020). It consists of three integrated interventions detailed as follows-

- **School-based intervention (Youth Aware of Mental Health)**—This intervention consists of a universal mental health promotion programme in schools within intervention villages aimed at preventing depression, reducing suicidal ideation, and promoting mental health among students in grade 9 who are between 14 and 16 years of age.
- **Community storage of pesticides**—This intervention consists of establishing community storage boxes placed in the Village Council office premises or at a central location. Each farming household is offered a locker at this facility free of charge and the family is encouraged to store all pesticides in this box. A trained attendant (facility manager) was stationed at the community storage facility and will document the use of the boxes on a day-to-day basis.

- **Community health worker (CHW) training in identification, support, and referral of persons with suicidal risk and behaviour**—This intervention consists of training and a follow-up programme for CHWs in the intervention villages to identify people at risk of self-harm and suicide and to support and refer such persons to appropriate local services. The training is based on the World Health Organization Mental Health Action Programme (mhGAP), Self-harm/Suicide module, initially designed to be used by medical practitioners in low-income and middle-income countries.

The interventions selected for the SPIRIT program are evidence-based and align with the recommendations of the World Health Organization for effective suicide prevention strategies (WHO, 2014). These recommendations emphasize three key areas: restricting access to means for suicide, enhancing coping skills among young people to manage daily life stressors, and early identification and management of individuals at risk of suicide, with ongoing follow-up to ensure continuity of care. By incorporating these WHO recommendations, the SPIRIT program aimed to implement a comprehensive and evidence-based approach to suicide prevention in the Mehsana district of Gujarat, India tailored to the specific social and cultural context of the community.

Following a rigorous, multi-faceted formative assessment process, involving a combination of quantitative needs surveys and in-depth, qualitative discussions with a diverse array of stakeholders—including community members, local leaders, subject matter experts, and policymakers. This collaborative approach allowed the team to gain invaluable, nuanced insights into the unique needs, perspectives, and existing resources within the community. These insights were then systematically leveraged to carefully tailor the intervention, ensuring it resonated with the community's values, preferences, and infrastructure. This iterative process continued throughout the implementation phase, allowing the program to dynamically evolve by deeply embedding the project within the social and cultural fabric of the community. This ensured the intervention's relevance, acceptability, and ultimately, its effectiveness in addressing the suicide prevention efforts.

This chapter provides a comprehensive overview of the Youth Aware of Mental Health (YAM) program, focusing on its adaptation and implementation. It details the contextual modifications made to fit the local environment and highlights the strategies employed to engage and educate the youth.

School-Based Training Program: Youth Aware of Mental Health (YAM)

YAM is a mental health promotion and universal suicide prevention program for young people. The findings from the SEYLE study highlight the effectiveness of the YAM program in reducing mental health issues like depression and the risk of suicidal ideation in the European context positioning it as a universal prevention program (Wasserman et al., 2012). Structured around a 5-h workshop spread over three weeks, YAM consists of interactive sessions that allow young people to understand mental health and its related challenges. The program is delivered through role-plays, discussions, and educational materials, aiming to empower young people by developing their skills in problem-solving and emotional regulation and encouraging positive behaviours and attitudes towards mental health issues (Wasserman et al., 2018).

The program adopts a youth-centric approach that engages participants, making the learning process both relatable and impactful (Lindow et al., 2020). The program's opening session focuses on exploring mental health issues, identifying signs and symptoms of stress and crisis, reducing stigma, and promoting coping mechanisms and help-seeking behaviour thus promoting mental health literacy. It also emphasises that mental health problems can emerge from day-to-day challenges. This foundational knowledge empowers adolescents to take proactive steps towards managing their mental well-being. This also promotes a supportive network for adolescents grappling with mental health challenges and enhances their understanding of how to provide support or seek help by dispelling myths about mental health issues.

YAM strategically uses supporting materials such as dilemma cards, booklets, and posters to enhance the learning experience and ensure retention of the program's key messages. Each participant receives a booklet covering crucial themes such as mental health awareness, self-help advice, understanding stress and crisis, recognizing signs of depression and suicidal thoughts, ways to help a friend in distress and guidance on seeking help. Additionally, a series of six posters is displayed in the classroom to reinforce the content and is left after the final session for later use by the youth.

Dilemma cards enhance decision-making activities by providing structured scenarios that encourage adolescents to practice responding to challenging situations. Each card presents a relatable dilemma, prompting participants to pause, reflect on their emotions, and consider how feelings influence their decisions. This process builds self-awareness, linking cognitive perceptions with emotions and helping participants recognize that some decisions are healthier than others. Adolescents actively engage in experiential learning, connecting procedural and conditional knowledge to real-life applications. The cards complement role-play sessions by offering context-specific scenarios, building emotional reflection, and enhancing problem-solving skills. Additionally, the role-plays and activities are carefully customized to address the challenges and situations relevant to the adolescents' social context, enabling them to practice problem-solving and coping skills in a supportive environment.

The final session aims to help participants process their emotions and reinforce cognitive processes through reflective exercises. It is tailored to the needs of the specific group of youth, considering their questions and concerns, and serves as a summary of what they have learned during the length of the program.

Features of the YAM Program

YAM focuses on how different people feel, the possible reasons for their actions, and thus enable to understand what kinds of support one might need in each situation. YAM facilitators are trained to promote dialogue, serve as mediators, and refrain from providing solution or imposing their own beliefs while engaging with young people. The program offers young people conversation and skills to think about if they encounter mental health issues in their daily lives, as opposed to attempting to modify their way of life. The core dimensions of the YAM program are discussed below:

a. ***Development of Practical Skills.*** YAM focuses on developing practical skills such as emotional understanding and regulation, coping mechanisms, and problem-solving through group activities like solving dilemmas and role-plays. This approach allows young people to explore various challenges encountered in daily life situations, find and propose solutions learning from different perspectives of their peers. The program provides a safe space for navigating these challenging scenarios, which were covered across various sections of the program including sudden trauma, domestic violence aftermath, school dropout due to discrimination, bullying, parental divorce, relationship issues, academic failure, parental unemployment, financial debts, and other stressful situations.

Furthermore, YAM helps young people recognize the importance of seeking support when facing challenges. Other than seeking help from their peers, young people are also provided with a vetted community resources list to reach out to other help-providing services by professionals, youth-centric organisations and psychosocial support services in the communities. This ensures access to resources for professional assistance and guidance when needed. Additionally, this promotes help-seeking from specialists in cases where the individuals are facing crisis and are at higher risk of engaging in self-harm.

b. ***Challenging Traditional Teacher-Student Dynamics.*** One of the key aspects of YAM is its effort to challenge traditional teacher-student dynamics and promote equal participation among young people. Through this approach, the program creates an inclusive and participatory learning environment where every voice is heard and valued. By involving an external facilitator, a judgment-free environment is created that encourages open discussion of issues like academic pressure, bullying, relationship issues, substance abuse, family issues, caste-based discrimination, etc., without fear of repercussions. Such a setting proved especially effective for capturing adolescents' attention, enhancing understanding, retention, and active participation, and allowing them to open up about their challenges and seek possible solutions collectively.
c. ***Empowering Youth and Acknowledging Autonomy and Safe Spaces.*** YAM employs active learning techniques (such as small group work and role-plays) and focuses on situations from real life that are significant to the students and can induce mental health challenges. They are provided with the tools they need

to think about, express, and talk about their stressors and mental health issues through various activities. By positioning youth as experts in their own lives and valuing their insights and experiences, YAM acknowledges their autonomy in discussions about the life events that affect their mental health. This approach is non-judgmental and allows youth to navigate complex emotions and situations without fear of correction, preaching, or criticism. Rather than forcing adolescents to make life adjustments as per existing normative behaviour, YAM equips them with tools to handle these challenges with a logical mindset as they arise in every domain of their lives, nurturing a sense of personal agency and empowerment.

YAM places a strong emphasis on peer interactions and discussions, creating a safe space for youth to share their experiences, challenges, and concerns. Through activities and group discussions, the program promotes peer support, encouraging relationships, empathy, and understanding among youth. By establishing a reliable support system within their peer group and utilizing and promoting the use of psychosocial resources as required, youth are better equipped to navigate the complexities around mental health.

d. ***Recognizing the Influence of Broader Cultural and Societal Factors.*** The YAM program aims to address the youth's immediate environment, including their families, friends, and schools, which plays a crucial role in shaping their mental health. It explores the impact of broader cultural and societal factors on youth mental health, recognizing that these factors can significantly shape an individual's well-being. To address this, YAM contextualizes role plays and discussions that explore family dynamics, peer relationships, and interactions with teachers and school staff. Since the YAM program is associated with the interactions and connections between different microsystems, such as the relationship between the family and school environments, it plays a crucial role in understanding and addressing the complex interplay between different social settings that influence youth mental health. By facilitating open discussions and promoting a participatory approach, the program encourages individuals to seek help when needed within their own social network and community. This also facilitates support-seeking from other conventional approaches such as psychotherapeutic interventions available in their vicinity (mentioned in the community resource list) by breaking the stigma associated with mental health in these low-resource settings.
e. ***Incorporating task sharing for mental health.*** The YAM program adopts a task-sharing approach by training young adults from the community as certified YAM instructors and helpers to deliver the program to youth groups over three weeks. These non-school personnel facilitate peer learning, providing a safe, non-judgmental space for youth to discuss daily life challenges while building trust, respect, and confidentiality.

Instructors undergo a structured 4.5-day YAM Instructor Course, which includes workshops, role-plays, simulations, and debriefings. This training equips them with facilitation skills, youth-centred perspectives, and strategies to manage sensitive topics. Debriefings after practice sessions enable feedback, troubleshooting, and content refinement to improve delivery. By emphasizing an understanding of youth reactions, needs, and the social contexts of stress and crises, the program ensures effective tailoring. Through task sharing, YAM leverages community capacity to deliver impactful, youth-focused mental health interventions.

Adaptation

The adaptation process for the YAM program was carried out to align with the theoretical bases, optimizing for differences in modality, and ensuring that processes like logistics, engagement, building rapport and trust, and safety are preserved (Wu et al., 2023). The program was adapted in collaboration with the experts from the MHiM and Karolinska Institute, Sweden in a structured manner (*Youth Aware of Mental Health*). Aside from language-related adjustments, the program's adaptations mostly involved adding more culturally relevant activities and examples to each of its sections based on a series of consultations with the experts from MHiM.

The other consultations of the program involved various stakeholders including parents, teachers, school administrators, and representatives from Civil Society Organizations. They were consulted for gathering feedback on program feasibility and acceptability in the rural Indian context. These experts were selected owing to their experience working or engaging with young people across multiple domains. Stakeholders were consulted on the various elements of the program such as intervention tools like slides, posters, roleplays, booklets, program content, language, delivery methodology, style, trainers, and related logistics. These consultations were done explicitly in the context of the rural and public school setup. Additionally, this engagement allowed reviewing potential adaptations to match the cultural norms.

In addition to expert consultations, focus group discussions were conducted with youth participants during the pilot where they shared their reflections on ease of understanding and experiences while receiving the sessions. Insights and experiences gathered from these consultations and discussions were integrated into the program. The focus was on enhancing the quality of content, process, and delivery of the sessions. This iterative improvement process was essential for building the abilities of the implementation team as YAM trainers and supervisors, ensuring a continuous enhancement of the program.

Implementation

Following the Instructor Course, trained instructors handled the delivery of the YAM program in the study schools. A pair of instructors and helpers conducted sessions to ensure the effective delivery of all program components. The intervention was implemented in smaller groups of 20–25 participants to support quality and facilitate engagement. Instructors were closely supervised to ensure adherence to program guidelines and effective communication of the content. This monitoring helped maintain consistency and fidelity to the program's principles and methods. It also involved tracking participant engagement and attendance to assess the program's reach and effectiveness. Instructors were trained to identify participants in need of additional support and to refer them to appropriate mental health professionals or support services. This referral pathway ensured that participants received the necessary help to address their mental health needs.

Evaluation

The study was initiated in June 2018 as a baseline period while the interventions were rolled out in the villages in a staggered manner from November 2019 to January 2022 followed by a 12-month follow-up phase till January 2023. The main objectives of the parent study were to detect the reduction in suicidal behaviour between the intervention and control arms. While for sub-objectives such as the YAM program the evaluation consisted of mixed methods guided by the RE-AIM implementation framework. Quantitative measures included the Suicidal Ideation Attributes Scale (SIDAS) and the Patient Health Questionnaire-9 (PHQ-9) to assess changes in suicidal ideation and depression symptoms among young adolescents across 12 months from the intervention delivery in the school setting. Qualitative assessments included focus group discussions and semi-structured interviews with YAM instructors and participants to gather in-depth insights into the program's acceptability, feasibility, and perceived impact.

Process measures documented the proportion of schools that approached and those that implemented the intervention, as well as the proportion of adolescents who received the YAM program. The YAM program, implemented as part of SPIRIT in collaboration with 47 public schools, successfully reached and trained 2,474 young students aged 14–16 in 9th grade in rural areas of Gujarat, India. Guided by the RE-AIM implementation framework, the program proved considerable reach and elevated levels of acceptability in the school setting. The YAM intervention was delivered as part of a comprehensive, integrated package rather than being researched as a singular strategy. This is following previous research in suicide prevention space that suggests that integrated approaches are often more effective compared to isolated interventions in addressing complex issues like suicide (Ayer et al., 2022; Caine et al., 2018; Decker et al., 2018).

Challenges

Through the implementation of the YAM program, we identified several context-specific challenges that affected its effectiveness. One of the key observations was that YAM is designed as a one-time intervention. While this effectively introduces mental health concepts, the lack of follow-up sessions, boosters, or periodic refreshers limited the opportunity to reinforce the learning over time. This highlighted the need for a multi-point intervention to ensure sustained impact as also highlighted in the findings of the focus group with the instructors on the implementation-related inquiry.

In the case of Indian youth, especially in rural areas, the limited understanding of mental health concepts and limited emotional vocabulary posed a challenge, as they required additional preparatory work to fully engage with the approach and content. Another gap observed was the limited availability of ongoing support and referral pathways for young people after they have received the intervention. Without integrating a mechanism for sustained care within the school ecosystem, the program's long-term impact remained constrained.

Cultural and infrastructural factors also presented challenges. Gender-based restrictions in some schools made it difficult to implement mixed-gender discussions. Additionally, many schools lacked the basic infrastructure, such as sufficient classrooms, to facilitate small group sessions, which are a critical part of YAM's interactive delivery.

Engaging school administrators proved critical, with some scepticism about the program's purpose and content occasionally hindering implementation. This challenge was further amplified by the stigma surrounding mental health, leading some adolescents to hesitate to participate openly due to fears of judgment or ostracism. The program highlighted the complexities of implementing a whole-school approach, particularly within India's diverse education system, which encompasses hierarchical administrative structures from district to block levels and varied school types in rural areas. These barriers underscore the importance of overall buy-in at all administrative levels and addressing stigma across stakeholders to ensure effective integration of mental health initiatives within the school ecosystem.

The COVID-19 pandemic challenged the program's implementation overall in a unique manner. Mobility restrictions imposed due to multiple waves of the pandemic and obstructed academic activities presented unforeseen hurdles. Temporary restrictions were implemented on accessing schools since the sudden increase in workload and pressure from district and school administrations demanded the completion of the curriculum. As a result, the implementation of the program occurred in multiple waves, depending on school availability and permissions.

Additionally, the program faced the challenge of student attrition and dropouts after the first wave of the pandemic, as supported by other research studies (UNFPA, 2020; UNICEF, 2020). This adversely affected the program's overall objective of reaching vulnerable youth, especially during the uncertain times of the pandemic when the mental well-being of young individuals was significantly impacted.

Despite these challenges, the implementation process successfully overcame obstacles through proactive measures, allowing for the completion of the program and providing support to vulnerable youth during trying circumstances.

Conclusion

The YAM program offers a structured model for addressing adolescent mental health, particularly in the context of suicide prevention. Building emotional regulation, problem-solving, and help-seeking behaviours, equips youth to navigate mental health challenges effectively. Its task-sharing approach, which trains non-school personnel to deliver structured interventions, provides a scalable and cost-effective solution, particularly in resource-constrained settings.

The program highlights the importance of integrating mental health promotion into educational systems, leveraging existing structures to reach vulnerable populations. The success of such initiatives relies on policies that allocate resources for mental health training, strengthen referral networks, and build cross-sector collaboration between health, education, and community organizations, with a whole-school approach that integrates mental health into the school environment.

While the conceptual framework of the YAM program is rigorous, its implementation requires further refinement and strengthening surrounding support systems, especially for low-resource settings. Key areas for improvement include establishing sustained support and referral pathways and adapting program content to diverse cultural and contextual settings.

Future research should focus on evaluating the program's effectiveness across varied settings, particularly in rural and underserved areas, and on examining its long-term impact on adolescent mental well-being. Studies on scalability, cost-effectiveness, and the development of sustainable support systems are essential to guide broader implementation and inform evidence-based policy decisions.

References

Aggarwal, S., Patton, G., Bahl, D., Shah, N., Berk, M., & Patel, V. (2020). Explanatory style in youth self-harm: An Indian qualitative study to inform intervention design. *Evidence-Based Mental Health, 23*(3), 100–106.

Arun, P., & Chavan, B. (2009). Stress and suicidal ideas in adolescent students in Chandigarh. *Indian Journal of Medical Sciences, 63*(7), 281–287.

Ayer, L., Nickerson, K., Grumet, J. G., & Hoover, S. (2022). Effective suicide prevention and intervention in schools. In *Youth suicide prevention and intervention: Best practices and policy implications* (pp. 31–40). Springer International Publishing Cham.

Balaji, M., Mandhare, K., Nikhare, K., Shah, A. K., Kanhere, P., Panse, S., Santre, M., Vijayakumar, L., Phillips, M. R., & Pathare, S. (2023). Why young people attempt suicide in India: A qualitative study of vulnerability to action. *SSM-Mental Health, 3*, 100216.

Bhosle, S., Zanjad, N., Dake, M., & Godbole, H. (2015). Deaths due to hanging among adolescents—A 10-year retrospective study. *Journal of Forensic and Legal Medicine, 29*, 30–33.
Bunney, W., Kleinman, A., Pellmar, T., & Goldsmith, S. (2002). *Reducing suicide: A national imperative*. National Academies Press.
Caine, E. D., Reed, J., Hindman, J., & Quinlan, K. (2018). Comprehensive, integrated approaches to suicide prevention: Practical guidance. *Injury Prevention, 24*(Suppl 1), i38–i45.
Chowdhury, K. (2024). Student suicides in Kota's 'coaching factories' point to india's broken education system. *The Diplomat*. https://thediplomat.com/2024/02/student-suicides-in-kotas-coaching-factories-point-to-indias-broken-education-system/
Cramer, R. J., & Kapusta, N. D. (2017). A social-ecological framework of theory, assessment, and prevention of suicide. *Frontiers in Psychology, 8*.
Decker, M. R., Wilcox, H. C., Holliday, C. N., & Webster, D. W. (2018). An integrated public health approach to interpersonal violence and suicide prevention and response. *Public Health Reports, 133*(1_suppl), 65S–79S.
Durkheim, E. (2005). *Suicide: A study in sociology*. Routledge.
Engel, G. L. (2012). The need for a new medical model: A challenge for biomedicine. *Psychodynamic Psychiatry, 40*(3), 377–396.
Eriksson, M., Ghazinour, M., & Hammarström, A. (2018). Different uses of Bronfenbrenner's ecological theory in public mental health research: What is their value for guiding public mental health policy and practice? *Social Theory & Health, 16*, 414–433.
Gray, S., & Otto, M. (2001). Psychosocial approaches to suicide prevention: Applications to patients with bipolar disorder. *The Journal of Clinical Psychiatry, 62*, 56–64.
Gulbas, L. E., Hausmann-Stabile, C., De Luca, S. M., Tyler, T. R., & Zayas, L. H. (2015). An exploratory study of nonsuicidal self-injury and suicidal behaviors in adolescent Latinas. *The American Journal of Orthopsychiatry, 85*(4), 302–314.
Jaiswal, A. (2024). 122 medical student suicides and 1,270 dropouts in past 5 years: NMC. *The Times of India*.
John, A., Glendenning, A. C., Marchant, A., Montgomery, P., Stewart, A., Wood, S., Lloyd, K., & Hawton, K. (2018). Self-harm, suicidal behaviours, and cyberbullying in children and young people: Systematic review. *Journal of Medical Internet Research, 20*, e129.
Khasawneh, A., Madathil, K. C., Dixon, E., Wiśniewski, P., Zinzow, H., & Roth, R. (2020). Examining the self-harm and suicide contagion effects of the blue whale challenge on YouTube and Twitter: Qualitative study. *JMIR Mental Health, 7*(6), e15973.
Klonsky, E. D., Pachkowski, M. C., Shahnaz, A., & May, A. M. (2021). The three-step theory of suicide: Description, evidence, and some useful points of clarification. *Preventive Medicine, 152*(Pt 1), 106549.
Kushner, H. I., & Sterk, C. E. (2005). The limits of social capital: Durkheim, suicide, and social cohesion. *American Journal of Public Health, 95*(7), 1139–1143.
Lindow, J. C., Hughes, J. L., South, C., Minhajuddin, A., Gutierrez, L., Bannister, E., Trivedi, M. H., & Byerly, M. J. (2020). The Youth Aware of Mental Health (YAM) intervention: Impact on help-seeking, mental health knowledge, and stigma in US adolescents. *The Journal of Adolescent Health: Official Publication of the Society for Adolescent Medicine, 67*(1), 101.
Ministry of Health and Family Welfare, GOI. (2022). *National suicide prevention strategy*.
Moizee, S. (2023). Why are Dalit students dying by suicide at India's prestigious universities? *The Quint*.
Mueller, A. S., Abrutyn, S., Pescosolido, B., & Diefendorf, S. (2021). The social roots of suicide: Theorizing how the external social world matters to suicide and suicide prevention. *Frontiers in Psychology, 12*, 621569.
Mungekar, B. (2023/2024, March 9). Data on caste-related deaths at educational institutes is telling. *Hindustan Times*.
Naslund, J. A., & Deng, D. (2021). Addressing mental health stigma in low-income and middle-income countries: A new frontier for digital mental health. *Ethics, Medicine, and Public Health, 19*.

NCRB. (2012). *Accidental Deaths & Suicides in India 2011.*
NCRB. (2023). *Accidental Deaths & Suicides In India 2022.*
O'Connor, R. C., & Kirtley, O. J. (2018). The integrated motivational-volitional model of suicidal behaviour. *Philosophical Transactions of the Royal Society of London. Series B, Biological Sciences, 373*(1754), 20170268.
Pathare, S., Shields-Zeeman, L., Vijayakumar, L., Pandit, D., Nardodkar, R., Chatterjee, S., Kalha, J., Krishnamoorthy, S., Jain, N., & Kapoor, A. (2020). Evaluation of the SPIRIT Integrated Suicide Prevention Programme: Study protocol for a cluster-randomised controlled trial in rural Gujarat, India. *Trials, 21*(1), 572.
Ratnayake, P., & Hyde, C. (2019). Mental health literacy, help-seeking behaviour and wellbeing in young people: Implications for practice. *The Educational and Developmental Psychologist, 36*(1), 16–21.
Sedgwick, R., Epstein, S., Dutta, R., & Ougrin, D. (2019). Social media, internet use and suicide attempts in adolescents. *Current Opinion in Psychiatry, 32*(6), 534–541.
Senapati, R. E., Jena, S., Parida, J., Panda, A., Patra, P. K., Pati, S., Kaur, H., & Acharya, S. K. (2024). The patterns, trends and major risk factors of suicide among Indian adolescents-a scoping review. *BMC Psychiatry, 24*(1), 35.
Sidhartha, T., & Jena, S. (2006). Suicidal behaviors in adolescents. *Indian Journal of Pediatrics, 73*(9), 783–788.
Sinha, D., Srivastava, S., Mishra, P. S., & Kumar, P. (2021). Predictors of deliberate self-harm among adolescents: Answers from a cross-sectional study on India. *BMC Psychology, 9*(1), 197.
Stewart, S. M., Eaddy, M., Horton, S. E., Hughes, J., & Kennard, B. (2017). The validity of the interpersonal theory of suicide in adolescence: A review. *Journal of Clinical Child and Adolescent Psychology: The Official Journal for the Society of Clinical Child and Adolescent Psychology, American Psychological Association, Division 53, 46*(3), 437–449.
Tossani, E. (2013). The concept of mental pain. *Psychotherapy and Psychosomatics, 82*(2), 67–73.
Tsui, Y.Y.-Y., & Cheng, C. (2021). Internet gaming disorder, risky online behaviour, and mental health in Hong Kong adolescents: The beneficial role of psychological resilience. *Frontiers in Psychiatry, 12*, 722353.
UNFPA. (2020). *Impact of the COVID-19 pandemic on family planning and ending gender-based violence, female genital mutilation and child marriage.*
UNICEF. (2020, June 11). *COVID-19 may push millions more children into child labour—ILO and UNICEF*
Verma, L., Garg, V. K., & Meena, S. K. (2021). Analysis of medico legal deaths in adolescence: An Autopsy based study at coaching city, Kota. *The Official Publication of Indian Academy of Forensic Medicine, 43*(2), 126–129.
Wasserman, C., Hoven, C. W., Wasserman, D., Carli, V., Sarchiapone, M., Al-Halabí, S., Apter, A., Balazs, J., Bobes, J., & Cosman, D. (2012). Suicide prevention for youth—A mental health awareness program: lessons learned from the Saving and Empowering Young Lives in Europe (SEYLE) intervention study.
Wasserman, C., Postuvan, V., Herta, D., Iosue, M., Värnik, P., & Carli, V. (2018). Interactions between youth and mental health professionals: The Youth Aware of Mental health (YAM) program experience. *PLoS ONE, 13*(2), e0191843.
WHO. (2014). *Preventing suicides: A global imperitive.*
WHO. (2021). Suicide worldwide in 2019: Global health estimates.
Wu, E., Lee, Y. G., Vinogradov, V., Kali, S., Yelkeyev, A., Goddard-Eckrich, D. A., Dasgupta, A., & Hess, L. (2023). Intervention adaptation and implementation method for real-world constraints and using new technologies. *Research on Social Work Practice, 33*(5), 562.
Youth Aware of Mental Health. Retrieved 17 April 2024 from https://www.y-a-m.org/

Nikhil Jain is a medical practitioner and public health researcher specializing in social epidemiology and mental health economics. His areas of interest include community mental health, mental health systems, and suicide prevention implementation science research.

Isha Lohumi, a mental health researcher, works in the Centre for Mental Health Law and Policy (CMHLP) at the Indian Law Society, Pune. She has been involved in many research projects focusing on suicide prevention, implementation sciences, and adolescent mental health.

Soumitra Pathare is a consultant psychiatrist and the Director of the Centre for Mental Health Law and Policy at Indian Law Society Pune. He played a key role in drafting India's Mental Health Care Act, 2017 and the National Mental Health Policy, 2014. which takes a rights-based approach to mental healthcare. He has served as a WHO consultant in many low and middle-income countries (Botswana, Seychelles, Lesotho, Samoa, Vanuatu, Eritrea) assisting them in drafting and implementing mental health legislation and national mental health policy. He is Co-Director of SPIRIT (an implementation research project on suicide prevention in Gujarat funded by NIMH, USA) and PI of CASP (a suicide prevention project in collaboration with Government of Chhattisgarh funded by Mariwala Health Initiative), co-Lead on Outlive (a youth suicide prevention project funded by Comic Relief, UK) and co-Lead on ENGAGE (a suicide prevention gatekeeper training for school teachers implementation research project in Chhattisgarh funded by Grand Challenges Canada) He enjoys travelling, meeting new people and dreams of being a cheese maker one day.

Chapter 10
Psychosocial Intervention for Farmers' Distress in Maharashtra: Study of Users' Satisfaction with Services and Mental Health Awareness in the Community

Sunayana Swain and U. Vindhya

Abstract The magnitude of farmers' suicides in recent decades in India indicates a public health issue of grave concern. underscoring the need for psychosocial support to farmers in distress. This chapter presents the findings of a study that assessed the efficacy of the Vidarbha Psychosocial Support and Care Program (VPSCP) located in Yavatmal district in the state of Maharashtra, the epicentre of farmers' suicides, to alleviate the psychological consequences of agrarian distress and ensure the delivery of mental health care services. Using a quantitative survey method, data were collected on (a) 119 respondents across 27 villages in two blocks of Yavatmal district on their post-intervention clinical status, and their satisfaction with the services provided by VPSCP and (b) two comparative groups of 135 and 132 respondents from the intervention and non-intervention villages respectively to assess their mental health awareness. The findings revealed more than 50% of the community reporting minimal to nil symptoms at the time of the survey; 79% as highly satisfied with the services of VPSCP; and a significant effect of the intervention on fostering awareness about mental health and illness in the intervention villages in comparison to the non-intervention villages. The findings suggest that VPSCP has been largely effective in providing individualized, community-focused services; ensuring early identification of symptoms; establishing and maintaining supportive relationships between the service users and health care workers; and creating mental health awareness for stigma-reduction.

This paper is drawn from an endline assessment study by U. Vindhya and Sunayana Swain, funded by Tata Education and Development Trust [Grant Cost Centre Code: HEA/SBI/TEDT/119], and conducted in 2018.

S. Swain (✉)
School of Public Policy and Governance, Tata Institute of Social Sciences, Hyderabad, India
e-mail: sunayana.swain@tiss.ac.in

U. Vindhya
Independent Researcher, and Former Professor, Tata Institute of Social Sciences, Hyderabad, Telangana, India

U. Vindhya (ed.), *Psychosocial Interventions for Social Issues in Contemporary India*,
https://doi.org/10.1007/978-981-96-6553-2_10

Keyword Agrarian distress · Psychosocial intervention for farmers' suicide · Community health workers · Mental health awareness

Introduction

It is estimated that around 16,000 farmers in India die by suicide per year, making farmers' suicides a public health issue of grave magnitude in recent years (National Crime Records Bureau [NCRB], 2018). In the years between 1995 and 2018, nearly 400,000 farmers have been reported to have died by suicide, which amounts to 48 farmer suicides per day (cited in Kannuri & Jadhav, 2021). According to recent NCRB data, a total of 10,881 persons involved in the farming sector have died by suicide in 2021, out of which 5318 were farmers/cultivators and 5563 were agricultural labourers. This figure accounts for 6.6% of total suicides (1,64,033) in the country (NCRB, 2021).

Furthermore, it is small and marginal farmers that have been found to be disproportionately affected, with the majority belonging to the backward castes (Kannuri & Jadhav, 2021), an overwhelming majority, around 90% of them, being male (Jadhav et al., 2019); and the highest number of suicides seen among cash crop growers, notably cotton farmers (Mitra & Shroff, 2007; Sharma, 2021). The suicide mortality rate among farmers is thus higher than the national suicide rate, and yet, these numbers are still considered as an underestimation of the actual figures (Nagaraj, 2008).

Of the ten top states in India reporting farmers' suicides, Maharashtra in the west with nearly 20% of total farmers' suicides in the country, is ranked the highest on the list followed by states like Karnataka and Andhra Pradesh in the south, and Punjab and Haryana in the north (NCRB, 2019). Within Maharashtra, the region of Vidarbha recorded the maximum number of farmers' suicides with Yavatmal among the 11 districts in the region reporting the highest number between 2001 and 2015 with the suicide mortality rate being 252 farmers' suicides per 10,000 persons registered in 2015 alone (Neelima, 2018). Between 2020 and 2021, Vidarbha region recorded more than 5000 farmers' suicides, contributing to 50% of the deaths in Maharashtra (Deshpande, 2022; Maitra, 2022).

While agrarian distress in the form of drought, floods, and crop failures combined with exploitative land revenue collection has been known to exist since colonial times (Talule, 2021), the neglect of agriculture since the 1980s by the state, followed by the launching of neo-liberal economic policies in the 1990s, further eroding the institutional support to agriculture, are said to be structural factors largely responsible for the phenomenon of farmers' suicides in recent decades (Reddy & Mishra, 2009). Factors such as increasing costs of agricultural production on the one hand, and falling prices of farm commodities on the other, both said to be spin-offs of trade liberalization and corporate globalization policies, combined with inadequate sources of credit, and increased dependence on noninstitutional credit sources such as private moneylenders, and increasing indebtedness of farmers have reportedly led to an agrarian crisis, pushing farmers to the perception that suicide is the only and ultimate solution to their distress (Das, 2011; Deshpande & Arora, 2010; Guha & Das, 2022; Jadhav et al., 2019; Meeta & Rajivlochan, 2006; Merriott, 2017; Vasavi, 2009). In addition to these structural factors, mental health consequences of the agrarian crisis such as alcoholism, depression, and anxiety, have acted as precipitating factors (e.g., Bomble & Lhungdim, 2020), underscoring the need for providing psychosocial support and counselling to farmers in distress (Dongre & Deshmukh, 2012) as well as building a case for strengthening the primary health care services (Pandya et al., 2020).

There have been a few initiatives launched both by the state and non-governmental organizations to address the issue of farmers' suicides in the region. These included, for instance, the Vidarbha Stress and Health Program (known by the acronym VISHRAM), a community-based mental health programme, run by two NGOS, Sangath and Prakriti, from 2013 to 2015, and aimed at the rural community in general in Amravati district of Vidarbha (Shidhaye et al., 2017); and two state-run schemes—the Baliraja Chetana Abhiyan and the Prerna Prakalp Project—introduced in July and October, 2015 respectively as dedicated programmes for alleviating the distress of farmers and reducing farmers' suicides in Vidarbha and Marathwada districts in particular. In addition, there was also the Sukhi Baliraja initiative, introduced by the Tata Trusts in 2008 in six suicide-affected districts of Vidarbha, as a holistic livelihoods strategy, and offering a livelihoods basket including interventions such as—sustainable agriculture, community-based micro-finance, collective agricultural marketing, promoting of poultry, dairy development and fisheries—for sustainable income generation and reducing agrarian distress.

VISHRAM addressed the mental health risk factors (depression and alcohol use disorders) for suicide, by enhancing mental health literacy through a model involving collaboration between three tiers of healthcare providers—village-based community health workers, health counsellors working in primary healthcare centres or rural hospitals, and facility-based general physicians or visiting psychiatrists (Shidhaye et al., 2016). In an impact assessment study of this programme, it was found that its implementation was significantly associated with equitable contact coverage, that is, there was a significant increase in proportion of people with depression seeking treatment, and in mental health literacy, such as the understanding and framing of depression as a mental health problem, and increased help-seeking (Shidhaye et al., 2017).

The Baliraja Chetana Abhiyan, introduced by the state government of Maharashtra aimed at creating awareness among farmers about government sponsored welfare schemes, appointing of nodal officers to supervise implementation of government schemes, setting up of skill development, employment, and entrepreneurship guidance centres, organizing health camps, counselling to minimize stress among farmers, and even conducting mass marriages for their daughters. The Prerna Prakalp Project, on the other hand, was a dedicated mental health service for farmers and entailed working in tandem with the District Mental Health Programme in district and sub-district hospitals in 14 districts in Vidarbha and Marathwada regions, that had high incidence of recorded farmer suicides in the state. The project was aimed at early identification and assessment of farmers and their family members for signs of mental illness, making referrals to district hospitals for further treatment if required, providing counselling services, psychiatric consultations and medicines free of charge, setting up of a helpline by name of *Manobal*, and training of ASHA (Accredited Social Health Activists) workers to help identify those with signs of psychological distress, encourage them to seek treatment, and to connect them to psychiatrists in the district hospitals (Jadhav et al., 2019). Though there have not been any impact evaluation studies of these government programmes, media reports point to limitations such as constant vacancies and inadequate staff, irregular supply of medicines, the sheer distance between the villages and district hospitals, and the additional workload for ASHA workers, that were found to be acting as barriers hampering the functioning and outcomes of the state-run programme (e.g., Barnagarwala, 2018; Wal, 2020).

It is therefore in this context that a multi-pronged intervention called the Vidarbha Psychosocial Support and Care Program (VPSCP) to alleviate the psychological consequences of adverse socio-economic circumstances and ensure the delivery of mental health care services to those in need in Yavatmal district in Maharashtra, was conceived, designed and implemented by the Tata Education and Development Trust. The VPSCP began catering to the farmers' community in Yavatmal district of Vidarbha region in 2016. The authors were commissioned by the Trust to conduct an endline assessment study of the VPSCP, and the present paper draws from this larger project of evaluation of VPSCP services, conducted in September–November 2018. Based on the field visit to know and understand first-hand the implementation and impact of the programme and analysis of the data gathered therein, the paper reports the findings of the quantitative segment of the assessment.[1] In particular, the present paper highlights three specific dimensions of impact of the project: (a) current mental health profile of those identified by VPSCP as people with mental illness (PWMI); (b) users' satisfaction with the services of VPSCP; and (c) levels of awareness in the community about mental health.

Estimates of mental disorders in India point to the enormous magnitude of the problem—about 150 million persons are in need of mental health care (Gururaj et al., 2016). A growing body of research points to the association of mental disorders both as causal and consequential factors with socio-economic vulnerabilities such as poverty and food insufficiency (e.g., Gururaj & Isaac, 2004; Gururaj et al., 2016; Lund et al., 2011; Patel & Kleinman, 2003), urbanization, migration, housing; gender disadvantage, low education, social exclusion and few and scattered forms of social support, loss, trauma and displacement due to disasters and civil violence (e.g., Chandra & Satyanarayana, 2010; Shidhaye & Patel, 2010; Desjarlais et al. 1995). While vulnerable groups report high rates of mental health conditions, resources and services for mental disorders however, are disproportionately low compared to the burden of these disorders (Chatterjee et al., 2009; Kallivayalil & Enara, 2022; Kururvilla & Jacob, 2007; Saxena et al., 2007).

[1] *The qualitative research segment of the project was earlier published as* Vindhya, U., Swain, S., Kapse, P., & Sule, N. (2022). Farmers' suicides and psychosocial intervention. *Psychology and Developing Societies, 34*(1), 104–124.

The psychosocial and economic correlates of mental health, the large mental health burden and the poor resource availability build therefore, a strong case for the adoption of a community mental health approach. Advocates of this model underscore the view that the huge burden of unmet mental health needs cannot be addressed by a mere extension of the existing traditional psychiatric and psychological. Rather, it is visualized as going beyond a treatment-oriented approach and includes vital features such as promotion of well-being, removal of stigma, and providing psychosocial support to those in need (Campbell & Burgess, 2012; Nelson et al., 2001).

Adopting the template of a community mental health approach, the VPSCP aimed to address the widespread agrarian distress in the region through four major objectives and processes: assessment, training, outreach, and multisectoral linkages. The psychosocial support services conceptualized and implemented by VPSCP thus included (a) capacity building of community health workers on provision of psychosocial care and support; (b) identification, making referrals to medical or psychiatric services close by, and follow-up care of people with mental illness (PWMI); (c) community education through awareness-raising programmes for village panchayat members, school and college students about mental health and illness, to break down misconceptions and stigma about mental illness; and (d) multisectoral linkages with state welfare and livelihood support programmes. Table 10.1 shows the range of activities of health and social justice perspectives through its emphasis on and socially and economically disadvantaged populations by making available necessary and humanized health care and support to those in need.

In addition, the VPSCP aimed to collaborate with the Prerna project of the District Mental Health Programme to provide free psychiatric consultations and medicines to PWMI. The range of services provided by VPSCP therefore sought to demonstrate its underlying commitment to public health and social justice perspectives through its emphasis on and socially and economically disadvantaged populations by making available necessary and humanized health care and support to those in need.

From its initiation in 2016 till 2018 when the project drew to a close,[2] VPSCP worked in 64 villages in the two blocks of Yavatmal and Ghatanji in Yavatmal district, considered to be, as mentioned earlier, a high-risk district for farmers' suicide in Maharashtra and indeed in India.

[2] Following the submission of the endline assessment report in December 2018, the VPSCP was given an extension for two more years. However, this paper is confined to the period of 2016–2018 for which the assessment was done.

Table 10.1 Scope of VPSCP, April 2016–March 2018

S.No	Component/sub-component/indicator	
1	**Sensitization and capacity building of stake holders**	**Number**
1.1	No. of ANM[3] trained/sensitized	193
1.2	No. of ASHA[4] trained/sensitized	562
1.3	No. of Awareness/Sensitization programs at Gram Panchayat[5]	342
1.4	No. of members who attended awareness programme at GP level	4004
1.5	No. of schools covered in Awareness program on Mental health	20
1.6	No. of students participated in awareness program on mental health	996
1.7	No. of new household visited to build awareness and identification of PWMI	9148
2	**Identification, referral, treatment, and follow-up care of PWMI**	
2.1	No. of OPD/ Clinic organized (Health Camp)	7
2.2	No. of people participated in Health Camp	251
2.3	No. of people screened for mental illness	23,233
2.4	No. of PWMI identified	1644
2.5	No. of PWMI enrolled in the programme	1106
2.6	No. of clients enrolled on the programme outside catchment	18
2.7	No. of (New) PWMI referred for the Pharmacological Treatment	509
2.8	No. of (New) PWMI received Pharmacological Treatment	223
2.9	No. of Persons enrolled with Severe Mental Disorders	170
2.10	No. of persons enrolled with Common Mental Disorders	553
2.11	No. of person enrolled with Other Mental Disorders (Epilepsy, Mental Retardation, Alcohol)	127
2.12	No. of PWMI undergoing psychosocial intervention	3324
2.13	No. of family members undergoing psychoeducation	3149

Source Tata Education and Research Trust, 2018

[3] ANM refers to Auxiliary Nurse Midwifery, village level female health worker in India.

[4] ASHA refers to Accredited Social Health Activist, community health worker, under National Rural Health Mission, Ministry of Health and Family Welfare, India.

[5] Gram Panchayat refers to formalized local self-governance system at village or small-town level in India.

Table 10.2 Sample size of the present study

	Domain	Sample
1	Post-intervention clinical status of PWMI	119*
2	Satisfaction with VPSCP services	119*
3	Mental health awareness	267**

*$N = 1274$; Using Cochran's Formula with correction, CI = 95%, $p = 0.5$, $e = 0.05$
** $N = 23{,}905$; Using Cochran's Formula with correction, CI = 95%, $p = 0.5$, $e = 0.05$

Method

Sample

1. A representative sample ($n = 119$) was drawn from the larger population of identified PWMI in order to assess their post-intervention clinical status, reasons for discontinuation of the VPSCP services and their satisfaction with VPSCP services.
2. Two comparative groups ($n_1 = 135$; $n_2 = 132$) were drawn from villages where the VPSCP was operational and where it was not in order to assess the impact of VPSCP in creating mental health awareness among the community. The sample size was calculated using the Cochran's formula. However, the collection of data had to be limited to size lesser than the computed size because of the time-bound nature of the project (Table 10.2).

Instruments

Post-intervention clinical status of PWMI. The Primary Health Questionnaire (PHQ-9), a nine-item standardized questionnaire was used for evaluation of the post-intervention clinical status of PWMI and a nine-item schedule to assess the factors contributing to the continuation or discontinuation of treatment by the PWMI.

Users' Satisfaction. A 24-item scale adapted from the *Mental Health Service Satisfaction Scale* (Mayston et al., 2017) and *Verona Service Satisfaction Scale* (Ruggeri & Dall'Agnola, 1993) was used to measure the users' satisfaction with VPSCP services. Four categorical questions in the scale pertained to the user's knowledge regarding the services of VPSCP: (1) the source of information about the programme (2) whether they have availed any services, (3) and if yes, the type of service availed and (4) the ways in which the VPSCP services helped them. The remaining were 20 statements with a 4-point scale ranging from 1 (*Strongly Agree)* to 4 (*Strongly Disagree)* pertaining to the users' satisfaction with lower scores indicating higher satisfaction with the services. The satisfaction of users pertained to the type and quality of services and care provided by VPSCP; perceived impact of the services on psychosocial coping mechanisms; and perceived improvement in functionality and reduction of psychological distress from the perspective of the user.

Mental Health Awareness. For determining the mental health awareness of the sample, a 22-item questionnaire adapted from the *Knowledge, Attitude and Practice Questionnaire for Health Workers (Department of Psychiatry, NIMHANS, Bangalore);* and the *ICMR evaluation study of DMHP* was used. For each correct response (*Yes*), the participant received a score of 1 and a 0 for an incorrect response (*No*). Item numbers 1, 2, 4, 11, 12, 13, 16, 22 were reverse scored. Higher scores indicated high level of mental health awareness.

Location of the Study and Procedure

Yavatmal district is one of the 11 districts in Vidarbha region of the state of Maharashtra and consists of 16 tehsils or revenue blocks and 2137 villages (District Census Handbook, 2011). Declared as a drought-prone area because of erratic and inadequate rainfall, it is regarded as the epicenter of agrarian distress in the country (Fig. 10.1).

The study was conducted in the two blocks—Yavatmal and Ghatanji—of Yavatmal district, wherein the VPSCP intervention programme was implemented. While the intervention was implemented in 64 villages of the two blocks of Yavatmal and Ghatanji, the assessment was carried out in 27 villages—12 in Yavatmal and 15 in Ghatanji, including in four non-intervention villages in Ghatanji block. Five research assistants (two women and three men), recruited for the purpose, all of whom had a postgraduate degree and were fluent speakers of Marathi, the local language, gathered

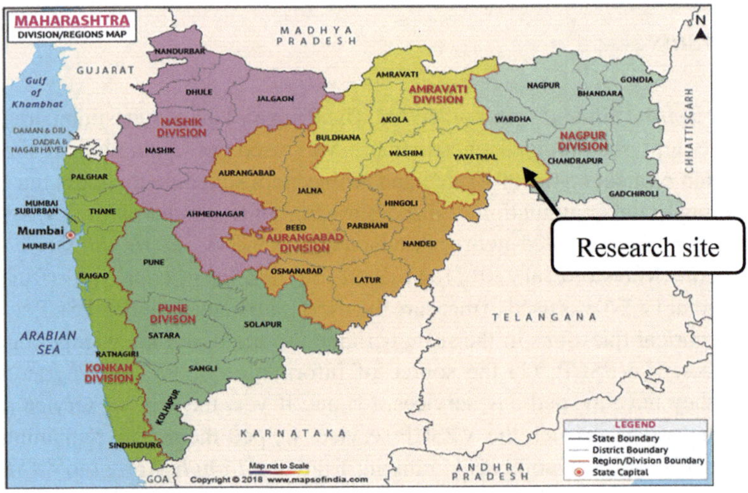

Fig. 10.1 Map of Maharashtra showing the research site. *Source* https://www.mapsofindia.com/maps/maharashtra/regions.html

the quantitative data using the structured interview schedule for socio-demographic data and the questionnaires on satisfaction with the services and awareness about mental health.

Ethical guidelines such as obtaining informed consent, ensuring confidentiality of the responses, anonymity of the study participants and their right to withdraw at any stage of the research process were followed.

A software tool, Statistical Package for Social Sciences (SPSS 19.0) was used to analyse the data.

Findings

Socio-Demographic Characteristics and Post-Intervention Clinical Status of PWMI

A socio-demographic profile of the surveyed sample of 119 PWMI users indicates the following in terms of the categories of age, gender, education, marital status, income and occupation (Table 10.3).

The PHQ-9 was administered on 119 respondents to determine the present clinical status of PWMI. The established norms to determine the clinical status are as follows (Table 10.4).

A frequency analysis of the categories across the respondents revealed that 54.6% of the respondents presented with minimal or no symptoms of depression (Fig. 10.2) at the time of the assessment, indicating that more than half of the representative sample had currently minimal or no symptoms of depression.

Results of the assessment of the post-intervention clinical status of the PWMI revealed that 35% of the respondents indicated that they had discontinued the services due to their recovery which is a positive indicator of the effectiveness of the programme (Fig. 10.3). Another 35% of the respondents reported 'other reasons' such as non-availability of medicine, side effects of the medication, lack of accompanying person to the hospital that led to discontinuation. The government-run Prerna Project, as mentioned earlier, provided free psychiatric medicines to the farmer communities. However, the Project stopped its services in 2017, and the non-availability of free medicines has been cited as one of the biggest factors in the discontinuation with the services. Ten percent of the respondents indicated non-availability of time as a factor, citing inability to afford loss of even a day's work resulting in loss of wages, as the reason for dropping out of the program, underscoring the economic vulnerability of the community. Ten percent of respondents discontinued because they reported not seeing any improvement in the mental health condition of the PWMI. Long distance to the facility was another reason with five percent reporting it as the reason for discontinuation. Given that the government hospital where psychiatrists were available was located at a distance of 60–70 kms from the villages, a visit to the hospital for consultation meant taking off an entire working day, thereby

Table 10.3 Socio-demographic characteristics of PWMI [$N = 119$]

	Characteristics	Classes	Percentage distribution
1	Age (in years)	18–29	31.1
		30–44	31.1
		45–59	27.7
		60+	10.1
2	Sex	Male	58
		Female	42
		Total	100
3	Educational status	Not literate	20.2
		Primary school	37.8
		Secondary school	21.8
		High school	14.3
		College	5.9
4	Monthly household income (in Indian Rupees)	Less than 1000	6.7
		1001–3000	58.8
		3001–5000	26.1
		5001–10,000	7.6
		Above 10,000	0.8
5	Occupation	Farmer	48.7
		Daily wage labourers	47.9
		Unemployed	3.4
6	Marital status	Married	73.1
		Unmarried	13.4
		Widow/Widower	10.1
		Separated	3.4

Table 10.4 Norms for PHQ 9

Score	Depression severity	Comments
1–4	Minimal	Monitor; may not require treatment
5–9	Mild	Use clinical judgment (symptom duration, functional impairment) to determine necessity of treatment
10–14	Moderate	
15–19	Moderately severe	Warrants active treatment with psychotherapy, medications, or combination
20–27	Severe	

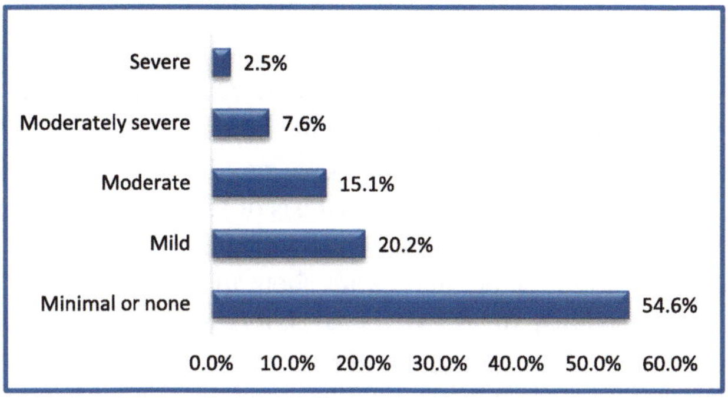

Fig. 10.2 Intensity of symptoms

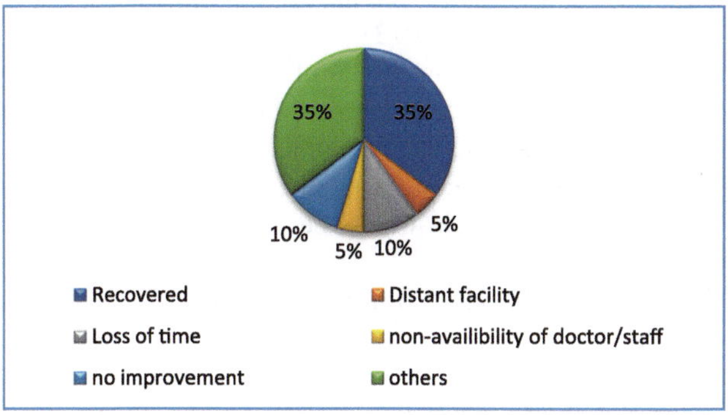

Fig. 10.3 Reasons for discontinuation of services

discouraging the people to access the services. Five percent respondents pointed to the non-availability of doctor/staff as a reason for discontinuation. As part of the District Mental Health Programme (DMHP) there is one psychiatrist posted at the district hospital in Yavatmal who caters to the entire district, making it a huge task for the single mental health professional to fulfill the requirements of the communities. Hence the factor of not able to spare time owing to loss of wage earnings, combined with inaccessibility to adequate healthcare, both due to distance and non-availability of doctor and medicines contributed to the poor help seeking behavior of the people.

Users' Satisfaction with Services

This section presents the results of the survey on satisfaction with VPSCP services conducted to elicit users' satisfaction in three domains: (a) the type of services (b) competencies and attitudes of the staff and (c) perceived impact of these services on the users' functionality and well-being. A 20-item questionnaire was administered across the sample of 119 respondents to determine the levels of satisfaction, along with the following four categorical questions: (a) Source of information about VPSCP; (b) Whether the users received any kind of services from VPSCP; (c) Kind of service availed from VPSCP; and (d) Feedback to the services availed.

Source of information. The frequency analysis of responses to the question from which source they had received information about VPSCP showed that the majority of the respondents i.e. 83.2% became aware about the VPSCP services as a result of the home visits made by the VPSCP counsellors and frontline health workers, making it the most effective strategy of creating awareness about the presence and availability of a service such as VPSCP in the community (Fig. 10.4). The positive role of community health workers serving as peer supporters and caregivers in the community, marking a move away from the role of an 'expert' to that of a catalyst and facilitator, providing information and creating support systems, has been emphasized in earlier literature too (e.g., Davar, 2012).

Type of service received. Out of the 99.3% of respondents who reported receiving some kind of service from VPSCP, the majority of services (76.6%) received referred to the category of provision and supply of medicines (Fig. 10.5).

With 99.3% of respondents having availed some or the other kind of services offered by VPSCP, further analysis was done to understand the responses to the services rendered.

Perceived Benefits of the VPSCP Services. A frequency analysis (Fig. 10.6) done to determine the responses of the people who have received services from VPSCP indicates that the most reported category referred to acquisition of new coping skills (32.8%) with improved ability to function coming a close second (26.1%), followed by emotional relief (14.3%), and clarity in problem solving (12.6%). The other benefits were associated with help received from the VPSCP staff in facilitating hospital visits, and assistance in securing their entitlements and welfare benefits from the government.

Overall satisfaction with VPSCP services. The satisfaction of the users with the VPSCP services was measured on a 4-point rating scale with responses ranging from

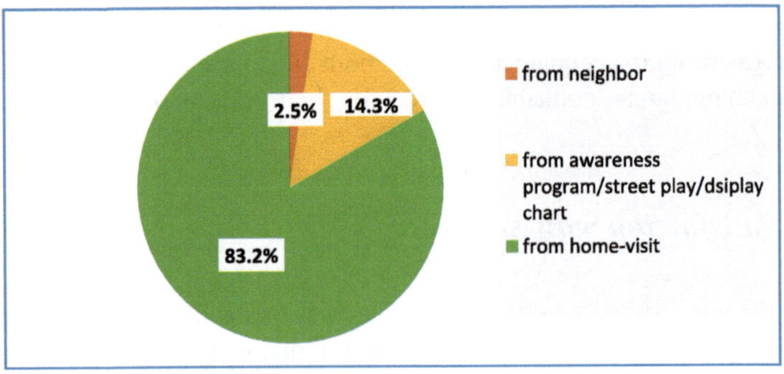

Fig. 10.4 Source of information

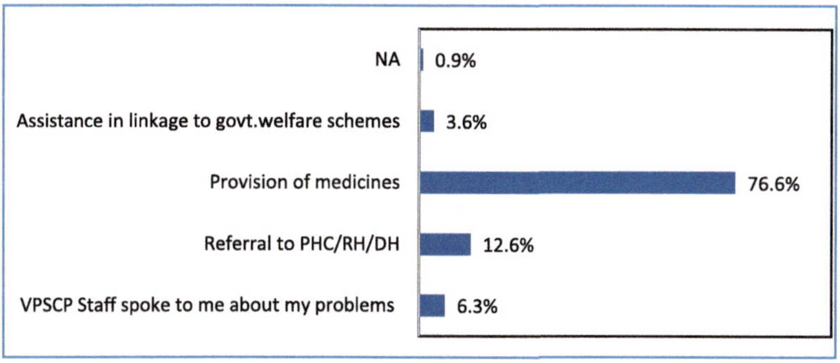

Fig. 10.5 Type of service received from VPSCP

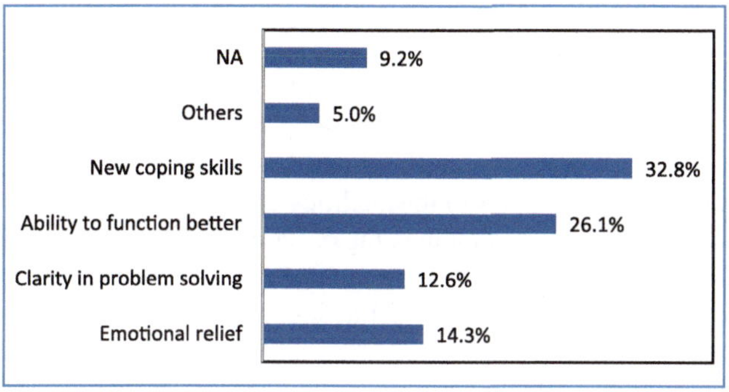

Fig. 10.6 Perceived benefits of VPSCP services

Strongly Agree to Strongly Disagree, with scores ranging between 20–80. Based on the scoring method, higher the score indicated less satisfaction with the services and low score referred to better satisfaction. The following norms were developed with the help of optimal binning (Table 10.5).

The descriptive analysis revealed that mean satisfaction of the users was 36.61 (SD = 7.49), with the mean score being in the highly satisfied category. Based on the norms, a frequency analysis was carried out. The results revealed that 79% of the users were highly satisfied, and 21% were moderately satisfied with the services provided by VPSCP.

Dimensions of Satisfaction of Users. The dimensions of satisfaction related to (a) the skills and attributes of the health workers (VPSCP counselors, frontline health

Table 10.5 Norms for overall satisfaction

Norms	Description
20–40	Highly Satisfied
41–60	Moderately Satisfied
61–80	Less Satisfied

workers), (b) facilities provided by the VPSCP and the associated public health institutions, and (c) the impact of the program as perceived by the users.

Dimension 1—Skills and Attributes. Satisfaction of the users with skills and attributes referred to the competency of the VPSCP staff working on the intervention sites, interpersonal skills such as active listening, and providing relevant support to those coping with psychological distress. In the Satisfaction with VPSCP Services Scale, nine items pertained to measuring the competencies of the VPSCP workers in the intervention sites. The maximum score one user could give was 36 and minimum was 9, wherein higher the score indicated less satisfaction and lower scores implied more satisfaction. Based on the responses, the following norms were evolved where a score between 9–18 was regarded as highly satisfied, 19–27 as moderately satisfied and 28–36 as less satisfied. The mean score on this dimension is 16.95 ($SD = 3.27$). A frequency analysis of the scores showed that 78.2% were highly satisfied on this dimension and 21.8% were moderately satisfied.

Dimension 2—Facilities. This dimension referred to the adequacy of the interface of the VPSCP services with the mental health services provided by the District Hospital such as information sharing, follow up on the treatment plan, referrals to hospitals, and accompanying the families to the hospital. There were six items on the scale that measured the adequacy of the facilities. Hence the maximum one could rate this dimension was 24 with minimum being 6. Based on the responses, the following norms were evolved where a score between 6–12 was regarded as highly satisfied, 13–18 as moderately satisfied and 19–24 as less satisfied. The analysis showed the mean score being 11.49 (SD = 2.39). The percentage of users that rated the adequacy of the facilities as highly satisfied was 74.8% while 25.2% were moderately satisfied.

Dimension 3—Perceived impact of the services. The third dimension is the perceived impact of the VPSCP in totality with reference to reduction in symptoms, decline in relapse rate, better chances of engaging in livelihood activities like farming, manual labor, etc. The dimension has four items with maximum score being 16 and minimum being 4. The norms for this particular dimension were 4–8 being highly satisfied, 9–12 showed moderate satisfaction and 13–18 as highly satisfied, with higher score indicating less satisfaction and less score meant higher satisfaction. The mean score was found to be 7.67 (SD = 2.17). The frequency analysis revealed that 75.6% of the respondents were highly satisfied, 21.8% were moderately satisfied and 2.5% were less satisfied with the perceived impact of the program. The results are depicted graphically in Fig. 10.7.

The ratings of the respondents on the three dimensions are a combination of variety of factors. The multitude of factors that contribute to the quality of the services as perceived by the users are a manifestation of number of variables involved and as in the case of skills and attributes, it can relate to the characteristics of the frontline health workers. Relevant skills of the staff included identifying people with psychosocial distress or mental illnesses, providing counselling and appropriate care, and making referrals if required to the nearest health facility. With majority of the users reporting as being highly satisfied with the skills and attributes dimension, it can be said that the training of the health workers has been effective in setting the stage for building

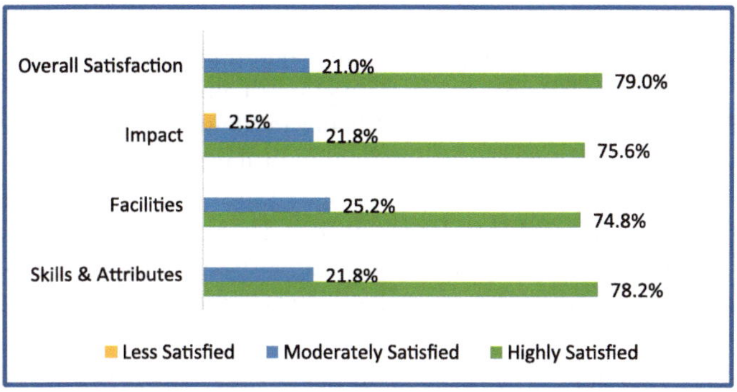

Fig. 10.7 Users' satisfaction with VPSCP services

of rapport and earning the trust of the community members; providing a listening ear to their concerns; and suggesting a plan of action.

The Facilities dimension referred largely to the acessibility to the mental health services of the District Hospital. The VPSCP facilitated the process of referrals, and hospital visits including follow-ups, with the VPSCP providing transportation to the community in case of referrals. It is pertinent to point out in this context that the DHMP set up under the aegis of the National Mental Health Programme (NMHP) of India had been present in the district of Yavatmal prior to the intervention of VPSCP. The DMHP envisaged a decentralized community based approach that aimed at developing effective partnerships and active collaborations between the district mental health team, and various stakeholders such as the primary health care teams, community based organizations, non-governmental organizations, users, family groups and various government departments to deliver a comprehensive and sustainable mental health care service that ensured accountability and focused on the local needs with regard to mental health (Goel, 2011; Murthy, 2011).

However, research evidence in this area has indicated that despite initiatives such as the DMHP, it has belied its initial promise in terms of its functioning, effectiveness and impact (Chatterjee et al., 2009; Jacob, 2001; Murthy, 2011; Shidhaye et al., 2015). Evaluations of the DMHP have shown that the reach of the programme is to a large extent limited in practice with its implementation in only 127 of 640 districts in India and inadequate utilization of funding allocated (e.g., Hans & Sharan, 2021). Reasons for the disappointing performance of the DMHP have been stated to be a 'top-down', 'one size fits all approach' to service delivery, inability to include diverse realities, poor governance, lack of a robust mentoring framework (Shidhaye et al., 2015); ill-paid and overburdened primary health care personnel (Goel, 2011); and disproportionate reliance on psychiatric and psychopharmacological management (Jain & Jadhav, 2009) with minimal engagement with community health workers, psychosocial counselling, access to livelihood and employment generation programs, support groups and family-based interventions (Goel, 2011). Given this context, the role of the VPSCP to bridge the gap to an extent in the district is significant, however modest in scale it might be, compared to the magnitude of the problem.

As for the Impact dimension, the perception of the users was reflected in the individual's prognosis and general well-being in tangible terms like reduction of symptoms, lesser relapse rate, increased ability of the user to engage in productive work and wage-earning. The small percentage of users who reported as being less satisfied with the impact could be perhaps attributed to factors ranging from individual ones such as non-adherence to medication to larger structural constraints such as lack of means to purchase psychiatric medicines. It must be noted here that free medication was provided under Project Prerna till 2017, after which the supply of medicines ceased. Hence, although the VPSCP could facilitate the treatment process through its referrals, it could not help when it came to providing psychiatric medicines free of cost.

Overall, a large percentage of users reported high levels of satisfaction in all the dimensions of VPSCP services, revealing that the program is well-received by the community and the program has effectively succeeded in fulfilling its remedial objective.

Awareness About Mental Health in Intervention and Non-Intervention Villages

Five intervention (V1) and five non-intervention (V2) villages across the blocks of Ghatanji and Yavatmal were selected randomly, with a sample of 135 ($n_1 = 135$) from V1 and a sample of 132 ($n_2 = 132$) from V2 were selected. A socio-demographic profile including age, gender, educational qualification, occupation, monthly income and marital status of the sample of both categories surveyed is presented in Table 10.6.

Based on the responses in the Awareness about Mental Health Scale, the scores of the respondents ranged between 4 to 21. By following optimal binning, the scores were classified into three levels as shown in Table 10.7.

A cross-tabulation was performed to assess the levels of awareness about mental health in the communities of the Intervention and Non-Intervention villages (Fig. 10.8).

It is seen that in the Intervention villages, 76.3% had good awareness about mental health, whereas the sample in Non-intervention villages showed comparatively differential scores with 4.5% revealing poor awareness about mental health, 43.2% showing average levels, and 52.3% with good awareness. In contrast, 76.3% of the sample in the Intervention villages showed high awareness, and 23% average awareness about mental health. To determine the difference in the level of awareness in the community members of the Intervention and Non-Intervention villages, the total score on the Mental Health Awareness Scale was determined and a Student's *t*-Test was done.

Table 10.6 Socio-demographic profile of respondents in intervention and non-intervention villages

S.No	Characteristics	Classes	$N_2 = 267$	
			Intervention ($n_1 = 135$)	Non-Intervention ($n_2 = 132$)
1	Age	15–29	39 (28.9%)	40 (30.3%)
		30–44	50 (37%)	48 (36.4%)
		45–59	35 (25.9%)	28 (21.2%)
		60+	11 (8.1%)	16 (12.1%)
2	Sex	Male	75 (55.6%)	73 (55.3%)
		Female	60 (44.4%)	59 (44.7%)
3	Educational status	Not literate	18 (13.3%)	12 (91.1%)
		Primary school	46 (34.1%)	36 (27.3%)
		Secondary school	35 (25.9%)	53 (40.2%)
		High school	25 (18.5%)	13 (9.8%)
		College	11 (8.1%)	18 (13.6%)
4	Monthly household income	Less than 1000	18 (13.3%)	20 (15.2%)
		1001–3000	75 (55.6%)	86 (65.2%)
		3001–5000	22 (16.3%)	20 (15.2%)
		5001–10,000	12 (8.9%)	5 (3.8%)
		Above 10,000	8 (5.9%)	1 (0.8%)
5	Marital Status	Married	114 (84.4%)	95 (72%)
		Unmarried	18 (13.3%)	32 (24.2%)
		Widow/widower	3 (2.2%)	5 (3.8%)
6	Occupation	Farming	95 (70.4%)	54 (40.9%)
		Others	39 (28.9%)	76 (57.6%)
		Farming & others	1 (0.7%)	2 (1.5%)

Table 10.7 Norms for awareness about mental health

Score range	Level of mental health awareness
0–7	Poor
8–14	Average
15–22	Good

The results showed a statistically significant difference in the mental health awareness scores between the Intervention villages ($M = 15.94$; SD = 2.38) and non-Intervention villages ($M = 14.20$; SD = 3.87, t (265) = 4.53, $p < 0.01$). The differences can be attributed to the outreach initiatives of the VPSCP—street plays, corner meetings, posters and other publicity material—that seem to have had a significant effect on increasing awareness and fostering positive attitudes about mental health in the community.

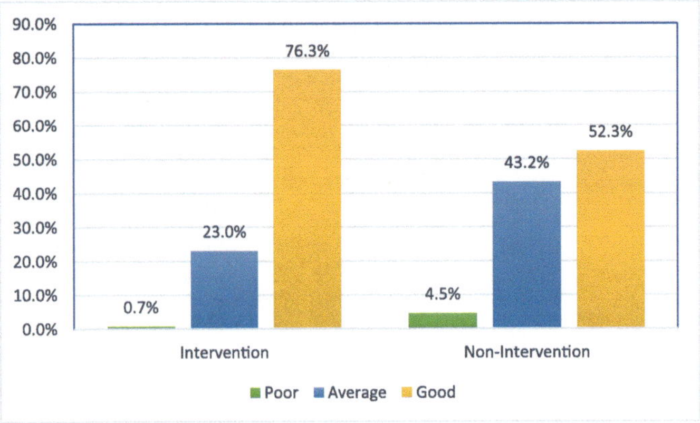

Fig. 10.8 Mental health awareness across Intervention and Non-intervention villages

Significant differences between the two categories of villages—intervention and non-intervention—showed in the following items with the respondents in the intervention villages revealing better awareness about mental health and illness.

- Mental illness is not contagious, and that it is curable
- Mentally ill need support and care from the community and family, should be taken to the nearest health centre for treatment, and that mental health problems can be discussed with a counsellor, and treated by effective and safe drugs
- Excessive alcohol dependence or drug abuse are likely factors leading to mental health problems, and symptoms like irregularity in sleeping patterns and eating habits need to be identified
- Quality of mental well-being depends on ability to meet daily demands of life, the way people value themselves, and on their interpersonal relationships
- Awareness about suicidal ideation, and the understanding that socio-economic factors can be a major contributory factor to mental health problems.

Discussion

Despite the modest reach of the VPSCP intervention, its relevance and usefulness need to be located in the larger context of inadequate availability of comprehensive mental health services and low awareness of mental health and illness in India. Community-based mental health programmes characterised by identification of those in need of mental health care and treatment, psychosocial rehabilitation, follow up, awareness creation, stigma reduction and advocacy, and interventions such as livelihood support have emerged in recent years to address the critical gap in mental health services. Developing community mental health services has been a key recommendation of the WHO (2010) in addition to deinstitutionalization of mental health care and integration of mental health into general health care. The community mental health approach is visualized as going beyond a treatment-oriented approach and includes key aspects such as promotion of well-being, removal of stigma, and providing psychosocial support, and rehabilitation of those in need (Campbell & Burgess, 2012).

As only around 20% of all districts in the country have included mental health services in public primary care facilities, the responsibility of implementation of community-based mental health programs has largely been shouldered so far by NGOs (Balagopal & Kapanee, 2019; Murthy, 2011; Patel & Thara, 2003; Thara et al., 2008). In such a context, the intervention program of VPSCP to a large extent has been effective in providing individualized, community-focused approaches to services; establishing and maintaining supportive relationships between those accessing the services and the health care workers; and creating mental health awareness in order to reduce stigma, and help in early identification of symptoms. As expressed by a community member, "*The people now know to how to look out for symptoms especially if one is suicidal, who to go to in case of emergency, what to do to help each other*" [interview excerpt]. Such views indicate that the VPSCP was to some extent at least effective in creating and facilitating pathways to better help-seeking behaviour in the community. Although it may be speculative to attribute the downward trend, (as depicted in Fig. 10.9) in farmers' suicide in the district in recent years to the VPSCP intervention alone, the graph below does present an optimistic picture.

To reiterate the findings, first, the study showcased the efficacy of a community-based mental health intervention in terms of sustained benefits like improvement in mental health state with minimal or no symptoms in those identified as PWMI. However, the reasons the participants cited as reasons for discontinuation of the VPSCP services—non-availability of medication, long distance to the district hospital, lack of availability of psychiatrist, and sheer inability to spend time in commuting for a consultation (that often meant loss of daily wage earnings), not only dent the impact of an intervention such as the VPSCP, but are also a telling pointer to the limitations of public healthcare planning and delivery of services in our country. Similar findings were reported by a survey conducted by the Mahila Kisan Adhikar Manch (MAKAAM), which clearly implicate the public health system and its inadequacies in meeting the health needs of the people (Jadhav et al., 2019). A

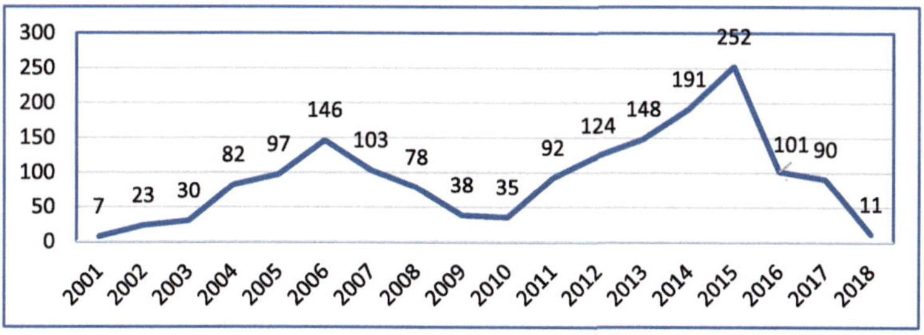

Fig. 10.9 Trend of reported suicides of farmers, 2001–2018, Yavatmal District. *Source* https://yavatmal.gov.in/farmer-suicide/

majority of the survey respondents reported either consulting private health facilities or preferring not to take any treatment at all and cited the following obstacles in consulting the public health sector: distance from the village to the government health facility; unavailability of psychiatrists and medicines; and lack of support from ASHAs and ANMs. Terming the findings as reflecting an "almost collapsed" (p. 19) public healthcare system, Jadhav et al (2019) point to the meagre budgetary allocations to public health, and even budget cuts with every year, the major imbalance in doctor- and ANM-population ratio, driving patients to seek treatment in private hospitals, and that make health care expenditure into a crucial and major burden, compounding farmers' distress.

Second, the study findings revealed the high levels of satisfaction of users with the VPSCP services and in particular with the home-based counselling and psychosocial support services that enabled prompt recognition of PWMI, and better awareness about mental health and help-seeking behavior. This finding is a significant and promising indicator of the role front-line health workers can play through the network of psychosocial support provided through regular home visits, follow-up, and individual care. The emphasis laid on engaging with health workers and lay volunteers is in line with the community mental health paradigm that views the need for such an engagement to be embedded in the local socio-cultural networks. Such an approach, according to the community mental health model, helps to deliver expanded services in resource-poor contexts with few trained personnel, to increase the reach of these services through community participation, enhance the possibility of effective prevention, care, treatment and local advocacy, and to provide better access to practical, emotional and material support for those with mental health concerns who need such care (Campbell & Burgess, 2012).

Finally, the study found a significant difference in attitudes and perceptions about mental health and illness between the intervention and non-intervention villages, indicating a positive effect of the intervention on increasing awareness and reducing stigma about mental illness, and fostering positive attitudes about mental health.

These findings are also in line with recent studies that underscore the necessity of multi-sectoral interventions. For instance, a recent review of 56 studies done in the United States and Australia that attempted to identify the key components of interventions addressing the issue of suicide of farmers found that programs that combined mental health literacy, peer and paraprofessional support, community-based and agro-ecological interventions were more efficacious than stand-alone mental health interventions (Younker & Radunovich, 2022).

In conclusion, given the inadequate resources in the public health care sector, these activities of VPSCP of engaging in capacity building of health workers in identification of mental health concerns, maintaining linkages with government health facilities on the one hand, and interface with livelihood support programmes for income generation opportunities on the other, ensured the positive impact of the project. The findings thus underscore the vital need for psychosocial interventions such as the VPSCP for managing and reducing psychosocial distress in the agrarian context.

References

Balagopal, G., & Kapanee, A. (2019). *Mental health care in community settings: Discussions on NGO approaches in India.* Springer.

Barnagarwala, T. (2018). Maharashtra: Lack of staff ail mental health programme for farmers. *The Indian Express,* April 12. https://indianexpress.com/article/cities/mumbai/prerna-prakalp-lack-of-staff-ail-mental-health-programme-for-farmers-5133832/

Bomble, P., & Lhungdim, H. (2020). Mental health status of farmers in Maharashtra, India: A study from farmer suicide prone area of Vidarbha region. *Clinical Epidemiology and Global Health, 8*(3), 684–688.

Campbell, C., & Burgess, R. (2012). The role of communities in advancing the goals of the Movement for Global Mental Health. *Transcultural Psychiatry, 49*, 3–4.

Chandra, P., & Satyanarayana, V. (2010). Gender disadvantage and common mental disorders in women. *International Review of Psychiatry, 22*(5), 513–524. https://doi.org/10.3109/09540261.2010.516427

Chatterjee, S., Pillai, A., Jain, S., Cohen, A., & Patel, V. (2009). Outcomes of people with psychotic disorders in a community-based rehabilitation programme in rural India. *British Journal of Psychiatry, 195*(5), 433–439.

Das, A. (2011). Farmers' suicide in India: Implications for public mental health. *International Journal of Social Psychiatry, 57*(1), 21–29.

Davar, B.V. (2012). Gender and community mental health: Sharing experiences from our service program. In B. S. Chavan, N. Gupta, P. Arun, A. Sidana, & S. Jadhav (Eds.), *Community mental health in India.* Jaypee Brothers.

Desjarlais, R. et al. (1995). *World mental health: Problems and priorities in low-income countries.* Oxford University Press.

Deshpande, R. S., & Arora, S. (2010). *Agrarian crisis and farmer suicides.* Sage.

Deshpande, A. (2022). Vidarbha continues to record higher farmer suicide. Retrieved on May 15 2023 from https://www.thehindu.com/news/national/other-states/vidarbha-continues-to-record-higher-farmer-suicides/article38310096.ece

Dongre, A. R., & Deshmukh, P. R. (2012). Farmers' suicides in the Vidarbha region of Maharashtra, India: A qualitative exploration of their causes. *Journal of Injury and Violence Research, 4* (1), 2–6. https://doi.org/10.5249%2Fjivr.v4i1.68

Goel, D. S. (2011). Why mental health services in low- and middle-income countries are under-resourced, under-performing: An Indian perspective. *National Medical Journal of India, 24*(2), 2011.

Guha, P., & Das, T. (2022). Farmers' suicides in India. *Economic and Political Weekly, 57*(5), 13–16.

Gururaj, G., Varghese, M., Benegal, V., Rao, G. N., Pathak, K., Singh, L. K. (2016). National mental health survey of India, 2015–16: Prevalence, pattern and outcomes, *NIMHANS Publication no. 129.* National Institute of Mental Health and Neurosciences.

Gururaj, G., & Isaac, M. K. (2004). Psychiatric epidemiology in India: Moving beyond numbers. In S.P. Agarwal (Ed.), *Mental Health an Indian Perspective—1946–2003* (pp. 37–61) Ministry of Health and Family Welfare.

Hans, G., & Sharan, P. (2021). Community-based mental health services in India: Current status and roadmap for the future. *Consortium Psychiatricum, 2*(3), 63–72.

Jacob, K. S. (2001). Community care for people with mental disorders in developing countries: Problems and possible solutions. *British Journal of Psychiatry, 178*, 296–298.

Jadhav, N., Aher, B., & Sudhindra, D. (2019). Public health system is failing the farmers. *Economic and Political Weekly, 54*(10), 17–19.

Jain, S., & Jadhav, S. (2009). Pills that swallow policy: Clinical ethnography of a community mental health program in northern India. *Transcultural Psychiatry, 46*, 60–85.

Kallivayalil, R. A., & Enara, A. (2022). Mental health in an unequal world: The role of social determinants. *Indian Journal of Social Psychiatry, 38*, 3–6.

Kuruvilla, A., & Jacob, K. S. (2007). Poverty, social stress & mental health. *The Indian Journal of Medical Research, 126*(4), 273–278.

Lund, C., De Silva, M., Plagerson, S., Cooper, S., Chisholm, D., Das, J., Knapp, M., & Patel, V. (2011). Poverty and mental disorders: Breaking the cycle in low-income and middle-income countries. *The Lancet, 378*(9801), 1502–1514.

Maitra, P. K. (2022). Six farmers die by suicide in Vidarbha in past 24 hrs. Retrieved on May 29 2023 from https://www.hindustantimes.com/cities/mumbai-news/six-farmers-die-by-suicide-in-vidarbha-in-past-24-hrs-101662205449667.html

Mayston, R., Habtamu, K. H., Medhin, G., Alem, A., Fekadu, A., Habtamu, A., Prince, M., & Hanlon, C. (2017). Developing a measure of mental health service satisfaction for use in low-income countries: a mixed methods study. *BMC Health Services Research, 17* (183), 1–13. https://bmchealthservres.biomedcentral.com/articles/10.1186/s12913-017-2126-2

Meeta, & Rajivlochan (2006). *Farmer's suicide: Facts and Possible Policy Interventions.* Yashwantrao Academy of Development Administration.

Merriott, D. (2017). Factors associated with the farmer suicide crisis in India. *Journal of Epidemiology and Global Health, 6*, 217–227.

Mitra, S., & Shroff, S. (2007). Farmers' suicides in Maharashtra. *Economic and Political Weekly, 42*(49), 73–79.

Murthy, S. R. (2011). Mental health initiatives in India (1947–2010). *National Medical Journal of India, 24*(2), 98–107.

Nagaraj, K. (2008). Farmers' suicides in India: Magnitude, trends, and spatial patterns. *Macro-scan*, http://www.macroscan.org/anl/mar08/anl030308Farmers_Suicides.htm

National Crime Records Bureau. (2016). *Crime in India.* Ministry of Home Affairs, Government of India.

National Crime Records Bureau. (2018). *Crime in India.* Ministry of Home Affairs, Government of India.

National Crime Records Bureau. (2021). *Crime in India.* Ministry of Home Affairs, Government of India.

Neelima, K. (2018). *Widows of Vidarbha.* Oxford University Press.

Nelson, G., Lord, J., & Ochocka, J. (2001). *Shifting the paradigm in community mental health.* University of Toronto Press.

Pandya, A., Shah, K., Chauhan, A., & Saha, S. (2020). Innovative mental health initiatives in India: A scope for strengthening primary healthcare services. *Journal of Family Medicine and Primary Care, 9*(2), 502–507.

Patel, V., & Thara, R. (Eds.). (2003). *Meeting the mental health needs of developing countries: NGO innovations in India.* Sage.

Patel, V., & Kleinman, A. (2003). Poverty and common mental disorders in developing countries. *Bulletin of the World Health Organization, 81*(8), 609–615.

Reddy, N., & Mishra, S. (2009). *Agrarian crisis in India.* Oxford University Press.

Ruggeri, M., & Dall'Agnola, R. (1993). The development and use of the Verona Expectations for Care Scale (VECS) and the Verona Service Satisfaction Scale (VSSS) for measuring expectations and satisfaction with community-based psychiatric services in patients, relatives and professionals. *Psychological Medicine, 23*(2), 511–523.

Saxena, S., Thornicroft, G., Knapp, M., & Whiteford, H. (2007). *Lancet, 370*(9590), 878–889.

Sharma, A. (2021). *A deepening mental health crisis among children: Altruistic suicides in crisis-prone regions in Maharashtra.* Social and Political Research Foundation, https://sprf.in/mental-health-crisis-among-children-altruistic-suicides-in-crisis-prone-regions/

Shidhaye, R., & Patel, V. (2010). Association of socio-economic, gender and health factors with common mental disorders in women: A population-based study of 5703 married rural women in India. *International Journal of Epidemiology, 39*, 1510–1521.

Shidhaye, R., Raja, A., Shrivastava, S., Murhar, V., Ramaswamy, R., & Patel, V. (2015). Challenges for transformation: A situational analysis of mental health care services in Sehore district, Madhya Pradesh. *Community Mental Health Journal, 51*(8), 903–912.

Shidhaye, R., Gangale, S., & Patel, V. (2016). Prevalence and treatment coverage for depression: A population-based survey in Vidarbha, India. *Social Psychiatry and Psychiatric Epidemiology, 51*, 993–1003.
Shidhaye, R., Murhar, V., Gangale, S., Alridge, L., Shastri, R., Parikh, R., Shrivastava, R., Damle, S., Raja, T., Nadkarni, A., & Patel, V. (2017). The effect of VISHRAM, a grass-roots community-based mental health programme on the treatment gap for depression in rural communities in India: A population-based study. *The Lance Psychiatry, 4*, 128–135.
Talule, D. C. (2021). Suicide by Maharashtra farmers: The signs of persistent agrarian distress. *Economic and Political Weekly, LVI, 51*, 46–55.
Thara, R., Padamavati, R., Aynkran, J. R., & John, S. (2008). Community mental health in India: A rethink. *International Journal of Mental Health Systems, 2* (1), 11.
Vasavi, A. R. (2009). Suicides and the making of India's agrarian distress. *South African Review of Sociology, 40*(1), 94–108.
Wal, A. (2020). Seasons of trouble. *The Caravan*, April 20. https://caravanmagazine.in/health/maharashtra-governments-efforts-to-provide-mental-health-care-amid-farmer-suicides
Younker, T., & Radunovich, H. L. (2022). Farmer mental health interventions: A systematic review. *International Journal of Environmental Research in Public Health, 19*(244), 1–30. https://doi.org/10.3390/ijerph19010244

Sunayana Swain currently working as faculty in the School of Gender and Livelihoods, Tata Institute of Social Sciences, Hyderabad campus, has had her academic foundation in the discipline of Psychology, earning a Doctoral degree from University of Hyderabad. Various aspects of her work have been published in journals of international and national repute. She has also contributed to open learning resources on Gender and Psychology. She has collaborated on multiple research projects on Gender, Rural Development, Public Policy, Education and has worked with organizations such as the World Health Organization (South East Asia), Tata Trust, Campaign for Tobacco-Free Kids-Global Health Advocacy Incubator (Washington DC), Department of Women Development and Child Welfare, State Prison Department, Government of Telangana, and Telangana Social Welfare Residential Educational Institutions and others.

U. Vindhya Independent Researcher, and Former Professor, Tata Institute of Social Sciences, Hyderabad, Telangana, India.

Chapter 11
Social-Psychological Dynamics and Interventions for Intergroup Conflict

Roomana N. Siddiqui

Abstract India is a country known for its social diversity characterized by peaceful co-existence of groups sharing each other's traditions, customs and ways of living. However, the peaceful coexistence gets ruptured at times on account of caste, religion, linguistic and regional divisions. As our society is hierarchically organized, where often one group enjoys greater privileges and access to resources (e.g., economic, political, educational opportunities, access to health care) it leads to flashpoints and sometimes to full blown communal tension. In India the genesis of communal violence has generally revolved around religious and caste narratives. In the wake of such violence, precious lives get lost, many innocent people are displaced and there is widespread destruction of property and resources. Such violent acts create a persistent threat in a community from those perceived as "the other." This not only creates a divide in society but permanently scars the human psyche and ruptures the very fabric of the society. A vicious cycle of violence is formed resulting in fear, anger, disillusionment and mental trauma. In order to restore normalcy and help people cope with the trauma of violence interventions are needed not only at the social and political levels, but also at the psychosocial level. Most of the interventions so far in India have been made by civil society organizations for rebuilding and restoring of trust and social bonding and specifically to rehabilitate those affected by social violence. Not much has been achieved however, at the level of psychosocial intervention. Psychologists in India have either responded to social conflict and violence rather late, or engaged academically to understand the complex social reality. This paper presents an overview of the nature of intergroup relations and conflict in India along with a brief review of the interventions made both by civil society organizations and academics for restoring peace in society.

Keywords Diversity · Intergroup relations · Conflict · Socio-psychological interventions

R. N. Siddiqui (✉)
Department of Psychology, Aligarh Muslim University, Aligarh, India
e-mail: roomana17@gmail.com

U. Vindhya (ed.), *Psychosocial Interventions for Social Issues in Contemporary India*,
https://doi.org/10.1007/978-981-96-6553-2_11

Introduction

India is a complex blend of diversity with about 1400 dialects and 18 officially recognized languages, several religions, caste and ethnic groups. It is one of the largest democracies where diverse groups live in unity, perhaps unparalleled anywhere in the world. This cultural pluralism, unlike the west, exists in a framework of interconnectedness. However, in this age of identity politics the differences between groups have been highlighted to reap political benefits. These political opportunisms have strained the syncretic culture of the country. Even in an age where the divide between religious and ethnic groups appears to be unbridgeable with increasing hate and violence escalating against each other one does regularly come across many instances which is a testimony to the fact that the divide is not permanent. It is these instances of bonding that helps us as a society to overcome any tension of an intergroup nature. Even in polarised times people have demonstrated that they do not only identify themselves in terms of their narrow group identity.

A few recent instances draw our attention to the prioritization of harmony and co-existence over conflict. Despite attempts being made to sharpen the lines of communal polarization, a Muslim builder in Ahmedabad, undertook the task of renovating a dilapidated 500-year-old Hanuman temple (Wangchuk, 2018). "I have grown up seeing the temple in its vibrant glory. I offer namaz five times a day, but as I passed by the temple, its dilapidated condition pained me. I contacted the priest and offered to renovate it. He happily agreed," said the buider. It is the spirit of co-existence and harmony which helps to prevail the winds of strife and prejudice for each other. Similarly, even at a time of heightened communal tension between Hindus and Muslims the Sikh and Hindu community members helped Muslims repair an old mosque in Nathowal village in Punjab. They even got a second storey added to it and most of the expenses (around 75%) was born by non-Muslims (Subramanian, 2017). In Kharagpur's Puratan Bazar (West Bengal) the Muslim community cancelled its Muharram[1] procession to save a Hindu life (Raja, 2017). In 2017 the club organising this procession raised 50,000 rupees but decided to cancel the event and donate the entire money to a mobile recharge shop owner of the Hindu community, who was suffering from Hodgkin's lymphoma, a cancer of the immune system. In a similar spirit a temple near Tirur cancelled its annual festival to condole the death of a local Muslim (Aranha, 2018). A very touching display of unity and compassion between families belonging to different faiths, was witnessed in the city of Mumbai where an extraordinary bond helped transcend religious boundaries for a life-saving cause.

Rafiq Shah's wife was suffering from kidney problem and was getting treated in one of the dialysis clinics where he came across Dr. Rahul Yadav, an Ayurveda practitioner from Ghatkopar. Due to blood group mismatches, it resulted in a bridging of faiths leading Girija, the mother of Dr. Rahul Yadav, to selflessly donate her kidney to Rafiq Shah, and Shah's wife, Khushnuma, reciprocating by donating her kidney to Yadav (Sabrang India, 2024).

[1] Muharram, a sacred day for Muslims, is a religious event which is celebrated to commemorate the sacrifice of Prophet's grandson, by taking out a procession.

These are just some of the instances of display of inter-faith harmony witnessed across the length and the breadth of the country but the question that these stories raise is, what enabled people to rise up to the occasion and come together in a show of trust and compassion for each other? Going by the *contact hypotheses* (Allport, 1954) contact between groups reduces prejudice but for this to happen there needs to be an optimal condition for intergroup contact (Pettigrew, 1998). Groups need to engage with each other in cooperative relationships. Since in day-to-day civic life people do interact and engage with each other the group identity gets decategorized. In de-categorization, the attributes of the group are down played in preference to the qualities of the individual members. The strategy involves encouraging personalized interactions between individuals while making their personal identities more salient relative to their social identities (Brewer & Miller, 1996). This people- to- people contact enables them to overcome prejudice.

A journey into the old cities of India gives a sense of how this social psychological reality was preserved by the planners of the city where the ordinary citizens did not get influenced by narrow personal, social or economic interests. Despite separatist insurgency in Kashmir, a Hindu temple and a Muslim shrine have stood close to each other in Manzgam, which is 100 km from Srinagar. Though Kashmir saw large scale exodus of Kashmiri pandits, there was no violence in this village and it was peaceful. Residents attribute this harmony to the two 600-year-old shrines present in that region. The Muslim shrine was named after the fifteenth century Sufi Baba Qiyaamud-Din whose teachings of peace are still being followed by Kashmiris, irrespective of their faith, while the Hindu temple was dedicated to a revered Hindu deity Mata Kheerbhawani. It is a regular feature that every year both the communities visit these sacred spaces to celebrate each other's festivals. In the words of one of the activists of that region "This is a decades-old divine bond no one can break" (IANS, 2016). In several cities, different religious spaces have existed side by side or in close proximity to each other and people have shown sensitivity and respect for each other's tradition and have also actively participated in these traditions. In the army, one of the most respected institutions of the country, whenever there is a mixed unit a *sarva dharmasthal* (common prayer hall) is provided where people from all religious backgrounds meet for various religious functions and ceremonies. Similarly, different communities come together to celebrate each other's important customs in Bidar in Karnataka. It is a key feature of the tradition in the village that the Muslims celebrate Dussehra and the Hindus partake in Ramzan (Subramanian, 2017). In the holy month of Ramadan, a Vishnu Temple in Kottakkal, Malappuram hosted a mass Iftar dinner for their local Muslim brethren with the explicit purpose of spreading the message of peace and harmony among the younger generation (Aranha, 2018). These instances from across the length and breadth of the country highlight the embracing of each other's reality by different social groups. However, this coming together of diversities has its own share of problems. This paper seeks to provide a glimpse of the social psychological reality of intergroup relations and conflict in India. It also looks into the interventions for overcoming the conflicts.

Multiculturalism in India: Unity in Diversity

As a country with a conglomeration of different groups, India has had a long history of cultural diversity (Chandra & Mahajan, 2007). Along with a vast geographical spread, India's richness of diversity in terms of region, language, caste, religion or culture makes it seem like a salad bowl where each has its distinct presence; and the coming together of such diversity is what makes it unique. Sociological scholarship on multiculturalism in India refers to its rich historical experience that includes both conflicts and attempts at negotiation (e.g., Oommen, 2007). A distinctive feature that has also long informed the multi-cultural history and traditions in India is co-existence, despite being a very multi religious, multi linguistic and multi-cultural society (Mahajan, 2010). Coexistence entails the presence of distinct elements (e.g., traditions, customs and practices) of several cultures in the life of individuals belonging to different cultural groups. They exist side by side without any attempt towards assimilation (Mishra et al., 1996; Tripathi & Mishra, 2016). It is this coming together that accounts for harmony in society.

Etymologically, harmony means 'joint'. It is the "binding together" and being in sync with one another in the context of communities of different thoughts and belief—be it social, economic, political and religious. It simply means living with unity and mutual reciprocity, beyond caste, creed, religion and class barriers. The multiculturalism propagated by the west presupposes the integration of diverse groups as against assimilation but the uniqueness in India is that the elements of different cultures have been integrated or synthesized to produce a syncretic or composite culture (Chandra & Mahajan, 2007). Societies that are multi-cultural and are characterized by a composite culture have ample opportunities for sharing cultural spaces. Singh et al. (2017) investigated shared spaces in contemporary India and reported. that diversity was not necessarily a precursor for conflict, and despite differences, people live with each other in an atmosphere of congeniality. The common spaces offered opportunities to collaborate with members of different religious group, be interdependent, engage in acts of reciprocity, mutual celebration and this enabled people to mutually respect different religions (Singh et al., 2023). This sentiment was corroborated by a study conducted in Northern India where majority of the participants preferred a composite cultural ideology in comparison to monocultural or multicultural ideology (Tripathi et al., 2023). Co-existence was the preferred acculturation strategy of the non-dominant groups in India (Mishra et al., 2017). In case an important norm of Hindus or Muslims were violated by members of the opposite group the most preferred reaction was conciliation rather than retaliation and retribution (Tripathi et al., 2018). This reflects the sensitivity and respect which people have for each other's culture.

Multiculturalism is associated with preference for 'integration'. People of different religious groups, caste, language and ethnicity, despite having their own distinctiveness, share many things as they lived in close proximity to each other. In their day-to-day interaction they do get exposed to different cultures. Exploring how Hindus and Muslims relate to each other's culture, Bano and Mishra (2011) reported a distinct preference for integration and co-existence amongst members of both the religious groups with least preference given to assimilation strategy. Contact between the two groups was a key factor as integration strategy and cultural security played an important role for Muslims but for Hindus, only those who had contact with Muslims preferred integration and co-existence intercultural strategy. Thus, it was clear that integration and cultural security positively related with multiculturalism if there were contact between communities. There is no dearth of evidence for "co-construction" (interdependence) of identities based on mutual respect and support for each other (Tripathi & Mishra, 2016). The pluralistic orientation was always an integral part of the Indian psyche and is still relevant even when relations appear to be strained between groups.

Understanding Intergroup Relations: A Socio Psychological Perspective

Intergroup relations have attracted the interest of researchers from various field. As intergroup relations have implications for the wellbeing of both individuals and society it has been a fertile area of research by social psychologists. Several theories have been postulated to understand intergroup dynamics. The relative deprivation theory (Gurr, 1970; Runciman, 1966) postulates that individuals feel deprivation if they perceive a discrepancy between what they have and what they are entitled to. At the core of the theory is comparison which is made between what one has and what one thinks they should get. This develops into a sense of unfairness, resulting in anger and resentment due to the subjective evaluations of unfairness. This feeling of injustice which members of one group have in comparison to the other, leads to resentment and conflict. Thus, this theory enables us to understand the origins of discontent in an intergroup context.

The realistic conflict theory, on the other hand postulates that intergroup conflict is due to incompatible goals. The classical research of Sherif et al. (1961) was seminal in the understanding of intergroup hostility and prejudice. The core assumption of his theory is that intergroup behavior and attitude will reflect the interest of the ingroup in comparison to the other group. While examining intergroup conflict, Sherif et al. (1961) argued that when groups are competing for scarce resources it leads to intergroup conflict. This finding became the basis of the realistic conflict theory (Sherif & Sherif, 1953).

The experiments by Sheriff established that when groups are competing for a goal then the group competition increases intragroup cooperation and cohesiveness. It is this ingroup solidarity that becomes the basis of negative prejudice towards the other group. Fascinated by this finding Tajfel and colleagues (Tajfel, 1982) investigated the minimal conditions necessary for ethnocentric bias to occur. The findings led to the emergence of the social identity theory (SIT) (Tajfel & Turner, 1986) that states that individuals' perceptions and interactions in intergroup contexts are influenced by their memberships in social categories. Thus, the minimal condition for intergroup behavior was a mere categorization of people in groups, referred to as ingroup and outgroup. This process of self-categorization and other-categorization is responsible for increasing the intergroup differences.

The self-categorization theory (Turner, 1987) is an expansion of the social identity theory. A major premise of self-categorization theory (SCT) is that social and personal identity are not the extreme points of a continuum but they can simultaneously operate and consequently guide behavior and cognitions. The basic process of SCT is self-categorization, "an active, interpretative, judgmental process, reflecting a complex and creative interaction between motives, expectations, knowledge and reality" (Turner, 1999, p. 31). Based on self-categorization, people start perceiving more similarity amongst members of the group with which they associate and highlight the difference with other group. As categories containing the self are easily accessible it leads to positive distinctiveness.

Apart from explaining the intergroup dynamics at the attitude level, some theories have attempted to investigate the process of intergroup behavior. The Norm violation theory (De Ridder & Tripathi, 1992) attempts to understand the conditions under which two coexisting groups can develop negative intergroup behavior if their norm is violated by the other group. This theory addresses the question of what happens when the member of one group violates the norm of another group. The theory has identified certain contextual factors that account for escalation or de-escalation of violence. One such factor that was identified by the social dominance theory (SDT) (Sidanius & Pratto, 2012) was the hierarchical nature of society where some groups are in a dominant position while others are lower in the hierarchical structure. Intergroup oppression, discrimination, and prejudice are manifestations of efforts to maintain this social hierarchy (Sidanius & Pratto, 2012). According to the SDT theory (Sidanius et al., 1994), social dominance orientation (SDO) represents the "desire to establish and maintain hierarchically structured intergroup relations regardless of the position of one's own group(s) within this hierarchy" (Sidanius et al., 2017, p. 152) and the "extent to which one desires that one's ingroup dominate and be superior to out-groups" (Pratto et al., 1994, p. 742).

Stephan and Stephan's integrated threat theory (ITT) (1996) offers an explanation to the feelings of threat which members of group have in relation to the other group. The main assumption of ITT is that due to threat perception people develop prejudice and negative attitudes towards out-groups. Stephan and Stephan (1996) identified four types of threat: realistic threat, symbolic threat, negative stereotype, and intergroup anxiety. Realistic threats is on account of the economic, political power, and physical or material wellbeing. Symbolic threats are felt in relation to cultural differences in values, morals, and worldview between the in-group and the out-group. Negative stereotypes are the commonly held negative notions about out-group which causes fear of negative consequences and intergroup anxiety refers to apprehension and fear which members of in-group experiences at the time of interaction with members of the out-group.

Social Psychological Research on Intergroup Conflict in India: An Overview

India has prided itself as a unity in diversity but despite this claim there were schisms between groups on the basis of religion, caste and language. It is this diverse complexity of the socio-cultural landscape that made Indian researchers attempt to unravel the socio psychological dynamics of society. Communal outbursts have been a challenge for the country, with the historical event of partition of the country in 1947 becoming a major source of tension between the two dominant groups of Hindus and Muslims, and leading to a full-blown fare-up with millions losing their lives and property on communal lines. The large-scale communal riots in the aftermath of the partition led to one of the major psychological studies of social tension in India by Gardner Murphy (1953), that foregrounded the importance of psychological factors such as prejudice and religious bigotry, and the need to focus on them in the planning of peace initiatives. Subsequent research in the area of communal relations has found that the differential status between the Hindu majority and Muslim minority influences the inter-group attitudes and relations between them (e.g.,Chatterjee et al., 1967); fraternal deprivation being perceived by Muslims in relation to job opportunity, political freedom, and association with hostile attitude towards Hindus; attribution of blame on Hindus for riots and maintenance of greater social distance between the two groups (Naqvi, 1982; Tripathi & Srivastava, 1981).

The Hindu Muslim conflict in India is unique as rightly pointed by Sen (2005) because there is no foreign group that can be targeted and these two groups are tightly integrated. Hence most of the researchers investigated Hindu Muslim relations focused on various aspects of ethnocentric attitude and relations between them. Taylor and Jaggi (1974) reported ethnocentric attribution bias among Muslims and Hindus in perception of desirable and undesirable acts. Others reported that children develop religious identity and related biases very early in life (Mishra & Bano, 2003; Singh, 1979). Majeed and Ghosh (1981) reported that high caste Hindus and Muslims had positive attitude towards in group, but when it came to scheduled caste, they expressed negative evaluation towards their own group but evaluated both Hindus and Muslims favourably. Siddiqui (2011) reported that when Hindus and Muslims evaluated their in-group positively, they evaluated the out-group negatively, but those Muslims who evaluated themselves negatively they evaluated Hindus positively. On the contrary, negative evaluation of in-group by Hindus did not result in positive evaluation of Muslims. Ghosh et al. (1992) reported that Hindus ascribed more power to themselves but Muslims reported more positive in-group identity. Thus, it is clear from the empirical evidences that all groups do not engage in intergroup relations in the same manner. In fact, there are large variations in how people seek to relate to each other in any society (Berry, 1990). These variations can be seen in the relationship orientations of various groups in the Indian society (Mishra et al., 1996, 2017).

Attempts have also been made to examine the structural and psychological factors motivating collective action in a wide range of social contexts. Tripathi et al. (2018) for instance, examined how norms and emotions influence action tendencies in an intergroup context when groups do not share equal social position. As members are emotionally attached to their group the emotions elicited in the wake of any norm violation of a group evokes strong reaction tendency. According to the intergroup emotions theory (Mackie & Smith, 2002; Mackie et al., 2000) intergroup anger generates a desire to harm the offending group (Mackie et al., 2000; Yzerbyt et al., 2003), but in the case of fear the desire is to avoid the out-group and support the in-group (Dumont et al., 2003). Tripathi et al. (2018) also reported that reactions to any intergroup norm violations is influenced by the emotions evoked by the violation. The results revealed that anger was the dominant emotion experienced post norm violation in all situations, anxiety was the next in order of intensity followed by fear. These emotions further influenced the action tendencies, but it worked differently for Hindus and Muslims. Hindus being the majority preferred making a retaliatory reaction while angry. But this was not the case for Muslims. Ghosh et al. (1992) reported Muslims experiencing greater fraternal relative derivation (FRD) but low resource and retaliatory power compared to the Hindus. Crosby (1976) pointed out that a high level of FRD may lead to resentment which with time surfaces as anger. Muslims' preference for retribution over retaliation and conciliation when experiencing anger or anxiety reflects the fact that intergroup relations are governed by structural variables (Tripathi et al., 2018).

These are some of the attempts made by social psychologists to understand the antecedents of intergroup conflict. In the 1980s when communal violence had become a regular feature, Singh (1985) had appealed for an effective intervention and for a scientifically planned social policy to guide and improve intergroup relations in the country. However, the consequences of communal violence as well as intervention are understudied in mainstream psychology. Some recent studies have reported greater prevalence of mental health conditions among Muslims in the post-riot context (e.g., Farooqui & Ahmad, 2021). In addition to fundamentally altering quality of life for victims of communal violence, and even of those who have witnessed it, the impact of communal violence has far-reaching social psychological as well as mental health consequences (Bebaak Collective, 2022). However, much of the work on the aftermath of communal violence has been undertaken by civil society organizations and NGOs. What is required therefore is a nuanced understanding of how communal conflicts escalate and de-escalate in order for researchers to suggest effective interventions to overcome the pain and trauma of the 'social suffering' of communal riots (Kleinman et al., 1997).

Beyond the Conflict: Building Bridges Through Psycho Social Interventions

History is filled with stories of collective living where people from diverse background have come together to celebrate each other's differences but it is also true that some of the most violent conflicts have taken place due to this diversity. As a result, people have experienced adverse psychological consequences due to intergroup conflict. The field of social-psychology has to a large extent understood the determinants of inter-group hostility, stereotyping, and prejudice. As mentioned earlier, major theories of intergroup conflict, such as, relative deprivation theory (Runciman, 1966; Walker & Smith, 2002), realistic conflict theory (Sherif, 1967), social identity theory (Tajfel & Turner, 1979), social dominance theory (Sidanius & Pratto, 1999), and integrated threat theory (Stephan & Stephan, 2000) have highlighted the role of the 'other' and how it accounts for the reasons why conflicts take place. Although the major focus has been on understanding the dynamics of conflict, social psychologists have also proposed theories and methods for resolution of conflicts. These theories consider whether the conflict is intractable or tractable (Bar-Tal, 2013). Attempts were also made to investigate the nature of the intervention, be it at the prevention level, or at the level of resolution of an existing conflict through mediation, arbitration, avoidance, conciliation or negotiation. Some of these methods deal with issues that arise post-conflict and are critical for achieving what Galtung (1967) calls positive peace.

Erikson (1969) while analysing Gandhi's intervention observes that his 'Satyagraha', was an attempt to create inclusive identities. In the wake of a communal violence Gandhi took to fasting and ensured that his followers reflect on what went wrong in their relationship with the other. His 'satyagraha' was more than a mere protest. His intention was to condemn the agency involved in it but more so he wanted to drive home the point that if the oppressor and oppressed continued to maintain their anger and hatred for each other, the conflict will never be resolved. During the "satyagraha" he would start his meetings with prayers where people of all religious faiths participated and this not only created common cultural spaces but helped in understanding each other's perspective.

Violence leaves behind traumas which if not addressed get transferred across generations leading to a cycle of revenge (Gobodo-Madikizela, 2008). The collective memory of partition which saw mass killings in India and Pakistan is still an important escalatory factor in communal riots especially in the northern part of India. The historical memory of the partition even today colours the intergroup relations between the two prominent groups in India. Hence, it becomes imperative that psychological interventions need to be made to bring about closure of intense negative emotion that results in acts of violence. One such attempt was made in the aftermath of the Gujarat riots of 2002. Bhadra (2006) designed an intervention project called the Gujarat Harmony Project, under the aegis of National Institute of Mental Health and Neuro Science, (NIMHANS), Bangalore. On the basis of their extensive survey of refugee camps they observed that the perception of threat was very high amongst the refugees. They observed a heightened sense of suspiciousness among children and adolescents for each other, and heightened sensitivity about their religious affiliation, affecting the social relationship between the communities (Bhadra, 2006).

Immediately after the riots, children and adolescents reported greater incidents of traumatic reactions (Prince-Embury, 2008). The scale of psychological trauma and disturbances among the children and adolescents was so varied and intense that different initiatives were undertaken (Bhadra, 2012). The strategies were multi-pronged to ensure psychosocial support for the riot survivors. Many of the community volunteers were themselves survivors of the riots. Gradually, some people from the other nearby Hindu communities also got involved in facilitating the process of communal harmony and peace building through community mobilization and participation (Bhadra, 2012). During rehabilitation in the camp, the activities used were story-telling, creative writing, drawing, school drama/skit, play or games, etc. that are known as creative-expressive activities. These activities provided them an opportunity to vent their feelings which not only helped in healing but made them look for positive changes.

Psychosocial support helps to facilitate sustainable peace among community members through people-to-people contact, cooperation, open forum discussions and the development of trusting relationships through various common initiatives. These participatory methods become critical components in post disaster interventions (Bordoloi & Khoja, 2006; Hansen, 2008; IASC, 2007; Pyles, 2007). The Gujarat Harmony Project in the end conducted various multi-religious prayers and meetings, collective celebration of religious festivals, with Hindu communities arranging an iftar celebration (celebratory dinner indicating the end of the holy month of Ramadan) to host the Muslim communities and Muslim communities inviting Hindus to celebrate Diwali (the festival of light celebrated by Hindus) in their communities (Bhadra, 2006). It is this participation in the community events of each other that generated feelings of acceptance and helped at building trusting relationships among the common people. Thus, the objective of the project to promote psychosocial competencies among the children and adolescents for establishing harmonious living and sustainable peace was achieved (Bharath & Kumar, 2004). This project thus presents a comprehensive and participatory model for facilitating psychosocial recovery among trauma affected children, adolescents, and adults.

To conclude, interventions for macro-level and protracted intergroup conflicts such as the Hindu-Muslim one will have to neutralise prejudice, discrimination and to focus on how to inculcate the readiness to engage with others' needs in order to bring the warring groups on one platform for negotiations and deliberations. For any intervention to be effective it should take a holistic perspective of resolving immediate psychosocial problems along with building permanent relationships on the basis of mutual trust and respect (Siddiqui, 2019). It is when people dialogue with diversity or transact on the basis of their shared identity then it becomes easy to establish sustainable bonds between groups. This requires an understanding of the processes that create social fissures and divisions, and processes which help in nurturing relationships based on trust and mutuality. The challenge that psychologists face is to come up with methods that will not only achieve peace but sustain it over a period of time. It is thus clear that for people to come together those processes which have divided them in the spheres of shared existence needs to be addressed.

References

Allport, G. W. (1954). *The nature of prejudice.* Addison-Wesley.

Aranha, J. (2018, May 25). *Kerala temple sets example of communal harmony, serves Iftar this Ramzan*! https://www.thebetterindia.com/142918/kerala-vishnu-temple-iftar-ramadan/

Bano, S., & Mishra, R. C. (2011). Relational orientations of Hindu and Muslim adolescents in traditional and modern schools. In P. Singh, P. Bain, L. Chan-Hoong, G. Misra, & Y. Ohtsubo (Eds.), *Identity, multiculturalism and changing societies: Psychological, group and cultural processes* (pp. 219–230). Macmillan.

Bar-Tal, D. (2013). *Intractable conflicts: Socio-psychological foundations and dynamics.* Cambridge University Press.

Bebaak Collective. (2022). *Social suffering in a world without support: Report on the mental health of Indian Muslims.* Mumbai: Bebaak Collective.

Berry, J. W. (1990). Psychology of acculturation: Individuals moving between cultures. In R. Brislin (Ed.), *Applied cross-cultural psychology* (pp. 232–253). Sage.

Bhadra, S. (2006). *Life events among the survivors of disasters* (PhD Thesis). Department of Psychiatric Social Work, National Institute of Mental Health and Neuro Sciences (NIMHANS), Bangalore.

Bhadra, S. (2012). Psychosocial support for the children affected by communal violence in Gujarat, India. *International Journal of Applied Psychoanalytic Studies, 9*(3), 212–232.

Bharath, S., & Kumar, K. V. K. (2004). *Activity manual for teachers on health promotion using life skills approach.* NIMHANS.

Bordoloi, S., & Khoja, A. (2006). Development of a psychosocial questionnaire and a worksheet for teachers, parents, students and other school personnel to assess educational needs of survivors of the tsunami in Calang, Indonesia. In J. O. Diaz, R. Lakshminarayana, & S. R. Murthy (Eds.), *Advances in disaster mental health and psychological support* (pp. 153–163). Voluntary Health Association of India Press.

Brewer, M. B., & Miller, N. (1996). *Intergroup relations.* Open University Press.

Chandra, B., & Mahajan, S. (2007). *Composite culture in a multicultural society.* Pearson/Longman.

Chatterjee, B. B., Singh, P. N., & Row, G. R. S. (1967). *Riots in Rourkela: A psychological study.* Popular Book Service.

Crosby, F. (1976). A model of egoistical relative deprivation. *Psychological Review, 83*(2), 85–113.

De Ridder, R., & Tripathi, R. C. (1992). *Norm violations and intergroup relations.* Clarendon Press.

Dumont, M., Yzerbyt, V., Wigboldus, D., & Gordijn, E. H. (2003). Categorization and fear reactions to the September 11th attacks. *Personality and Social Psychology Bulletin, 29*(12), 1509–1152.

Erikson, E. H. (1969). *Gandhi's truth: On the origins of militant non-violence.* W.W. Norton & Company.

Farooqui, N., & Ahmad, A. (2021). Communal violence, mental health and their correlates: A cross-sectional study in two riot affected districts of Uttar Pradesh in India. *Journal of Muslim Minority Affairs, 41*(3), 510–521.

Galtung, J. (1967). *Theory and methods of social science research.* Columbia University Press.

Ghosh, E. S. K., Kumar, R., & Tripathi, R. C. (1992). The communal cauldron: Relations between Hindus and Muslims in India and their reactions to norm violations. In R. De Ridder & R. C. Tripathi (Eds.), *Norm violation and intergroup relations* (pp. 70–89). Clarendon Press.

Gobodo-Madikizela, P. (2008). Transforming trauma in the aftermath of gross human rights abuses: Making public spaces intimate through the South African Truth and Reconciliation commission. In A. Nadler, T. E. Malloy, & J. D. Fisher (Eds.), *The social psychology of intergroup reconciliation* (pp. 57–76). Oxford University Press.

Gurr, T. R. (1970). *Why men rebel.* Princeton University Press.

Hansen, P. (2008). Psychosocial interventions. In W. Agen (Ed.), *A handbook.* International Federation Reference Center for Psychosocial Support.

IANS. (2016, June 19). *A small village in Kashmir is teaching the rest of India a valuable lesson in communal harmony*. https://www.thebetterindia.com/58744/communal-harmony-hindu-muslim-kashmir-manzgam/
Inter-agency Standing Committee (IASC). (2007). *Mental health and psychosocial support in emergencies*. IASC.
Kleinman, A., Das, V., & Lock, M. M. (Eds.). (1997). *Social suffering*. University of California Press.
Mackie, D. M., Devos, T., & Smith, E. R. (2000). Intergroup emotions: Explaining offensive action tendencies in an intergroup context. *Journal of Personality and Social Psychology, 79*, 602–616.
Mackie, D. M., & Smith, E. R. (2002). Beyond prejudice: Moving from positive and negative evaluations to differentiated reactions to social groups. In D. M. Mackie & E. R. Smith (Eds.), *From prejudice to intergroup emotions: Differentiated reactions to social groups* (pp. 1–12). Psychology Press.
Mahajan, G. (2010). Responding to identity conflicts: Multiculturism and the pursuit of peaceful co-existence. *Peace Prints: South Asian Journal of Peacebuilding, 3*(2), 1–10.
Majeed, A., & Ghosh, E. S. K. (1981). Ingroup and outgroup evaluation in intergroup context. *Psychological Studies, 26*(1), 34–40.
Mishra, R. C., & Bano, S. (2003). Ethnic identity and bias in Hindu and Muslim children. *Social Science International, 19*, 52–64.
Mishra, R. C., Bano, S., & Tripathi, R. C. (2017). Intercultural relations in India. In J. W. Berry (Ed.), *Mutual intercultural relations*. Cambridge University Press.
Mishra, R. C., Sinha, D., & Berry, J. W. (1996). *Ecology, acculturation and psychological adaptation: A study of Adivasis in Bihar*. Sage.
Murphy, G. (1953). *In the minds of men*. Basic Books.
Naqvi, N. (1982). *Relative deprivation and attribution of blame in communal riots* (Unpublished manuscript). University of Allahabad, India.
Oommen, T.A. (2007). Multiculturism in twentieth-century India: Ambiguity and ambivalence. In B. Chandra & S. Mahajan (Eds.), *Composite culture in a multicultural society* (pp. 219–236). Pearson/Longman.
Pettigrew, T. F. (1998). Intergroup contact theory. *Annual Review of Psychology, 49*, 65–85. https://doi.org/10.1146/annurev.psy.49.1.65
Pratto, F., Sidanius, J., Stallworth, L. M., & Malle, B. F. (1994). Social dominance orientation: A personality variable predicting social and political attitudes. *Journal of Personality and Social Psychology, 67*, 741–763.
Prince-Embury, S. (2008). The resiliency scales for children and adolescents, psychological symptoms, and clinical status in adolescents. *Canadian Journal of School Psychology, 23*(1), 41–56.
Pyles, L. (2007). Community organizing for post-disaster social development: Locating social work. *International Social Work, 50*(3), 321–333.
Raja, V. (2017, October 6). *This Muslim Community wants to cancel Muharram procession to save a Hindu*. https://www.thebetterindia.com/117433/muslim-community-cancel-muharram-save-hindu-west-bengal-hindu-muslim/
Runciman, W. G. (1966). *Relative deprivation and social justice*. Routledge and Kegan Paul.
Sabrang India. (2024, January 13). Heartrending tales of communal harmony amidst polarised times. https://www.newsclick.in/heartrending-tales-communal-harmony-amidst-polarised-times.
Sen, A. (2005). Human rights and capabilities. *Journal of Human Development and Capabilities, 6*, 151–166.
Sherif, M. (1967). *Social interaction: Process and products: Selected essays of Muzafer Sherif*. Aldine.
Sherif, M., Harvey, O. J., White, B. J., Hood, W. R., & Sherif, C. W. (1961). *Intergroup conflict and cooperation: The robbers cave experiment* (Vol. 10). University Book Exchange.
Sherif, M., & Sherif, C. W. (1953). *Groups in harmony and tension; an integration of studies of intergroup relations*. Harper & Brothers.

Sidanius, J., & Pratto, F. (1999). *Social dominance: An intergroup theory of social hierarchy and oppression*. Cambridge University Press.

Sidanius, J., Cotterill, S., Sheehy-Skeffington, J., Kteily, N., & Carvacho, H. (2017). *Social dominance theory: Explorations in the psychology of oppression. In Cambridge handbook of psychology of prejudice* (pp. 149–187). Sibley C. Barlow. Publisher's Version.

Sidanius, J., & Pratto, F. (2012). Social dominance theory. In P. A. M. Van Lange, A. W. Kruglanski, & E. T. Higgins (Eds.), *Handbook of theories of social psychology* (pp. 418–438). Sage Publications Ltd.

Sidanius, J., Pratto, F., & Mitchell, M. (1994). Group identity, social dominance orientation, and intergroup discrimination: Some implications of social dominance theory. *Journal of Social Psychology, 134*, 151–167.

Siddiqui, R. N. (2011). Appraisal of outgroup in the context of intergroup relations: Role of personal and collective identity. *Pakistan Journal of Psychological Research, 26*(2), 167–182.

Siddiqui, R. N. (2019). The dilemma of harmony: From distrust to trust. In J. Pandey, R. Kumar, & K. Thapa (Eds.), *Psychological perspectives on diversity and social development*. Springer.

Singh, A. K. (1985). *Developing secularism and national integration in India*. Presidential address, Section of Psychology and Educational Sciences, 72nd Indian Science Congress Association, Lucknow.

Singh, M. P. (1979). Political arrival. *Seminar, 243*, 12–17.

Singh, P., Misra, G., Kapur, P., Mishra, A. K., & Siddiqui, R. N. (2017). *The shared spaces: Exploring the boundaries, barriers and bridges in contemporary India* (Project Report, Research Programme, ICSSR).

Singh, P., Misra, G., Kapur, P., Mishra, A. K., & Siddiqui, R. N. (2023). Towards deciphering shared spaces among religious groups in contemporary Indian society: Some illustrations and challenges. *Social Change, 53*(4), 469–485.

Stephan, W. G., & Stephan, C. W. (1996). Predicting prejudice. *International Journal of Intercultural Relations, 20*, 409–426.

Stephan, W. G., & Stephan, C. W. (2000). An integrated threat theory of prejudice. In S. Oskamp (Ed.), *Reducing prejudice and discrimination* (pp. 23–45). Lawrence Erlbaum Associates publishers.

Subramanian, A. (2017, March 2). This village in Bidar doesn't have any statues. *Bangalore Mirror.* http://timesofindia.indiatimes.com/articleshow/49266111.cms?utm_source=contentofinterest&utm_medium=text&utm_campaign=cppst

Tajfel, H. (1982). Social psychology of intergroup relations. *Annual Review of Psychology, 33*, 1–39.

Tajfel, H., & Turner, J. C. (1979). An integrative theory of intergroup conflict. In W. G. Austin & S. Worchel (Eds.), *The social psychology of intergroup relations* (pp. 33–47). Brooks-Cole.

Tajfel, H., & Turner, J. C. (1986). The social identity theory of inter-group behavior. In S. Worchel, & W. Austin (Ed.), *Psychology of Inter-group relations*. Nelson Hall.

Taylor, D. M., & Jaggi, V. (1974). Ethnocentrism and causal attribution in a south Indian context. *Journal of Cross-Cultural Psychology, 5*(2), 162–171.

Tripathi, R. C., & Srivastava, R. (1981). Relative deprivation and intergroup attitudes. *European Journal of Social Psychology, 11*(3), 313–318. https://doi.org/10.1002/ejsp.2401110306

Tripathi, R. C., Kumar, R., Siddiqui, R. N., & Bano, S. (2018). Emotional reactions to norm violations. *Psychology and Developing Societies, 30*(2), 1–28.

Tripathi, R. C., Kumar, R., Siddiqui, R. N., Mishra, R. C., & Bano, S. (2023). Ideological frames and reaction to norm violations. *Psychology and Developing Societies, 35*(1), 131–168.

Tripathi, R. C., & Mishra, R. C. (2016). Acculturation in South Asia. In D. Sam & J. W. Berry (Eds.), *The Cambridge handbook of acculturation psychology* (2nd ed., pp. 337–354). Cambridge University Press.

Turner, J. C. (1987) Introducing the problem: Individual and group. In *Rediscovering the social group: A self-categorization theory* (pp. 1–18). Blackwell.

Turner, J. C. (1999). Some current issues in research on social identity and self-categorization theories. In N. Ellemers, R. Spears, & B. Dossje (Eds.), *Social identity: Context, commitment, content* (pp. 6–34). Blackwell.

Walker, I., & Smith, H. J. (Eds.). (2002). *Relative deprivation: Specification, development, and integration.* Cambridge University Press.

Wangchuk, R. N. (2018, February 7). *Harmony over hate: This Muslim man from Ahmedabad is restoring a 500-year-old temple.* https://www.thebetterindia.com/130300/harmony-hate-muslim-man-ahmedabad-restoring-500-year-old-temple/

Yzerbyt, V., Dumont, M., Wigboldus, D., & Gordijn, E. (2003). I feel for us: The impact of categorization and identification on emotions and action tendencies. *British Journal of Social Psychology, 42*(4), 533–549.

Roomana N. Siddiqui is a professor in the department of psychology at Aligarh Muslim University. She is a social psychologist with interest in contemporary social issues that includes environmental issues, issues of identity, role of contact in intergroup relations and exploring the role of trust in intergroup harmony. She has worked on significant projects related to mass religious gatherings, identifying shared spaces in diverse societies and currently she is collaborating on an international project investigating cultural diversity and identities across Asia. She is on the editorial Board of reputed journals and is the South Asia representative of Asian Association of Social Psychology.

Chapter 12
Sustainable Peace: Thinking Through a Psychosocial Lens

Shobna Sonpar

Abstract This paper argues that in order to sustain peace, interventions must address more than an end to conflict and violence. At the level of conceptual analysis, the psychosocial perspective offers a systemic and systematic approach to the conditions that would make for sustainable peace in a given context. At the level of practice, it would suggest what kinds of interventions, in what domains, administered by who, will likely have meaningful impact. It would also indicate the limitations imposed by particular contexts on the success of psychosocial interventions, an important concern given the notorious chronicity of many situations of violent conflict. Psychosocial intervention conventionally has tended to be identified narrowly with mental health and individual wellbeing. But sustaining peace calls for a more radical understanding that embraces many domains relevant to peace, yet is based on psychological principles. These points are illustrated with examples from India as well as other parts of the world.

Keywords Sustainable peace · Peace-building · Protracted conflict

Societies where political violence has occurred have a long and arduous journey before peace and people's wellbeing are restored. These sites often see violent conflict recurring over and over again despite peace talks and accords. To build sustainable peace on the ground, the material, emotional and psychological needs of the people affected as individuals and as communities have to be addressed, and capacity has to be built to handle potential conflicts constructively.

This chapter adopts a psychosocial lens to examine peacebuilding processes and argues that incorporating such a perspective ensures a more durable peace. In this light, it elaborates on components of peacebuilding beyond conventional peacemaking. These components include dealing with the material and psychological wounds to individuals and communities affected by violent conflict, transitional justice, dialogue and reconciliation, and structural peacebuilding. It delineates the

---

S. Sonpar (✉)
Kullu, India
e-mail: shobnasonpar@yahoo.co.in

U. Vindhya (ed.), *Psychosocial Interventions for Social Issues in Contemporary India*,
https://doi.org/10.1007/978-981-96-6553-2_12

particular relevance of the psychosocial lens to peacebuilding, and describes how the psychosocial model has evolved, the interventions it encompasses, and the attempts to systematize the field. It also discusses how psychosocial programs contribute to peace and positive social change in post-conflict societies even when their goals are not explicitly identified with peacebuilding. To this end, the findings of a multi-site project (Hamber & Gallagher, 2015) undertaken by the International Conflict Research Institute (INCORE) are discussed including the case study undertaken in the Indian state of Jammu & Kashmir. The chapter does not aim to present an exhaustive or comprehensive review about interventions at a global level but cites relevant examples to illustrate the concepts under discussion.

The Psychosocial Model

The psychosocial model emerged from the work of the Psychosocial Working Group (PWG) which was set up in 2000 as a consortium of international humanitarian agencies and academic institutions working in the field of psychosocial interventions in complex emergencies such as armed conflict. Faced with a wide diversity of perspectives and interventions in areas of armed conflict, the PWG formulated a conceptual framework to assess impacts on the affected population, their psychosocial needs, and to guide culturally sensitive interventions (Strang & Ager, 2003).

This model emphasizes the close interconnection between the *psychological aspects of experience* (thoughts, emotions, behavior) and *wider social experience* (relationships, traditions, norms, culture) (Strang & Ager, 2003). It recommends that interventions be directed toward promoting psychosocial wellbeing in the three interrelated domains of human capacity (the physical and mental health of persons as well as their knowledge and skills), social ecology (the social connections and support networks that people share), and cultural capital (the culture, values, norms that are the context that influences how people experience, understand and respond to events).

This model is seen as limited by practitioners and scholars from the global South critiquing Western models of care and intervention (Abeyasekara et al., 2008; Galappatti, 2003; Salih & Samarasinghe, 2006). Abeyasekara and Amarasuriya (2008) propose a psychosocial framework that includes economic circumstances and the political factors affecting people's lives. This framework, the Psychosocial Assessment of Development and Humanitarian Intervention (PADHI) program at the Social Policy Analysis and Research Centre at the University of Colombo, Sri Lanka (2008), was developed empirically to understand local understandings of the concepts of wellbeing and distress, and incorporate these in development and humanitarian intervention. It proposes three dimensions of analysis. The first addresses the domains of wellbeing. The second dimension identifies power and identity as factors that mediate wellbeing. The third dimension identifies systems and institutions as key to enabling or undermining the achievement of wellbeing. These operate at levels that range from the micro (family, informal social groups), to the meso (religious or other community bodies, health and education services, NGOs, local government bodies, militias) and to the macro (economic, political, judicial, legislative, and so on). With psychosocial wellbeing at its core, the framework provides a comprehensive psychosocial lens to understand the needs of people and communities and to plan and evaluate interventions. It also affords a dynamic view into how tensions may develop between levels which constrain and limit psychosocial work. For instance, interventions to address gender-based violence at the micro level may come into conflict with forces suspicious of such interventions at the meso level such as religious or other community bodies.

Peacebuilding and the Psychosocial Lens

In the past five decades, scholars have shown that ending violent conflict involves attending to the psychological needs and emotions of the people involved and changing the relationship between adversaries towards greater trust and cooperation and (Nadler et al., 2008). Yet these aspects of conflict and post-conflict contexts often do not enter the peacemaking deliberations.

Economists from the 1960s had similarly discounted the role of emotional and psychological factors assuming that humans were reasonable actors operating in a rational world. In the 1970s, psychologists like the Nobel prize winning Daniel Kahnemann began to challenge these assumptions and showed empirically that human beings have all sorts of biases and illusions and are influenced by things that happen inside them over which they have no control and of which they are not even aware. But these 'irrational' behaviours are also quite predictable, and economists have since adjusted their models to account for these systematic human quirks (Kahnemann, 2011; Ripley, 2019).

In discussing the centrality of emotional and psychological processes in the genesis and remedy of political violence, Majumdar (2020) points out that the findings from neuropsychological and cognitive research make irrelevant the assumed distinction between intelligent reasoning and emotional irrationality since all behaviours are influenced by emotional systems and cues which are closely associated with cognitive processes. She also highlights how emotions are inherently social and relational and at the centre of how communities are organized, function and communicate.

In the context of peacebuilding, attention to 'the psychological aspects of experience' and to 'wider social experience' is relevant on several counts. First, people in contexts of political violence suffer grievous losses of many kinds, violations of physical, sexual and mental nature that are emotionally scarring, and an emotional climate of constant fear and insecurity. In Kashmir, around 1996–2002 when political violence due to militancy and counter-militancy was at its height, the emotional climate was palpably one of intense fearfulness and loss underneath which was simmering anger, together with a social climate of distrust, suspicion and disconnection, and an overwhelming sense of helplessness and humiliation (Sonpar, 2000). Such impacts are not undone automatically when violence abates.

Secondly, the social fabric of the community is damaged in ways that are similar to the tissues of the body and mind, resulting in a loss of 'communality' (Erikson, 1976). Somasundaram (2007, 2014), describing the conflict situation in Sri Lanka, used the term 'collective trauma' to describe the negative impact on social processes, networks, relationships, institutions, dynamics, capital and resources.

Thirdly, such collective trauma damages the integrity of the cultural system on which people depend for meaning and direction (DeVries, 1996). Extreme violent events cause a rupture in the basic meaning structures that inform our vision of ourselves and our world. It entails the breakdown of a social and moral symbolic order based on trust, goodwill, compassionate interconnectedness and its replacement by a malevolent order based on fear, suspicion, and violence. Extreme violence 'unmakes' the internalized, culturally constituted webs of trust based on social norms, world views and moral conventions (Robben & Suarez-Orozco, 2000).

Fourthly, when conditions as described above are protracted, societies adapt so as to fulfil psychological needs for safety, mastery and positive identity, to handle stress, and to manage relations with perceived adversaries. Bar-Tal (2007) describes this as the 'sociopsychological infrastructure' that emerges as an adaptation to violent and protracted conflict, which itself becomes a big part of the problem impeding the restoration of peace. This sociopsychological infrastructure is characterised by collective narratives and memories of loss and victimization, 'chosen traumas' and 'chosen glories' (Volkan, 2001) often reaching far back in history. These narratives selectively represent one's own identity group positively, and help satisfy the need to understand what is happening in a coherent frame. Alongside, there is a sense of collective victimhood often used to justify their own acts of violence and revenge. A set of assumptions and beliefs, consistent with the collective narratives that are circulating, and characterized by black and white thinking, begins to emerge. In describing the elements of 'extreme political traumatisation', Hamber (2015) draws attention to the discursive distortions marked by the rhetoric of dehumanization, deceptive public discussion, and language aimed at creating exclusion and sometimes provoking direct violence. These orient current and future relations with perceived adversaries and thus constitute significant obstacles in reconciliation.

Fifthly, while hope can become an instrumental pathway towards conflict resolution in the context of ongoing conflict (Bar-Tal et al., 2017), high levels of fear and anger override hope as the primary emotional and cognitive orientation thus becoming an obstacle in peacebuilding. Indeed, intervention models to break cycles of violence start with dealing with the traumatic emotions of grief and anger following violation, and steer the ensuing narrative away from revengeful violence towards the establishment of justice and the possibility of reconciliation (Botcharova, 2001). Further, mentalization (Fonagy et al., 2002), the ability to accurately read one's own subjective state and that of the other, is inhibited under conditions of severe physical and psychological unsafety. This capacity is significantly related to being able to control emotions, to be reflective rather than reactive, to negotiate rather than fight, and to empathise with the other. Thus the importance of considering emotional regulation strategies in the context of post conflict peacebuilding (Halperin & Pliskin, 2015; Halperin et al., 2011, 2014).

Since the emotional life of individuals and societies has not been seen as relevant, policy discussions and conflict resolution efforts in India and Asia have largely ignored the aspect of emotional grievances, frustration, fear, humiliations, anger, as well as hope and resilience that are omnipresent in communities exposed to political violence (Majumdar, 2020).

In her study of youth in Kashmir, Majumdar (2020) found that the emotional consequences of living in a long-drawn conflict context had significant ominous potential in that their ability to cognitively reappraise emotional experience was affected. This related to their belief that the world was a vile place, as well as their support for violence as a remedy. Her findings suggest a role for extremist ideology in such circumstances, the extreme ideas providing the solace of righteousness and simplicity in a complex and dangerous world. The emotional processes were intermeshed with identity processes such that in-group identity became stronger while other groups were viewed negatively and as potentially dangerous. Thus the dominating narrative among Kashmiri youth centred around the violent and persecutory Other and the victimized Us. These findings echo the conclusions reached from a study of former militants in Kashmir (Sonpar, 2007).

In the absence of attending to the 'psychosocial', the wounds of violent conflict, combined with lack of justice and accountability, the stresses of life in post-conflict contexts, and ongoing socio-economic and political marginalisation, can contribute to a cycle whereby violence reasserts itself time and again.

Building Sustainable Peace

In order to be sustainable, peacebuilding involves working for 'negative peace' or the cessation of direct violence at one end, and working for 'positive peace', the building of a healthy society that seeks to correct the structural violence inherent in economic and social inequities that may have contributed to conflict in the first place (Galtung, 1969), at the other. Other processes addressing the material, emotional, psychological and relational impact of violent conflict are equally important as are the issues of accountability and justice All these components of peacebuilding may be summarized as follows.

1. ***Peacemaking or working towards the cessation of direct violence through peace accords and agreements***. This is a top down process and is usually the province of peacemakers—diplomats, politicians, security experts—who engage in negotiating agreements. The wellbeing of people rarely figures in these deliberations. They may give the illusion of settlement but psychosocial aspects are not addressed and the terms may not be acceptable to people. For instance, a popular civil resistance movement began in 2004 against international peacekeepers, the

UN Mission in Kosovo, for imposing an externally driven governance model deemed illegitimate and unacceptable to the Kosovar people (Dudouet, 2017).

An in-depth analysis of peacemaking over the years in the three Indian states of Andhra Pradesh (left wing extremists or the Maoists), Manipur (secessionist militancy, tribal hostilities) and Kashmir (secessionist militancy, 'proxy war' with Pakistan), reveals the obstacles to making peace due to factors such as political expediency by the government in power, the readiness of the state to use its coercive armed powers rather than sustain dialogue in good faith, and disruption by 'spoilers' invested in continuing the conflict. Interestingly, civil society inputs did happen notably in the Andhra case in which a citizens' committee drove the process (Centre for Humanitarian Dialogue & Delhi Policy Group, 2011).

2. ***Dealing with the material and psychological wounds to individuals and communities as a result of the violent conflict***. This means addressing the psychological traumas that people have undergone as a result of displacement, loss, atrocity as well as the collective trauma to communities where the social and material fabric is ruptured and victims and perpetrators of violence may have to coexist. Post-conflict societies have high rates of gender-based violence, crime, substance abuse in addition to mental health disorders. Attending to all this is essential to restoring psychosocial wellbeing and a peaceful community. The field of psychosocial intervention is typically associated with this aspect of the peacebuilding process now termed Mental Health and Psychosocial Support (MHPSS).

   As elaborated upon in later sections of this chapter, the field of MHPSS has seen a systematization under the Inter Agency Standing Committee (IASC) Guidelines and there has been an interrogation and recasting of what constitutes psychosocial support and the role of the 'outside' practitioner. While there are growing efforts towards intentionally integrating MHPSS and peacebuilding conceptually and in practice, it is also the case, as described in the INCORE study, that psychosocial interventions contribute to longer term impacts on peace and social transformation without these being explicit goals.

   Working with children and youth growing up in contexts of chronic political violence is a crucial area addressing the dangers of intergenerational transmission of trauma and continuing cycles of violence. Such interventions include peace education (Singh, 2018), an important area not covered in this chapter.

3. ***Transitional justice*** refers to macro-level approaches usually adopted by governments and sometimes other public bodies, like the UN or the Catholic church, that aim to address the systematic abuse of power by former regimes without endangering the democratic transitions that are underway. It encompasses a range of mechanisms and processes associated with society's attempt to come to terms with past legacies of violence in order to ensure accountability and serve justice. These include both judicial and non-judicial mechanisms—truth commissions, criminal prosecution, material and symbolic reparation, memorialization efforts, cultural and creative initiatives, preservation of archives, reform of history education, as well as legal and institutional reforms (International Centre for Transitional Justice, 2009).

Minow (1998) discusses transitional justice processes highlighting their underpinnings in the complex emotional and psychosocial issues around truth-seeking and truth-telling, remembering and forgetting, trauma and healing, vengeance and forgiveness, acknowledgement and apology, reparation and restorative justice.

The best known example is that of the South African Truth and Reconciliation Commission that was created by the South African parliament in 1995 with committees on human rights violations, amnesty and reparations. As described by Minow (1998), it was decided that to achieve national unity and a morally acceptable reconciliation, it was necessary that truth about past atrocities be publicly established by fair and official procedures, together with the identity of planners, perpetrators and victims. In order that a peaceful transition to democracy be achieved, amnesty was given to those who personally applied for it on the condition that they disclosed fully the facts of their politically motivated misdeeds.

4. ***Dialogue and reconciliation.*** Reconciliation is a process that aims towards mutual acceptance between groups that were in conflict such that they can find a way to live alongside one another and develop a degree of cooperation necessary to share society (Tankink & Bubenzer, 2017). This is a core aspect of peacebuilding usually involving sustained intergroup dialogue during which the participants grow to trust and understand one another, dispel prejudices, reflect on themselves, acknowledge harms done to one another and find a way of coexisting that is just and peaceful.
5. ***Structural peacebuilding.*** In order to sustain peace in the long term, the root causes of the conflict located in structural inequities and power asymmetries need to be addressed. Development is seen as one route towards this end. The other is non-violent collective action and civil resistance movements that seek to influence public policy and decision-making in the direction of social justice.

Psychosocial Interventions and the Inter-Agency Standing Committee (IASC) Guidelines on Mental Health and Psychosocial Support in Emergency Settings

While the post-Cold War period saw humanitarian interventions taking a psychosocial turn focusing on mental health (especially in the 80s and 90s), the assumption was that it was necessary to do 'trauma healing' in order to prevent cycles of violence from perpetuating. Thus the dominant conceptualization of suffering was in the idiom of psychopathology, especially post-traumatic stress disorder (PTSD). This biomedical trauma model applied to suffering arising from natural and manmade disasters has been criticized for ignoring the sociopolitical context, reducing complex human responses to clinical phenomena, being individual in focus and neglecting the wider impact on communities, ignoring cultural expressions of suffering, community strengths and ways of coping, and people's priorities (Ager, 1997; Bracken et al., 1997; Breslau, 2004; Pederson, 2002; Pupavac, 2002; Sonpar, 2008; Summerfield, 1999, 2004). The concept of trauma has since undergone change and is closer to the idea of sequential traumatization (Becker, 2004), a process in which situations arising from specific extreme events exert their own pressures that become a continuing traumatization. People thus experience different mental health impacts at different points in time and it is necessary to pay attention continually to the changing context and its implications.

A great variety of interventions including counselling, psychoeducation, interpersonal skills development, social expressive activities, creative arts, storytelling, mobilizing social networks, supportive practices for child development, vocational skills training, micro-credit groups, spiritual and grief work, livelihoods support, human rights interventions and so on all tend to be clubbed under the label ‘psychosocial’. Galappatti (2003) points out that although these fall broadly under the mental health, community-developmental and social justice domains of intervention, the programs rarely explicate the linkages between domain, strategy and outcome. The IASC Guidelines on Mental Health and Psychosocial Support (MHPSS) in Emergency Settings help plug this gap (Inter-Agency Standing Committee, 2007; Wessells & Ommeren, 2008).

The Interagency Standing Committee (IASC) was established by the UN General Assembly as an inter-agency forum for coordination, policy development and decision-making by the executive heads of key humanitarian agencies. The IASC Guidelines that was released in 2007 defines MHPSS as a composite term ‘to describe any type of local or outside support that aims to protect or promote psychosocial wellbeing and/or treat mental disorder’. The guidelines cover psychosocial concerns over all sectors of humanitarian work, recognize that a focus on traumatic stress and PTSD leads to the neglect of many other key mental health and psychosocial issues, and recommends that interventions in post-conflict settings should not only address problems but also strengthen resilience and coping of individuals and communities.

It suggests a layered system of complementary supports that meets the needs of different groups as illustrated in a pyramid of four levels. Level 1 at the base of the pyramid addresses the need for basic services, adequate governance and security which affect most of the conflict affected population. Although MHPSS workers do not deliver these directly, they can advocate that these services be put in place documenting their impact on human wellbeing and by influencing those responsible.

Level 2 of the pyramid of MHPSS addresses community and family supports. In a post-conflict situation, many people are affected by loss, displacement, family separation, as well as disrupted social networks and a social climate of fear, mistrust and hostility. Useful interventions at this level include assisted mourning and community healing ceremonies, family tracing and reunification, mass psychoeducation about constructive coping, formal and non-formal educational activities and supportive parenting programs, livelihoods activities, creative and sports activities, women’s groups and youth clubs.

Level 3 of the pyramid of MHPSS concerns the provision of focused support addressing the need of smaller groups of people who require more targeted individual or group intervention by trained workers who may not be professionals. Such interventions include the provision of basic mental health care by primary health care workers trained in psychological first aid, interventions addressing gender-based violence, human rights abuses like enforced disappearances and torture, and engaging specific groups like ex-combatants.

Level 4 at the top of the pyramid of MHPSS is for specialised services addressing the needs of the small percentage of the population whose suffering and difficulties in daily functioning warrants the services of mental health professionals like psychiatrists and psychologists.

Case studies using the IASC Guidelines indicate their usefulness as a coordination tool for stakeholders in identifying priority needs and planning intervention from a holistic perspective in contexts of political violence such as in Colombia (Echeverri & Castilla, 2008) as well as in the context of climate-change related emergencies such as in Bangladesh, Burkina Faso, Madagascar, Nigeria, Sierra Leone and Zimbabwe (Eaton et al., 2022). In contexts like Nepal where few organisations specialize in MHPSS and there is a lack of coordination and understanding between organisations, there is need to do comprehensive preparatory work in order to implement the guidelines effectively (Jordans et al., 2010). In order to make the guidelines accessible to community workers who may have difficulty reading and comprehending the guidelines, there have been efforts to use pictorial aids and 'high-visual' instruction materials in several post-disaster settings in Latin America and Southeast Asia (Diaz et al., 2008). In India, the IASC Guidelines have informed the development of the National Disaster Management Guidelines: Mental Health and Psychosocial Support in Disasters (National Disaster Management Authority & Rahbar, 2023).

Psychosocial Practices and Practitioners

From the above, it will be apparent that the need for psychosocial interventions requiring professional mental health experts such as clinical psychologists and psychiatrists, applies to a small segment of the affected population. Psychosocial practitioners can come from a variety of backgrounds and develop competency through training and supervision. The competencies required may be wide-ranging from being able to provide psychological first-aid to understanding and facilitating group work to engaging in liaison and advocacy work.

Increasingly, psychosocial support is not seen as a specific intervention belonging to certain projects, but is rather an approach informing all humanitarian and developmental interventions (Williamson & Robinson, 2006). In Sri Lanka, Galappatti and Salih (2006) find poverty-reduction programs ideally suited to enhance psychosocial wellbeing in the aftermath of political violence given the stressful nature of the experience of poverty with its restriction on people's ability to exercise choice, and the sheer hopelessness and humiliation associated with it. They developed a resettlement program where psychosocial principles were incorporated into the economic-developmental interventions. This involved the use of psychosocial workers to facilitate group meetings, understand group dynamics, address group conflicts, advocate on behalf of more vulnerable members, model perspective-taking, and generally be helpful in a non-intrusive way in the lives of the people involved.

The Gujarat Harmony Program (NIMHANS & CARE, India, 2003) brought the principle of psychosocial care as a central and essential part of an otherwise diverse array of interventions undertaken by 21 participating organisations that came together after the ethnic riots in Gujarat in 2002. These interventions encompassed livelihoods strengthening activities, women's groups, children's play and education, medical relief, social rehabilitation, legal help, constructions of shelters, ethnic reconciliation and so on. The principles of psychosocial care were seen as active listening, empathy, ventilation of feelings, social support, encouraging externalisation of interests, spiritual and recreational activities.

In their exhaustive review of empirical research into immediate and mid-term mass trauma intervention, Hobfoll et al. (2007) endorse five elements: the promotion of safety, calming, collective and self-efficacy, connectedness and hope. Interventions guided by these elements can be termed 'trauma aware' and can be applied at individual and community levels and inform a range of activities including those that are broadly economic-developmental.

There has also been much discussion of the position of the practitioner in terms of being an 'insider' or an 'outsider' along with the danger of imposing values and ways of understanding and acting that are at odds with the local milieu. 'Psychosocial accompaniment' has been suggested as a way of explicitly avoiding acting out the colonial pattern of 'helping' that culturally invades, depowers and disrespects those 'inside' (Watkins, 2021). An ethical approach to accompanying requires critical reflection on one's own positionality and its effects. It may require depowering and de-privileging oneself as much as possible in order to support the leadership and voices of those from within the community. This reorientation enables accompaniment to potentially become a mutual process of collaboration that over time transforms into committed solidarity for just relations.

Integrating MHPSS and Peacebuilding

The umbrella phrases of psychosocial intervention and peacebuilding conventionally cover widely diverging fields, a primary goal of the former being to improve the wellbeing of individuals and families whereas the latter focuses on communal and institutional processes (Hamber et al., 2014). Global definitions of peacebuilding do not sufficiently recognize the grievous impact of violent conflict on psychosocial wellbeing and that for positive peace MHPSS is essential. MHPSS practitioners focus on the wellbeing of individuals and families while not sufficiently taking into account that these take place within larger societal processes. Altering the wider social context is seen as the work of politicians and activists and beyond the remit of psychosocial practitioners (Hamber et al., 2014).

Bubenzer and Tankink (2017) discuss the integration of peacebuilding and MHPSS through a literature review and a mapping exercise and find that although the benefit of doing so was generally agreed upon, in practice organisations working in the field of peacebuilding and those in MHPSS rarely cooperate nor coordinate their efforts in an ecological way. The perceived gap seemed partly to be based on lack of knowledge and opportunity for engagement with the other field. The study also points to a number of myths, notably that MHPSS is a humanitarian activity whereas peacebuilding is political in nature, that MHPSS is about narrowly defined trauma and trauma healing, that an integrated approach would compromise the political 'neutrality' of MHPSS workers.

However, in the past decade more concerted efforts are being made to integrate peacebuilding and MHPSS. Also the Inter Agency Standing Committee has reported on integrating MHPSS and peacebuilding through a mapping exercise and has made recommendations for practitioners (IASC, 2024). Projects that intentionally integrate MHPSS with peacebuilding are also growing such as that described by Tankink et al. (2022) in northern Uganda.

Hamber et al. (2014) ask how psychosocial intervention in conflict and post-conflict situations might shape long-term collective social processes of peacebuilding and wider social change. To this end a project was undertaken by the International Conflict Research Institute (INCORE) at the University of Ulster with multi-disciplinary researchers from around the globe, who conducted cases studies in Guatemala, Northern Ireland, Mozambique, India, Sri Lanka, South Africa and East Jerusalem (Hamber & Gallagher, 2015). Two case studies from Northern Ireland and India are described below to illustrate the diversity of psychosocial practices on the ground and the kinds of impact these had on peace and social transformataion.

Northern Ireland Case Study

Reflecting on the psychosocial programs in post-peace agreement Northern Ireland, Gallagher and Hamber (2015) focus on the experience of young men who are a priority vulnerable group. Young men report higher levels of political and inter-community violence in a society that remains polarized and divided, and were more likely to participate in violence themselves. They face threats of paramilitary attacks and intimidation and are also in danger of paramilitary recruitment. This, along with high youth unemployment, is thought to contribute to high rates of suicide and harmful behaviours such as substance abuse.

The authors studied four psychosocial programs of which two were specifically targeted at victim survivors and had a trauma focus. Most of the young men attending these programs were from impoverished backgrounds and had low educational attainment. One psychosocial program engaged men who are young fathers dealing with a range of problems from addiction to being in trouble with the police to school suspension. The support group taught young men how to communicate, build interpersonal skills, and rebuild fragmented relationships with family and friends. Another program tried to address the isolation that men feel by providing a safe space for them to get help for a variety of problems ranging from mental health to anger management to sexual abuse. They used counselling, substance abuse awareness and self-esteem building techniques to get young men to realise their worth and build better lives for themselves.

A third psychosocial program, specifically for victim-survivors, offered care and support to anyone bereaved or traumatized through the violence irrespective of religious or political belief. It mainly used psychotherapy and counselling complemented with art, storytelling and drama, and also provided vocational training opportunities. The fourth program, also for victim-survivors, was a community-led organisation with a Christian ethos that tried to address the transgenerational effects of the conflict. It encouraged young people to address the feelings, prejudices and misunderstandings they may have as a result of the narratives circulating about the conflict. The project provided training in essential life skills and used art, drama, music and prayer to help youth.

All the programs placed importance on developing capacities as key to personal and eventual social change. They saw themselves as equipping young men to build their self-worth and be in control of their lives which placed them in a better position to deal with others, especially those different to themselves. The men themselves became the embodiment of social change, and could go on to catalyze change in society. Together with personal capacity development, there was also a focus on inter-community exploration of political issues and attitudes. Through exploring attitudes, learning about cultural identity and gaining an understanding of the past conflict, they became aware of their own often subliminal sectarian attitudes. This helped gain perspective on other narratives, arrive at a mutually shared understanding of the past, encourage empathy and cooperative interaction thus helping hitherto antagonistic groups build relationships. The young men emphasized the personal process bringing inner peace that translated into better relationships. The staff of the projects highlighted how such changes contributed to the collective process that in Northern Ireland meant narrowing the divide between Catholic and Protestant communities.

India Case Study

The India case study (Sonpar, 2015) was undertaken in 2010–2011 with the objective of determining the impact of psychosocial programming on peacebuilding, development and social transformation in the context of political violence in Jammu & Kashmir (JK). Psychosocial programming at that time was a little over a decade old in JK. The earliest interventions aimed to bring relief to orphans and widows, from which the field expanded to encompass mental health, community-developmental and social justice activities. In the initial years, a proliferation of non-governmental initiatives, and the perception that these had money-making rather than humanitarian intent, coupled with the fear of "outsider" influence on Kashmiri culture and values, contributed to a public wariness. They also struggled with the constraints inherent to working in a conflict zone such as lengthy delays and scrutiny in registering organizations, funding restrictions, and an ambiguous relationship with government agencies (Suri, 2003). The earthquake that devastated northern areas of Kashmir in 2005 brought in humanitarian aid that helped change perceptions. By the time of the present study, psychosocial programs run by international organisations as well as local initiatives were well-established. Thus one respondent in the study described the field as starting with a "passive" and traumatized population, to "NGOisation", and increasingly to community-led initiatives.

For the India case study, three projects were selected for in-depth analysis and another five were studied through interviews with their coordinating staff. The three main projects studied were (a) Help Foundation which provides help to under-privileged sections of Kashmiri society in the sectors of education, health and economic assistance, (b) Association of Parents of Disappeared Persons (APDP) which campaigns collectively for accountability and justice with regard to the enforced disappearance of their missing relatives, and (c) Athwaas Project in the Purkho Camp in Jammu which brought together women from the displaced Hindu Pandit community in a safe place where they could share their stories and lives, reflect and engage in activities for income-generation as well as participate in workshops for psychosocial healing, gender and domestic violence related awareness, and dialogues between Hindu and Muslim women. The other five organisations were the Coalition of Civil Society (working in the field of civil rights including enforced disappearances), Centre for Dialogue and Reconciliation (facilitating dialogue between civil society from different regions of JK, between Kashmiri Hindus and Muslims, and between Kashmiris in JK and Pakistan), Action Aid (that runs mental health programs, and is active in community mental health initiatives), and two organizations that focused on youth—MercyCorps (engaged in capacity building among youth for leadership and entrepreneurship) and Yakjah Reconciliation and Development Network (working among youth from different regional and religious backgrounds in JK to foster peaceful coexistence).

These programs were selected on the basis of diversity of sectors of intervention and representation of differences along lines of gender, age, ethnicity, and nature of traumas suffered. Most were also developed from local Kashmiri initiatives.

All the programs found it necessary to engage with the emotional and psychological impact of the years of political violence on the participants and psychosocial healing interventions were a significant part of their work. Indeed, several organizations not included in the study such as Medecins sans Frontieres have been active in providing mental health counselling, and building local mental health counselling capacity through training.

In the domain of development, it was found that these psychosocial programs contributed to economic well-being, educational improvement and the development of human capital. In families with low unstable incomes, even small amounts of regular financial assistance go a long way and the income generation modules of these projects led to a sense of empowerment among the participants. Across all the projects, the development of human capital was a major effect. Self-confidence, better communication and interpersonal skills, and discovery of latent talents and strengths, were important markers of personal growth for participants. Beyond the personal benefits, many participants also felt that it made them catalysts for social change. A significant number of participants described their experience in the project as a turning point in their understanding of society and of themselves as having social agency and efficacy.

The findings in the peacebuilding domain indicate that while the projects helped participants find 'inner peace', a major achievement in a context that is emotionally fraught and insecure, they also helped restore 'communality'. Many attributed the role of the projects in creating a caring community despite an emotional climate full of mistrust, suspicion and cynicism. It was also seen that in time there was constructive collaboration amongst many civil society organisations.

With respect to inter-group dialogue and reconciliation, the findings suggest the need for methodical and sustained efforts over a long period. They point to the difficulties inherent in such work where social identities are central and emotions associated with personal and community traumas run high. Workshops where displaced Pandit women and Kashmiri Muslim women came together were extremely emotional events and much genuine warmth was expressed along with the sharing and acknowledgment of one another's stories of suffering. But issues outside their control situated in their social group, as well as the larger sociopolitical context, made it difficult to follow up on the initial steps.

The role of the macro sociopolitical environment on the work of psychosocial programs was factored into the interventions undertaken by the Centre for Dialogue and Reconciliation (CDR). Its approach was to initiate dialogue at the grassroots level to understand ground realities and also with influential civil society actors, followed by lobbying and advocacy with the government or its institutions. It initiated civil society dialogue between different regions of JK and also between the civil society of JK and Pakistan-administered Kashmir and sustained these dialogues over several years. The former gave voice to large areas of the state that were hitherto neglected such as the border communities whose fields and homes were destroyed by shells and mines. The latter provided inputs to the Track One peace talks between India and Pakistan. In early stages, the dialogue dwelt on sharing experiences. When it expanded from personal tragedies to sociopolitical grievances, it became apparent that it was necessary to interface with the state. Thus advocacy became an important intervention. A strategy that was adopted was to commission research studies that were used to anchor dialogue to facts and to strengthen advocacy. Another intervention was to foster linkages between institutions. For instance, the chambers of commerce in Jammu and in Kashmir were involved in a dialogue that resulted in mutually agreed ways to prevent political agitations from getting regionally polarized and this initiative did bear positive results during subsequent agitations.

The role of the larger sociopolitical environment on psychosocial programs in the sector of human rights, justice and accountability is often constricting and even adversarial. The work of the APDP to put pressure on the government through a weekly public protest, and with the media to keep their concerns in the public eye, had been successful in that it was no longer easy for the state to disappear people with impunity though the work of seeking accountability in individual cases moved slowly. Public silence was also broken with respect to disappearances at the hands of militants. The finding of 2700 unmarked graves containing a total of 2943 bodies led to a successful campaign for government inquiry which was taken up by the State Human Rights Commission.

The attention of several psychosocial programs focused on youth recognizing that an entire generation of children born amidst political violence has now reached adulthood. The huge youth involvement in anti-government protests and rising prevalence of substance abuse triggered alarm. There is enormous disaffection among youth in JK and complex factors related to cycles of violence and intergenerational transmissions are at play. An attempt was made by CDR to introduce peace education in secondary schools and although over 200 teachers were trained in the curriculum that was developed, further progress was stalled in bureaucratic machinery. The two youth-related programs covered in this study generated much enthusiasm among participants leading the organisers to believe that conflict transformation lay in being able to channel the idealism of youth to alternatives perspectives and experiences. These programs successfully reached out to youth to impart leadership and negotiation skills, to train them to think critically and constructively about sociopolitical issues, to develop entrepreneurship capacity as well as to change attitudes in the direction of coexistence and harmony in place of prejudice and hostility. However, there was also an apprehension of the new-found enthusiasm and agency being shattered by an unyielding sociopolitical environment and institutions. Indeed, some of the young coordinators interviewed, who had started out with passion and commitment, showed signs of bitterness and burn-out by the wearying nature of battling what they describe as a brick wall.

Yet changes were happening that suggested greater engagement of people in citizenship practices that arguably deepen democracy. Gaventa and Barrett (2010) in a meta-case analysis of 100 research studies of citizen engagement in 20 countries of varied degrees of political stability and democratization, found that citizen participation through local association activities, social movements, campaigns, formal participatory governance, and so on had highly significant positive effects. An awareness of rights, knowledge of legal and institutional procedures, engaged action, organization skills, robust civic networks were all indicators of emerging democratic citizenship. Several of the psychosocial programs covered in the JK case study, particularly those in the social justice sector like APDP, also engaged in imparting knowledge of entitlements, rights, legal instruments and processes, the use of the Right to Information that allows transparency and accountability in government functioning, organising collective protests, initiating public interest litigation and so on. Arguably, psychosocial programs that further the practice of substantive citizenship could be considered political (Montero, 1998). However, the program staff interviewed insisted on calling these activities 'humanitarian', perhaps for strategic and security reasons of appearing political neutral.

Over time with the central government espousing an ideology at odds with Muslim-majority JK and fraught relations with Pakistan, the political situation on the ground changed. In 2019, JK lost its special constitutional status and statehood. It was divided into two Union Territories governed by the Centre. This was accompanied by the detention of local political and religious leaders for many months, curbs on the media and reporting, internet blackout, and swift punitive action for protest or dissent. Organisations working on human rights issues were particularly affected. The work of the JK Coalition of Civil Society is at a standstill and its coordinator who is also the Chairperson of the Asian Federation against Involuntary Disappearances is in prison as an undertrial under draconian counter-terrorism laws. The work of other organisations has also suffered due to curtailment of funds. Indeed, the work of the NGO sector and civil society in general in India has become fraught with the National Security Adviser declaring in 2021 that the new frontiers of war, or fourth-generation warfare, is civil society because civil society risks being subverted, suborned and manipulated to hurt national interests (Baru, 2021).

This case study highlights the vulnerability of psychosocial programs to macro political factors and policy changes over which they have no control. Writing about the Sri Lanka case, Samarasinghe (2015) notes that the end of the 30-year old war in 2009 that saw the defeat of the Liberation Tigers of Tamil Eelam (LTTE) was marked by many positive changes but the lack of accountability and justice for the thousands of civilians killed in the last few months of the war, the collapse of the rule of law, political killings and impunity for abuses continue to be matters of concern. A Presidential Task Force set up in 2009 was mandated to prepare plans for resettlement and rehabilitation in the northern Province. All NGOS had to register with them and special permission had to be obtained for certain activities deemed to be against national interest. Providing psychosocial intervention or documenting human rights violations were part of this list. At the time of the study in 2011 no organization in the North or the East had been granted permission for psychosocial intervention.

Drawing on the overall findings from the INCORE project and other similar studies, Hamber et al. (2014) show that psychosocial work has a very positive role to play in the peacebuilding process at three overlapping levels.

First, by addressing individual psychological needs and capacities it prepares individuals to engage in wider social processes like peacebuilding. Thus, the study of psychosocial programming in Northern Ireland for alienated young men who were vulnerable to violence indicated a personal transformation. This personal transformation was seen as a first step towards social transformation and peacebuilding work. Similarly, among Mayan women in the Guatemala case study (Lykes & Crosby, 2015) the various interventions led to burgeoning capacities to engage actively in local and national transformative processes. This aspect is akin to the concept of building psychological capital defined as an individual's positive psychological development characterized by efficacy, optimism, hope and resilience (Luthans & Youssef-Morgan, 2017).

Secondly, psychosocial interventions foster relationship building by challenging exclusion and separation. Hart and Colo (2014) focus on interventions with small groups of women in Bosnia & Herzegovina that initially involved listening, sharing stories and information that built trust and promoted individual healing. The sustained dialogue process that ensued enabled stereotyping and prejudice to decrease and as the women came together in joint economic and civic activities, the relations between hitherto hostile groups improved.

Thirdly, psychosocial interventions help create an expanded awareness and understanding at a cognitive, analytical level. Thus, the Mayan women in Guatemala

(Lykes & Crosby, 2015) gained an understanding of their predicament in terms of gender and also in terms of belonging to a stigmatized indigenous community. They were 'conscientised' (Freire, 1970) to the forms of gendered and racialized violence that was their everyday experience and this helped raise their voice in the community and political arena.

Transitional Justice

Transitional justice measures can play an important psychosocial role in restoring an affected community's sense of the existence of a social-symbolic moral order and in repairing intergroup relations. In Sri Lanka, following the end of the war with the LTTE, the government established a Lessons Learnt and Reconciliation Commission as a mechanism for accountability and for reconciliation. Samarasinghe (2015) describes how this process provided space for people to air their grievances and for their suffering to be acknowledged. In its recommendations, the Commission talks about redress to the next of kin of those killed, investigation into enforced disappearances, ensuring detentions and arrests are done within a legal framework, implementation of a language policy ensuring equality of access and opportunity and active measures towards reconciliation. The Commission recognizes that people's suffering needs to be addressed through counselling, justice mechanisms, compensation and acknowledgment if peace and reconciliation are to happen. It also notes that these can happen only through systemic changes in the law and state structures, and through a process of integration. However, while the government tries to implement its reconciliation plans, the realities on the ground in the North and East are ominous. With emergency and antiterrorism laws still in place, media and political opponents somewhat repressed and the military dominating the areas once ruled by the LTTE, the task itself has become ambivalently fraught.

Reflecting on what transpired in East Timor, Le Touze et al. (2005) ask if there can be healing without justice. They suggest that some of the social instability and civic upheaval including gender-based violence and crime occur in part due to collective anger that past injustices have not been adequately redressed. In East Timor, although a truth and reconciliation commission had been set up to establish the truth of the human rights violations between 1974–1999, only perpetrators of minor violations were brought under its purview. A parallel Serious Crimes Unit was set up but these perpetrators, who were more powerful people, escaped to Indonesia.

The tension between the desire to build peace and leave the past behind, and the need to establish truth and acknowledge justice in relation to past human rights violations remains a constraint that all such truth commissions contend with. In India too, voices have been raised from time to time asking for truth commissions related to the Partition, the anti-Sikh riots of 1984, the Gujarat riots of 2002, Kashmir and so on. But as pointed out by Kurian (2023), in the context of the recent call for a Northeastern India Truth and Reconciliation Commission put forward by women's organisations in Northeast India, truth commissions are premised on fact finding and truth telling but those who are, or have been, in power will resist this fearing being implicated by the findings.

Becker (2005) points out that reconciliation, without truth, is picked up by politicians to gloss over the crimes of perpetrators in the aftermath of conflict. He gives the example of Chile where once the transition into peace began, victims' groups which had hitherto been at the forefront of the struggle, began to be seen as a threat to the process of democratization. He argues that the goal of reconciliation should not be harmony between erstwhile enemies, but an improved capacity to handle conflict in constructive, non-violent ways, and that instead of putting the past to rest, there must be a continuous engagement with what the past has taught us. Truth telling and transitional justice are part of this process not synonymous with it.

But such commissions also have positive outcomes. Discussing the value of the South African Truth and Reconciliation Commission, Gobodo-Madikizela (2008) describes how the public admission of guilt creates a new understanding between victims and perpetrators that helped heal broken relationships. When perpetrators express remorse they acknowledge the victims' suffering giving them back their dignity. Forgiveness from the victim can be a healthy response that allows both parties to move on. Using case examples from Tunisia, Colombia, Gambia and the Democratic Republic of Congo, the UN Office of the High Commissioner for Human Rights (2020) concludes that when a range of transitional justice measures are deployed in a manner that is context specific, nationally owned and focused on the needs of victims, societies can achieve positive transformation.

The case study by Lykes and Crosby (2015) in Guatemala with Mayan women survivors of sexual violence committed during the 36 year-long Guatemalan armed conflict shows how psychosocial projects may contribute to processes of transitional justice. These women participated in an explicitly feminist series of actions in support for their struggles for truth, justice and reparation. This fed into the wider processes of transitional justice instituted after the war such as the events associated with the project of Historical Memory and the Tribunal of Conscience. The Tribunal was structured as a mock trial with women survivors presenting their testimony before lawyers and judges, and with expert witnesses providing the context for these crimes to a general audience of around 800 people. This 'performance of pain' created a public space for women to tell their stories, to influence public opinion and to establish networks of solidarity in the lead up to the presentation of a formal legal case of sexual violence as a weapon of war to the Guatemalan courts. Achieving recognition and justice from the Guatemalan state and the army perpetrators of the violence was a key goal for women survivors.

Importantly, victims who testify in such truth commissions need concurrent and ongoing psychosocial support since the process of reopening wounds in recounting their experiences leaves many emotionally shaken and even re-traumatised. Hamber (2015) asks the important question of what is the relationship between how the individual's (often victim) process of coming to terms with mass atrocity (a micro perspective) relates to the collective or political process of finding ways of dealing with the past (a macro perspective). It is often the case that the individual's process is 'moving' at a different pace from what might be happening at the collective/political level. Further, it is important to acknowledge the reality that the psychological impact of extreme violence can never be totally alleviated and that collective processes can never fully meet all human needs. Also the manner in which transitional justice measures are implemented has to be ever-mindful of the emotional and psychological aspects of dealing with traumatic loss, violation and abuse. For instance, while symbolic reparations such as apology and memorialization can bridge the internal psychological world and social world for victims, the context has to be one that demonstrates adequate levels of recognition, responsibility and acknowledgement of the harm inflicted without indirectly providing justification for the offence.

Dialogue and Intergroup Reconciliation

Inter-group dialogue and reconciliation is another modality of peacebuilding often supplementing the macro measures of transitional justice undertaken by governments as described above, but also extensively used at the community level in a wide range of contexts.

Nadler et al. (2008) usefully distinguish between socioemotional and instrumental reconciliation. Socioemotional reconciliation aims to change the relationship between adversaries from a process of working through emotions and threats to identity that are the consequence of the pain and humiliation that the parties had inflicted on one another. Instrumental reconciliation aims to change adversarial relations into positive relations that will allow the parties to coexist without conflict and is a long-term process during which their contact with one another enables trust and positive attitudes to replace enmity and negative attitudes. Many such programs involve cooperative efforts to achieve instrumental goals important to both parties. Contact alone may not reduce intergroup tension but can be usefully combined, depending on the context, with the pursuit of superordinate goals, economic development, forgiveness, confidence building, education for mutual understanding, prejudice reduction and exploring cultures (Ryan, 1995).

The mohalla committees, citizens' committees for peace, set up in Dharavi in Mumbai (Barve, 2003) are a successful example involving elements of socioemotional and instrumental reconciliation. In an atmosphere leading to ghettoization of the Muslim community after the 1992–1993 Mumbai attacks, and an insidious campaign to foment communal discord, an effort was made to have dialogue between antagonistic groups to help deepen understanding of their diverse communities, address prejudice and stereotyping, and build a team which would work towards fostering community spirit at a local level. These citizens' committees for peace became the nodes for a network of programs to prevent violence, deal with civic problems, ensure communal harmony and good public-police relations. The committee members learned how to detect and negotiate conflict, and also advocate with the government for the needs of their communities. It spawned other projects to generate income, to provide vocational training to unemployed youth, set up sports and recreational facilities.

In the first of a series of dialogues between Kashmiri Muslim and Kashmiri Pandits aimed at reconciliation under the auspices of the Centre for Dialogue and Reconciliation (Sonpar, 2012), it was seen that what emerged first were two competing narrative strands representing each community's story. There was genuine engagement and courteous expression even though each narrative from one side evoked counter-complaint and defensive rebuttal from the other. The underlying need to maintain positive group identity was very apparent and conversation that moved toward own-group culpability in any way was quickly deflected. Kashmiri Muslims wanted acknowledgement of the discrimination and unfairness to which they had been subjected by the dominance of the Pandit community in education, employment, and socioeconomic status as well as the direct violence they had suffered by the militarization of the state. The Pandits wanted acknowledgement of the direct violence and displacement they had suffered, and also stated their desire for their cultural and religious sites to be respected and preserved. Although each party was able to articulate these needs, mutual defensiveness appeared as some participants argued in favour of more extreme ideological positions. Debating these positions felt like a slur on their identity. Others holding moderate views hesitated to speak up possibly to uphold group solidarity. It was recognized by the facilitators that this was a process that could not be hurried and that in order to contain the distress and negativity that would inevitably accompany more difficult confrontations, the trust in the group had to be further strengthened.

Bar-On (2005) discusses empirical criteria for reconciliation in practice from his experience of the long-running dialogue between Jewish and Palestinian participants of the Reflect and Trust Group. He points out that effective programs acknowledge the emotional complexities around the conflict and also attend to the power asymmetries. Where conflict has become 'intractable' one finds that identity has become monolithic in opposition to the Other and what is needed is a more complex representation of identities.

The Difficult Conversations Lab at Columbia University attempts to study real-life conflict in a controlled setting. An important finding was that people continue a conversation that has become angry and frustrating when there is a complexity to the conversation. This is because complexity leads to a fuller, more accurate story. Also when people encounter complexity they become curious and less closed-off to new information. They continue to listen (Coleman, 2021; Ripley, 2019). This and other research on the role of identity processes (Riek et al., 2008) including that of building superordinate identities, intergroup contact (Dovidio et al., 2008; Hewstone et al., 2008), and emotions and emotional regulation (Gunn & Wilson, 2011; Halperin & Pliskin, 2015; Halperin et al., 2011, 2014; Iyer & Leach, 2008) offer promising insights as to how dialogue between adversaries can be made fruitful.

Structural Peacebuilding

Issues of social injustice, political exclusion and economic grievance are ignored in many peace agreements and result in relapse into conflict in few years (Manchanda, 2006). Where socioeconomic deprivation overlaps with specific ethnic or regional groups, especially when these have been marginalized by prevailing power structures, the situation is ripe for violent conflict (Manchanda, 2006). Sustainable peace requires that both direct violence and such structural violence be addressed to use Galtung's (1969) distinction. Direct peacebuilding efforts aim to mitigate or prevent direct forms of violence while structural peacebuilding aims to create just social structures that ensure sustainable and equitable satisfaction of needs for all people (Christie, 2006). Structural peacebuilding is consonant with an emphasis on psychosocial wellbeing and the human capabilities approach to development (Kumar, 2006). However, this may not be the understanding that informs all development initiatives in the aftermath of violent conflict.

Governments often do embark on post-conflict development-related activities. Unfortunately, these may not be in tandem with other peacebuilding efforts that address the psychosocial traumas that individuals and communities have suffered. Policy makers may not be psychosocially aware and may seek quick and simple solutions that do little to address the extreme pain, loss and humiliation of victims. For instance, in Sri Lanka although the government has undertaken development and reconstruction activities in the north and east, there is little attention paid to how these are also contributing to minority fears and alienation (Samarasinghe, 2015).

In India, public policy has tended to see 'development' as the remedy for regions riven by political violence without acknowledgment or redressal for the suffering of the people due to structural violence and human rights violations. The government's special economic packages and schemes for development in Jammu & Kashmir and in the North East, both being sites of long standing violent insurgent conflict, were perceived to serve pacification rather than peacebuilding intent since they sidestep issues of justice, human security and dignity (DasGupta, 2012). In Jammu & Kashmir, the Indian Army's Operation Sadhbhavana is a product of the doctrine of sub-conventional warfare that gives a central place to winning the hearts and minds (WHAM) of people in counter insurgency operations. Its activities have included infrastructure development, health care and sanitation, veterinary camps, education, human resource development and national integration. It is reported to have had positive impact because of services provided to people in areas the civil administration could not reach (Anant, 2011). However, it has done so at the cost of undermining the civil administration. Through their ethnographic study of the project, Aggarwal and Bhan (2009) show how the discourse of democracy and development has been appropriated by the military for securing the border and controlling the civilian population. They caution that the rhetoric of 'disarming violence' though democracy and development may be used to consolidate militarization and to offset intensification of military violence for national security.

While development is one route toward structural peacebuilding, non- violent collective action is another. Anderson and Christie (2001) put the struggle for social justice at the centre of psychologically-based principles to guide policy development and activism for peace, and suggest that a liberation psychology is well-suited for such social transformation. Liberation psychology, originating in the work of Martin Baro in El Salvador (Martin-Baro, 1996), understands the psychology of impoverished and oppressed communities by conceptually and practically addressing the oppressive structures in which they exist (Lykes, 2000).

Structural violence is insidious since it is built into the fabric of the political, social and economic systems. A transformational praxis towards a just society necessarily includes 'conscientisation' (Freire, 1970) and collective action. Non-violent social movements that seek to transform political oppression, economic exploitation and the cultural narratives that support such domination and social exclusion may be considered structural peacebuilding (Montiel, 2001). Active non-violence in this view is behavior aimed at influencing public policy and decision making through group action. Her study of non-violent political transformation in three Southeast Asian countries—Cambodia, East Timor and Philippines—show how peace movements were created even under governments seen to be oppressive, undemocratic and socially unjust (Montiel, 2006).

It should be mentioned that in Latin America, the political violence in several countries spawned a unique tradition of community-based outreach and participatory psychosocial work that is grounded in social justice and human rights (Van den Berg et al., 2013), as well as 'action research' where intervention and research go hand in hand (Martinez & Eiroa-Orosa, 2010). An example of this tradition is a community approach to support people affected by violence and torture in post-conflict Guatemala. Using health as an entry strategy, the program aimed not just to relieve health-related symptoms but also to create structures within the community capable of fostering sociopolitical change (Berliner et al., 2006).

According to Dudouet (2017), peacebuilding and civil resistance are both approaches to conflict transformation sharing a commitment to social change and improved justice through peaceful means. One is 'resolutionary' and the other 'revolutionary' (Lederach, 1995). Conflict transformation is a comprehensive term referring to actions and processes that seek to address the root causes of conflict over the long term in pursuit of just peace by nonviolent means. It aims to transform negative, destructive conflict into positive constructive conflict. Civil resistance is defined as an extra-institutional conflict-waging strategy in which organized grassroots movements use various non-violent tactics and strategies such as strikes, boycotts, marches, demonstrations, non-cooperation, and other constructive resistance to fight perceived injustice without the threat or use of violence. It was perfected as a nonviolent practice and conceptually articulated as a clear strategy that could be planned and implemented under Gandhi's campaign for civil rights and national liberation. Because it is strongly linked with social and political change from below and grassroots empowerment, it is conducive to participatory democracy which is also the purpose of peacebuilding activities in post-conflict zones (Dudouet, 2017).

Civil resistance can be seen as a violence prevention and pre-negotiation strategy that can be used by oppressed groups, enabling them to wage necessary conflicts peacefully and thus put pressure on elites to redistribute power equitably (Curle, 1971). The methods of peacebuilding help translate the gains of civil resistance into mutually acceptable negotiated outcomes and reconcile polarized relations in the wake of a nonviolent struggle. Civil resistance is also required in post conflict societies to put pressure on all stakeholders to implement commitments to state reforms and social justice. Examples of the synergy between civil resistance and peacebuilding are seen in women's advocacy for peace in Liberia, post-revolutionary transformation in Tunisia, post-war mobilisation for positive peace in Nepal, genocide prevention through nonviolent resistance in Timor Leste and civil resistance to unpopular peacebuilding in Kosovo (Dudouet, 2017).

Conclusion

Montiel (2009) offers three propositions about peace psychology in Asia. First, peace and violence are both embedded in macro-levels beyond the individual—in history, politics and culture. Second, direct and structural peace are inter-related. She adds that the discipline of peace psychology takes an ethical position to pursue non-violence (direct peace) and to support more equal structural configurations (structural peace). Third, peace psychology remains attendant to that which is subjective at individual and group levels as well as cultural narratives that support peaceful and egalitarian structures. Psychosocial approaches to peacebuilding resonate with the above. In addition, the psychosocial model offers a systemic understanding of the interplay and tensions between individual level (micro), social-community level (meso), and the level of state, institutions and politics (macro), while keeping people's wellbeing at the heart. As described in earlier sections, psychosocial programs in the aftermath of violent conflict contribute to healing of individuals and communities, as well as to the building of psychological and social capital. In some contexts, social transformation towards an empowered and engaged citizenry that seeks justice and structural equity can become fraught in the clash with existing power structures. This poses a challenge to psychosocial programming in that their typical positioning as humanitarian, neutral and apolitical can be limiting. Even so, by centering on psychosocial wellbeing and fostering an empowered citizenry, a new way of doing politics emerges (Montero, 1998).

References

Abeyasekara, A., & Amarasuriya, H. (2008). *Proposing "psychosocial" as a framework for assessing development and humanitarian intervention in Sri Lanka.* Working Paper, SPARC, University of Colombo.

Abeyasekara, A., Amarasuriya, H., & Ferdinando, M. (2008). *A model for wellbeing: Proposing a psychosocial framework to understand wellbeing in Sri Lanka* (Working Paper, SPARC). University of Colombo.

Ager, A. (1997). Tensions in the psychosocial discourse: Implications for the planning of interventions with war-affected populations. *Development in Practice, 7*(4), 402–407.

Aggarwal, R., & Bhan, M. (2009). Disarming violence: Development, democracy and security on the borders of India. *The Journal of Asian Studies, 68*(2), 519–542.

Anant, A. (2011). *Counterinsurgency and Operation Sadhbhavana in Jammu & Kashmir* (IDSA Occasional Paper No. 19). Institute for Defence Studies and Analyses, New Delhi.

Anderson, A., & Christie, D. J. (2001). Some contributions of psychology to policies promoting cultures of peace. *Peace and Conflict: Journal of Peace Psychology, 7*(2), 173–185.

Bar-On, D. (2005). Empirical criteria for reconciliation in practice. *Intervention, 3*(3), 180–191.

Bar-Tal, D. (2007). Sociopsychological foundations of intractable conflicts. *American Behavioural Scientist, 50*(11), 1430–1453.

Bar-Tal, D., Halperin, E., & Pliskin, R. (2017). Why is it so difficult to resolve intractable conflicts peacefully? A sociopsychological explanation. In M. Galluccio (Ed.), *Handbook of international negotiation: Interpersonal, intercultural and diplomatic perspectives* (pp. 73–92). Springer International Publishing.

Baru, S. (2021, December 27). *State and civil society, from Karat to Doval.* Civil Society. www.civilsocietyonline.com. Accessed 20 May 2024.

Barve, S. (2003). *Healing streams: Bringing back hope in the aftermath of violence.* Penguin.

Becker, D. (2004). Dealing with the consequences of organized violence in trauma work. In *Berghof handbook of conflict transformation.* Berghof Centre for Constructive Conflict Management. At berghof-foundation.org. Accessed on 15 April 2024.

Becker, D. (2005). Reconciliation—The wrong track to peace? *Intervention, 3*(3), 167–179.

Berliner, P., Dominguez, M., Kjaerulf, F., & Mikkelsen, E. (2006). What can be learned from "crazy" psychologists? A community approach to psychosocial support in post-conflict Guatemala. *Intervention, 4*(1), 67–73.

Botcharova, O. (2001). Implementation of track two diplomacy: Developing a model of forgiveness. In R. G. Helmick, & R. J. Petersen (Eds.), *Forgiveness and reconciliation* (pp.279–304). Templeton Foundation Press.

Bracken, P., Giller, S., & Summerfield, D. (1997). Rethinking mental health with survivors of wartime violence and refugees. *Journal of Refugee Studies, 10*(4), 431–442.

Breslau, J. (2004). Culture of trauma: Anthropological views of post-traumatic stress disorder in international health. *Culture, Medicine and Psychiatry, 28*, 113–126.

Bubenzer, F. & Tankink, M. (2017). Introduction to special issue: Linking mental health and psychosocial support to peacebuilding in an integrated way. *Intervention, 15*(3), 192–198.

Centre for Humanitarian Dialogue and Delhi Policy Group. (2011). *Conflict resolution: Learning lessons from dialogue processes in India.* Centre for Humanitarian Dialogue.

Christie, D. J. (2006). What is peace psychology the psycholgy of? *Journal of Social Issues, 62*(1), 1–17.

Coleman, P. (2021). *The way out: How to overcome toxic polarization.* Columbia University Press.

Curle, A. (1971). *Making peace.* Tavistock.

DasGupta, S. (2012). Pacification is not peacebuilding: Why special economic packages and special legislation do not work. In J. B. Galvanick, H. J. Giesmann & M. Mubashir (Eds.), *Norms and premises of peace governance: Sociocultural commonalities and differences in Europe and India* (Berghof Occasional Paper No. 32, pp. 18–24).

DeVries, M. (1996). Trauma in cultural perspective. In B. A. van der Kolk, A. McFarlane, & L. Weisaeth (Eds.), *Traumatic stress: The effects of overwhelming experience on mind, body and society* (pp. 398–413). Guilford Press.

Diaz, P., De Prewitt, J., & Dayal, A. (2008). Words to action: Pictorial contextualisation of the IASC guidelines on mental health and psychosocial support in emergency settings. *Intervention, 6*(3), 327–333.

Dovidio, J. F., Gaertner, S. I., John, M., Halabi, S., Saguy, T., Pearson, A. R., & Riek, B. M. (2008). Majority and minority perspectives in intergroup relations: The role of contact, group representation, threat and trust in intergroup conflict and reconciliation. In A. Nadler, T. E. Malloy, & J. D. Fisher (Eds.), *The social psychology of intergroup reconciliation* (pp. 227–253). Oxford University Press.

Dudouet, V. (2017). *Powering to peace: Integrated civil resistance and peacebuilding strategies.* International Centre on Nonviolent Conflict.

Eaton, J., Nwefoh, E., & Duncan, J. (2022). Addressing mental health and wellbeing in the context of climate change: Examples of interventions to inform future practice. *Intervention, 20*(1), 107–113.

Echeverri, C., & Castilla, J. (2008). A case study in Colombia: Implementation of the IASC guidelines on mental health and psychosocial support in emergency settings. *Intervention, 6*(3), 284–290.

Erikson, K. (1976). Disaster at Buffalo Creek: Loss of communality as Buffalo Creek. *American Journal of Psychiatry, 133*(3), 302–305.

Freire, P. (1970). *Pedagogy of the oppressed.* Continuum Publishing Corporation.

Fonagy, P., Gergely, G., Jurist, E. L., & Target, M. (2002). *Affect regulation, mentalization and the development of the self*. Other Press.

Galtung, J. (1969). Violence, peace and peace research. *Journal of Peace Research, 6*(3), 167–191.

Galappatti, A. (2003). What is psychosocial intervention? Mapping the field in Sri Lanka. *Intervention, 1*(2), 2–17.

Galappatti, A., & Salih, M. (2006). Integrating a psychosocial perspective into poverty reduction: The case of a resettlement project in northern Sri Lanka. *Intervention, 4*(2), 127–145.

Gallagher, E., & Hamber, B. (2015). Addressing the psychosocial needs of young men: The case of Northern Ireland. In B. Hamber & E. Gallagher (Eds.), *Psychosocial perspectives on peacebuilding* (pp. 71–116). Springer.

Gaventa, J., & Barrett, G. (2010). *So what difference does it make? Mapping the outcomes of citizen engagements* (IDS Working Paper No. 347). Institute of Development Studies, Brighton.

Gobodo-Madikizela, P. (2008). Transforming trauma in the aftermath of gross human rights abuses: Making public spaces intimate through the South Africa Truth and Reconciliation Commission. In A. Nadler, T. E. Malloy, & J. D. Fisher (Eds.), *The social psychology of intergroup reconciliation* (pp. 57–75). Oxford University Press.

Gunn, G. R., & Wilson, A. E. (2011). Acknowledging the skeletons in our closet: The effect of group affirmation on collective guilt, collective shame and reparatory attitudes. *Personality & Social Psychology Bulletin, 37*(11), 1474–1487.

Halperin, E., & Pliskin, R. (2015). Emotions and emotional regulation in intractable conflict: Studying emotional processes within a unique context. *Advances in Political Psychology, 36*(Supplement 1), 119–150.

Halperin, E., Pliskin, R., Saguy, T., Liberman, V., & Gross, J. (2014). Emotional regulation and the cultivation of political tolerance: Searching for a new track for intervention. *Journal of Conflict Resolution, 58*(6), 1110–1138.

Halperin, E., Russell, A. G., Deveck, C., & Gross, J. (2011). Anger, hatred and the quest for peace: Anger can be constructive in the absence of hatred. *Journal of Conflict Resolution, 55*(2), 274–291.

Hamber, B. (2015). Dealing with painful memories and violent pasts: toward a framework for contextual understanding. In B. Austin & M. Fischer (Eds.), *Transforming war-related identities.* Berghof Handbook Dialogue Series No. 11. Berghof Foundation, Berlin.

Hamber, B. & Gallagher, E. (2015). *Psychosocial perspectives on peacebuilding*. Springer.

Hamber, B., Gallagher, E., & Ventevogel, P. (2014). Narrowing the gap between psychosocial practice, peacebuilding and wider social change. *Intervention, 12*(1), 7–15.

Hart, B., & Colo, E. (2014). Psychosocial peacebuilding in Bosnia and Herzegovina: Approaches to relational and social change. *Intervention, 12*(1), 76–87.

Hewstone, M., Kenworthy, J. B., Cairns, E., Tausch, N., Hughes, J., Tam, T., Voci, A., Hecker, U., & Pinder, C. (2008). Stepping stones to reconciliation in Northern Ireland: Intergroup contact, forgiveness and trust. In A. Nadler, T. E. Malloy, & J. D. Fisher (Eds.), *The social psychology of intergroup reconciliation* (pp. 199–226). Oxford University Press.

Hobfoll, S., et al. (2007). Five essential elements of immediate and mid-term mass trauma intervention: Empirical evidence. *Psychiatry, 70*(4), 283–315.

Inter-Agency Standing Committee. (2007). *IASC Guidelines on mental health and psychosocial support in emergency settings*. IASC.

Inter-Agency Standing Committee. (2024). *Integrating mental health and psychosocial support and peacebuilding: A mapping and recommendations for practitioners*. IASC.

International Centre for Transitional Justice. (2009). *What is transitional justice?* ICTJ.

Iyer, A., & Leach, C. W. (2008). Emotions in inter-group relations. *European Review of Social Psychology, 19*, 86–125.

Jordans, M., Upadhaya, N., & Tol, W. (2010). Introducing the IASC mental health and psychosocial support guidelines in emergency settings in Nepal: A process description. *Intervention, 8*(1), 52–63.

Kahnemann, D. (2011). *Thinking, fast and slow*. Penguin.

Kumar, S. A. K. (2006). A human development perspective. *Seminar*, No. 568 (Issue-Securing the insecure).

Kurian, A. (2023, July 12). Why India needs a truth and reconciliation commission. *The Wire*. http://thewire.in/rights/truth-and-reconciliation-in-india. Accessed 25 March 2024.

Lederach, J. P. (1995). *Preparing for peace: Conflict transformation across cultures*. Syracuse University Press.

Luthans, F., & Youssef-Morgan, C. M. (2017). Psychological capital: An evidence-based positive approach. *Annual Review of Organizational Psychology & Organizational Behaviour, 4*, 339–366.

Lykes, M. B. (2000). Possible contributions of a psychology of liberation: Whither health and human rights? *Journal of Health Psychology, 5*(3), 383–397.

Lykes, M. B., & Crosby, A. (2015). Creative methodologies as a resource for Mayan women's protagonism. In B. Hamber & E. Gallagher (Eds.), *Psychosocial perspectives on peacebuilding* (pp. 147–186). Springer.

Majumdar, S. (2020). *Youth and political violence in India: A social psychological account of conflict experiences from the Kashmir valley*. Routledge.

Manchanda, R. (2006). Conflicts and the politics of peace in South Asia. In R. N. Kumar & S. Muller-Rappard (Eds.), *Critical readings in human rights and peace* (pp. 65–94). South Asia Forum for Human Rights.

Martin-Baro, I. (1996). *Writings for a liberation psychology*. A. Aron & S. Corne (Eds.). Harvard University Press.

Martinez, M. A., & Eiroa-Orosa, F. (2010). Psychosocial research and action with survivors of political violence in Latin America: Methodological considerations and implications for practice. *Intervention, 8*(1), 3–13.

Minow, M. (1998). *Between vengeance and forgiveness: Facing history after genocide and mass violence*. Beacon Press.

Montero, M. (1998). Psychosocial community work as an alternative mode of political action. *Community, Work & Family, 1*(1), 65–78.

Montiel, C. J. (2001). Towards a psychology of structural peacebuilding. In D. J. Christie, R. Wagner, & D. Winter (Eds.), *Peace, conflict and violence: Peace psychology for the 21st century* (pp. 282–294). Prentice Hall.

Montiel, C. J. (2006). Political psychology of non-violent democratic transitions in Southeast Asia. *Journal of Social Issues, 62*(1), 173–190.

Montiel, C. J. (2009). Overview of peace psychology in Asia: Research, practice, and teaching. In C. J. Montiel & N. M. Noor (Eds.), *Peace psychology in Asia* (pp. 3–20). Springer.

Nadler, A., Malloy, T. E., & Fisher, J. D. (2008). Intergroup reconciliation: Dimensions and themes. In A. Nadler, T. E. Malloy, & J. D. Fisher (Eds.), *The social psychology of intergroup reconciliation* (pp. 3–12). Oxford University Press.

National Disaster Management Authority & Rahbar. (2023). *National disaster management guidelines: Mental health and psychosocial services in disasters.* National Disaster Management Authority, Government of India.

NIMHANS & CARE, India. (2003). *Workshop on issues and challenges in psychosocial care for persons living in conflict situations: Experiences from Gujarat riots.* Workshop proceedings.

Office of the United Nations High Commissioner for Human Rights. (2020). *Thematic paper: Peacebuilding, sustaining peace and transitional justice.* OHCHR.

Pederson, D. (2002). Political violence, ethnic conflict and contemporary wars: Broad implications for health and social wellbeing. *Social Science & Medicine, 55*, 175–190.

Pupavac, V. (2002). Therapeutising refugees, pathologising populations: International psychosocial programs in Kosovo. *New Issues in Refugee Research*, Working Paper No. 59. UNHCR.

Riek, B. M., Gaertner, S. I., Dovidio, J. F., Brewer, M., Mania, E. W., & Lamoreux, M. J. (2008). A social psychological approach to post-conflict reconciliation. In A. Nadler, T. E. Malloy, & J. D. Fisher (Eds.), *The social psychology of intergroup reconciliation* (pp. 255–273). Oxford University Press.

Robben, A., & Suarez-Orozco, M. (2000). Interdisciplinary perspectives on violence and trauma. In A. Robben & M. Suarez-Orozco (Eds.), *Cultures under siege: Collective violence and trauma* (pp. 1–42). Cambridge University Press.

Ripley, A. (2019). *Complicating the narratives.* https://thewholestory.solutionsjournalism.org/complicating-the-narratives-b91ea06ddf63. Accessed 14 February 2024.

Ryan, S. (1995). *Ethnic conflict and international relations.* Dartmouth Publishing Company.

Salih, M., & Samarasinghe, G. (2006). *Localising transitional justice in the context of psychosocial work in Sri Lanka.* SPARC, University of Colombo.

Samarasinghe, G. (2015). Rethinking psychosocial programming in post-war Sri Lanka. In B. Hamber & E. Gallagher (Eds.), *Psychosocial perspectives on peacebuilding* (pp. 117–145). Springer.

Singh, S. (2018). Education for peace through transformative dialogue: Perspectives from Kashmir. *International Review of Education, 64*(1), 43–63.

Social Policy & Analysis Research Centre, University of Colombo. (2008). *PADHI: A tool a guide a framework.* University of Colombo.

Somasundaram, D. (2007). Collective trauma in northern Sri Lanka: a qualitative psychosocial-ecological study. *International Journal of Mental Health Systems, 1*(5).

Somasundaram, D. (2014). Addressing collective trauma: Conceptualisations and interventions. *Intervention, 12*(Supplement 1), 43–60.

Sonpar, S. (2000). Kashmir: Trauma and psychological intervention. *Psychological Foundations—The Journal, 2*(2), 84–88.

Sonpar, S. (2007). *Violent activism: A psychosocial study of ex-militants in JK.* Aman Trust.

Sonpar, S. (2008). *Trauma, development and peacebuilding. Cross regional challenges: South Asia.* Paper presented at Trauma, Development and Peacebuilding Conference, New Delhi, India, September 9–11, 2008. International Conflict Research Institute (INCORE) & International Development Research Centre (IDRC).

Sonpar, S. (2012, February 10–12). Reflections on intercommunity dialogue, Jammu. Personal notes.

Sonpar, S. (2015). Transforming conflict, changing society: Psychosocial programming in Indian Jammu and Kashmir. In B. Hamber & E. Gallagher (Eds.), *Psychosocial perspectives on peacebuilding* (pp. 33–69). Springer.

Strang, A. B., & Ager, A. (2003). Psychosocial intervention: Some key issues facing practitioners. *Intervention, 1*(3), 2–12.

Summerfield, D. (1999). A critique of seven assumptions behind psychosocial trauma programmes in war-affected areas. *Social Science & Medicine, 48*, 1449–1462.

Summerfield, D. (2004). Cross-cultural perspectives on the medicalization of human suffering. In G. Rosen (Ed.), *Post-traumatic stress disorder: Issues and controversies* (pp. 233–245). Wiley.

Suri, A. (2003). *NGOs in Kashmir: Agents of peace and development?* (IPCS Research paper 2). Institute for Peace & Conflict Studies, New Delhi.

Tankink, M., & Bubenzer, F. (2017). Building sustainable peace through an integrated approach to peacebuilding and mental health and psychosocial support. *Intervention, 15*(3), 199–214.

Tankink, M., Otto, B., & Mangen, P. O. (2022). "Peace starts with peace of mind": Study of the intersection between post-conflict trauma, peacebuilding and economic development in Northern Uganda. *Intervention, 20*(1), 46–57.

Touze, D. L., Silove, D., & Zwi, A. (2005). Can there be healing without justice? Lessons from the Commission for Reception, Truth and Reconciliation in East Timor. *Intervention, 3*(3), 192–202.

UN Office of the High Commissioner for Human Rights (2020). Thematic paper: Peacebuilding, sustaining peace and transitional justice. https://www.ohchr.org/en/transitional-justice. Accessed 20 May, 2024.

Van den Berg, S., Akello, G., & Sonpar, S. (2013). The first decade of Intervention: Facts, figures and trends. *Intervention, 11*(1), 52–76.

Volkan, V. (2001). Transgenerational transmission and chosen trauma: An aspect of large group identity. *Group Analysis, 34*(1), 79–97.

Watkins, M. (2021). Towards a decolonial approach to psychosocial accompaniment from the "outside." In G. Stevens & C. Sonn (Eds.), *Decoloniality and epistemic justice in contemporary community psychology* (pp. 101–120). Springer.

Wessells, M., & Ommeren, M. (2008). Developing inter-agency guidelines on mental health and psychosocial support in emergency settings. *Intervention, 6*(3), 199–218.

Williamson, J., & Robinson, M. (2006). Psychosocial intervention or integrated programming for wellbeing? *Intervention, 4*(1), 4–25.

Shobna Sonpar Ph.D. is a clinical psychologist, psychotherapist and clinical supervisor for counsellors and psychotherapists. Her research interests have been in gender, social justice and political violence. Her research work includes studies of survivors of the displacement and violence of India's 1947 Partition, former militants in J&K, women's role in peacebuilding, the gendered impact of economic liberalization policies on psychosocial wellbeing, ragging in educational institutions in India and the impact of psychosocial programming on social transformation in J&K. She has also been associated with projects that build capacity for psychosocial support among community workers and community peacebuilding initiatives.

GPSR Compliance

The European Union's (EU) General Product Safety Regulation (GPSR) is a set of rules that requires consumer products to be safe and our obligations to ensure this.

If you have any concerns about our products, you can contact us on ProductSafety@springernature.com

In case Publisher is established outside the EU, the EU authorized representative is:

Springer Nature Customer Service Center GmbH
Europaplatz 3
69115 Heidelberg, Germany

Batch number: 08836269

Printed by Printforce, the Netherlands